To Peter mon ami
with gratitude

Jean-Marie

Susanne Binder (ed.)

The Macula

Diagnosis, Treatment and Future Trends

SpringerWienNewYork

Univ.-Prof. Dr. Susanne Binder
The Ludwig Boltzmann Institute of Retinology and Biomicroscopic Laser Surgery, Department of
Ophthalmology, Rudolf Foundation Clinic, Vienna, Austria

© 2004 Springer-Verlag/Wien
Printed in Austria
Springer-Verlag Wien New York is a part of
Springer Science + Business Media
springeronline.com

Typesetting: SNP Best-set Typesetter Ltd., Hong Kong
Printing: Druckerei Theiss GmbH, A-9431 St. Stefan

Printed on acid-free and chlorine-free bleached paper
SPIN: 10942024
Library of Congress Number: 2004104634

With 128 partly coloured Figures

ISBN 3-211-40691-3 Springer-Verlag Wien New York

For my Mother

Preface

Enormous developments have been made in ophthalmology during the last century. Higher precision and newer instrumentation in surgery as well as better examination methods and progress in microbiology have given us access to much more information about the pathological physiology and anatomy that we are confronted with in our various fields of expertise. As we have approached a new millennium we decided to capture some of these new ideas and incorporate them into a conference where we could share our work and benefit from each others' experiences. This book is based on contributions presented at the "2nd **International Conference on Vitreoretinal Diseases**" which was held in September 2002 in Vienna, Austria which focused on the retinal macula. The meeting was very fortunate to have the world's most renowned leaders in macular research attend and share their vast experience and expertise as well as their latest research and results. This meeting followed the "**First International Conference on Vitreoretinal Diseases**" which was held in Vienna, Austria in 1998, and focused on retinal transplantation and retinal microsurgery.

After the great success of the "2nd **International Conference on Vitreoretinal Diseases**" an overwhelming interest was expressed to gather all these new and innovative ideas that had been developed in a book in order to give colleagues and students access to a valuable collection of the information presented at the meeting.

This international meeting was administrated by, Mrs. Tilly and Mr. Sven Gerling, whose vast experience in the field of ophthalmology and personal contacts to most of our speakers helped tremendously in making it a very successful meeting. I would also like to acknowledge the medical staff of the Rudolf Foundation Hospital's Department of Ophthalmology and the Ludwig Boltzmann Institute for Retinology and Biomicroscopic Laser Surgery for their invaluable help and united efforts both before and during the meeting. Without the support of the medical director of the Rudolf Foundation Hospital, Dr. Wilhelm Marhold and the Executive City Counsellor for Public Health and Hospitals of Vienna, Prim. Dr. Elisabeth Pittermann-Höcker as well as the Mayor of Vienna, Dr. Michael Häupl and the Austrian Minister of Education, Mrs. Elisabeth Gehrer a meeting of this magnitude would never have been possible. Many pharmaceutical sponsors and exhibitors helped us to finance this event and I am truly very grateful to all of them.

Finally, I would like to express my utmost gratitude to my companion John and my son Christian for being so patient and tolerant as well as giving me so much of their support and their time.

Prof. Dr. Susanne Binder
Vienna, Austria, April 20, 2004

Contents

New instruments – intrasurgical tools

Retinal prosthesis

Macular photoreceptor organization

Modular substructuring – a consistent feature along all foveal cone elements

P.K. Ahnelt, Ch. Schubert, and E.M. Anger

Department of Physiology, Vienna Medical University, Vienna, Austria

Abstract

A precondition for maximum acuity and other optimizations of human and primate photopic visual function is the high density of the retinal foveolar cones. Spatial packing is near optimum in the all-cone foveal center but always deviations from ideal hexagonal order remain. Pattern analysis has allowed to demonstrate the presence of serially arranged lattice defects separating crystalline patches sharing similar axial orientation [18]. The present study demonstrates similar patchwork-like organizations in the initial portion of cone axons. It is proposed that these patterns are correlated with the batch-wise descendence and sequential stacking of cone cell bodies during mosaic condensations. The multitiered relocation of the primarily monolayered macular sensory epithelium compensates the diameter difference between somata and slender inner segments. Induced by the arrangement of somata this modular organization is projected upon the two dimensional aspects on both sides of the ONL: distally it appears as the inner/outer segment patches and proximally it leads to the bundling of cone axons below the nuclear layer. Thus discontinuities are an inherent element of foveal microarchitecture and may be sites of increased vulnerability to mechanical/osmotic stress and retinoschisis.

Introduction

Human and primate retinas are unique among mammals by providing a macular center with extreme minimization of the sensory units [4, 6]. Densities of more than 200.000 cone inner/outer segments/mm^2 at the center result from progressive centripetal condensation of a primordial all-cone region during pre- and postnatal stages. It has been noted that the foveolar lattice (subdued to gradual centripetal crystalline condensation) is not entirely hexagonal but that there is also positional noise [9]. The role of this noise for reduction of aliasing effects has been discussed [12, 24] and patchy aliasing has been observed using laser interferometric procedures [20]. We [3, 18] and others [5] have shown previously that defects of the adult foveal cone mosaic are not randomly distributed within the hexagonal lattice. Pattern analysis reveals linear series of errors resulting in tiling of the hexagonal areas into coherent patches. The patches share similar axial orientation, which differ from the neighbor areas by discrete angular steps of 12–15° (Fig. 1a). The mechanisms leading to these faults and sub structuring have been unclear. The present findings suggest that this low frequency component in the inner segment lattice is not due to random events. It rather reflects spatial constraints originating in the underlying cone cell body arrangement.

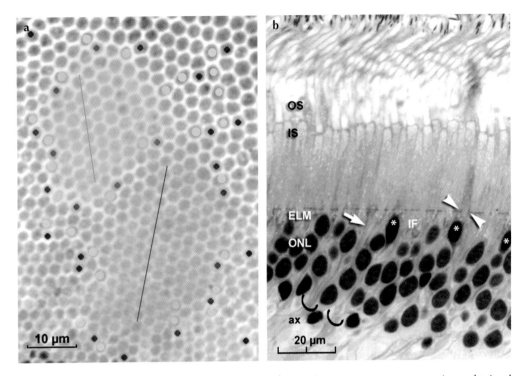

Fig. 1a. Human fovea. Schematic representation of cone inner segment cross sections obtained from a tangential semithin section. The majority of cones has direct 6 neighbors and thus forms a regular lattice. The hexagonal order is however subdivided in (color coded) domains that differ in axial orientation (indicated by straight lines) by 12–15 degrees. Borders between patches are sites of increased disturbances, larger size variances and high frequency of 5- (red) and >6-neighborship (yellow) patterns

Fig. 1b. Rhesus monkey fovea. Radial section, Toluidine blue stain, ca. Right border ca.130 μm from center. Cone cell bodies (ONL). tend to be arranged in descending sequences. Only the few initial cells (asterisks) remain close to the external limiting membrane (ELM). At the peripheral side of the oblique cone arrays thin inner fibers (IF) arise connecting them with the inner segments at the ELM. At the central side axons (ax) descend and assemble in bundles (open circles). Bundles leaving the outer nuclear layer bend towards the periphery

Materials and methods

Human eyes provided by the corneal transplant lab at the Vienna University Eye Clinic were immersed in 0,1 M phosphate buffered 4% paraformaldehyde (PF) or in a mixture of 1% glutaraldehyde/2% PF for 3–7 hrs post mortem. Monkey retinas were immersion fixed or perfusion fixed with GA/PF mixtures. After fixation for 1–24 hrs the retinas were dissected and processed as wholemounts or a central disc (Ø 10 mm) with the fovea and papilla was trephined and removed together with choroids and pigment epithelium.

Samples were either processed for cryosectioning or for semithin sections. Resin embedded samples were serially sectioned radially and tangentially with a Diatome Jumbo knife. Sections were photographed and aligned in consecutive image planes of *Adobe Photoshop* files to map soma arrangements, the course of inner fibers, of axons and pedicles.

Results

In the adult primate and human foveal center inner segment (IS) diameters are minimized (2,5 µm) and increase towards the periphery more than twofold [10]. The features described in the following are present in both human and primate foveas with some differences which mostly result from different foveal dimensions. These inner segment mosaics tend to establish highly regular lattices. Still, the mosaic contains non-hexagonal defects (positions with <6> neighbors). Beyond the foveolar center these lattice defects appear arranged in linear series (Fig. 1) which circumscribe crystalline domains [5, 18].

Foveolar cell bodies and inner fibers

In the center of the foveola cell bodies, fibers and axons are dispersed between voluminous Müller cell columns [2] and only few pedicles and interneurons are detectable at the foveolar floor [1]. Beyond this center the foveal cone cell bodies have a strong tendency for sequential radial and centrifugal stacking since they cannot minimize their diameters due to the unchanged nuclear volume. This leads to the multitiered arrangement wherein the somata remain connected to the inner segments via slender (1,3–1,8 µm) inner fibers. These fiber elements arise at the distal poles of the somata and accumulate with increasing length depending on their distance from the external limiting membrane. At ca. 100 µm eccentricity the sequences may include 8–12 somata/axons/inner fibers/inner segments. Due to the oblique displacement of consecutive somata the inner fibers (IF) ascend and assemble in bundles along the peripheral face of the soma (arrow in Fig. 1b). The IS mosaics which emerge from the slender inner fibers of these descended cone arrays have similar cross sections and tend towards self-organized (hexagonal) optimum tiling during centripetal migration. Along consecutive sections it becomes evident that in three dimensions the beaded patterns are in fact concentrically layered bundled arrangements. Thus when viewed tangentially these modules are sized similar to the iso-orientation patches present in the inner segment mosaics.

Most of foveal cones have outer fibers diameters which are by far smaller than the inner segments (2,2 µm) – When crossing the ELM the connecting fibers expand to become the base of the inner segments. Only a minor group of cones (asterisks in Fig. 2) retains their cell body's position directly underneath the external membrane requiring the shortest outer fibers. Consequentially the axons of these "resting cones" then take the longest course within the ONL. In these cones the soma diameter has direct influence on the base of the inner segment across the external limiting membrane and thus they tend to have larger inner segment cross sections (120%) and often higher staining affinity than their direct neighbors (Fig. 2), also in micrographs in [7, 19]. This in turn often leads to cone positions with 7, 8 or 5 neighbors instead of the 6 dominant in uniform regions. The lattice tension created by these cones may progress along to other cones with soma-at-top positions. This may create the linear series of non-hexagonal "cracks" in tangential section aspects of inner segment mosaics (Fig. 1a). At increasing eccentricities the discrepancy between inner segment diameter and soma size decreases. The tension is relaxed, the number of cone cell body tiers in the outer nuclear layer decreases. It is also is increasingly interspersed proximally by rod cell bodies which then dissolve the regularity of the all-cone mosaic.

Axon bundles

The "Fibers of Henle" constitute a prominent foveal sublayer. The axons begin already within the cone nuclear layer, reciprocal to the respective inner fiber's length. While a

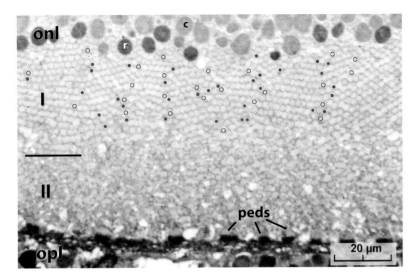

Fig. 2. Cross-sections of cone axons in Rhesus monkey fovea. Distal axons (arising from neighboring zones) appear highly organized into packages with upright elliptical shape. Axons from more central locations are positioned more proximally and do not display similar sub-organization patterns

few central cone terminals appear to remain at the foveal floor [1] most axons bend ± horizontally and take a radiating course of differing lengths [19, 21] towards the concentric ring of displaced pedicles. The axons emerge along the medial side of the cone soma series mirroring the distal outer fibers. The axons descend and accumulate along the central side of the cell bodies (Fig. 1B and schematized in Fig. 3). Since the dimension of the concentric synaptic pedicle zone is compensated by differential lengths of the cone axons their bundle piling up at the foveal rim. In radial cross sections (Fig. 2) of the axons at the rim two zones can be distinguished. A proximal sublayer (II) includes axons that have already descended far (up to more than 300 µm) from their somatal origin at the foveolar center. These axons are mixed with increasing proportions of glial tissue shortly before terminating as pedicles (ped) at the concentric outer plexiform layer. The distal region (I) includes axons which emerge from the somatal arrays of extrafoveolar cones. They are cut at a short distance after emerging from the ONL and most have similar diameters (0,7–1,3 µm). These groups of axon bundles attain optimized (hexagonal) packing order. As in the inner segment plane, patches appear to share similar axial orientation and are demarcated by non-hexagonal disturbances (colorized as in Fig. 1A).

Discussion

The term "foveal cone mosaic" generally refers to the strikingly regular patterns of condensed cone inner and outer segments, which nevertheless has been shown to include non-randomly distributed discontinuities [5, 18]. The less familiar and less understood part of foveal cones is the further course towards their synaptic terminals. It includes a two step transition. From a two-dimensional mosaic for image reception it is rearranged into to a three-dimensional somatal tiling, which then again spreads out to establish the concentric monolayered pedicle meshwork [19]. The present study points to the specific organization of cones as the likely primary source for the patchiness of the foveal mosaic.

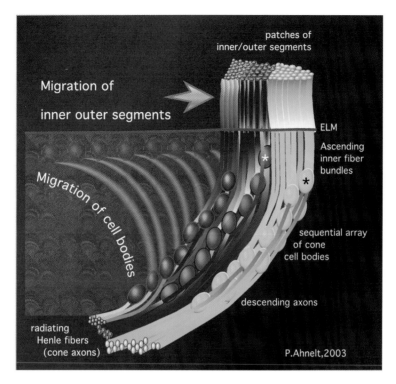

Fig. 3. Schematic summary of foveal modular organization. False colors indicate three cone arrays with their associated elements. Each array consists of three main components (Müller cells not included): grape-like arrangements of cell bodies alternate with two fibrous sheaths. Contributing reciprocal proportions. Axons accumulate proximally and inner fibers distally arising. The alternation of somas and fibers in the ONL is mirrored in modular packaging in the inner segment mosaic (beyond the ELM) and in the initial course of cone axon radiating centrifugally towards their pedicles. At the left of the first array the original position of its cell bodies before mosaic condensation is indicated (transparent ovals) as well as their presumed path (tapered rays) to their adult position

Fetal cones representing a monolayer with relatively large cubical inner segments undergo secondary concentric condensation and descent [8, 17]. Neighboring cell bodies do not appear to descend at arbitrary depths but rather adjoin closely below the previous soma creating a "perikaryal surf". Such series (with 3–12 somas) match the running length of inner segment patches. Somas are ensheathed by two fiber types a) inner fibers ascending to the inner segments and b) the axon bundles arising from the foregoing somata (Fig. 1B, Fig. 3). This stacking of cone cell bodies contributes substantially (up to >150 μm) to the profile of the foveal rim. For light directed at the central bouquet of cones this leaves an almost direct path with minimized scatter.

There are solutions for optimized continuous packing of a mosaic with decreasing diameters in both nature (e.g. sunflower seeds) as well as in geometrical grid deformation procedures [15]. However these cases are restricted to two-dimensional aggregates. Retinal design (or neural tissue in general) has to include input/output connections and therefore discontinuities are to be expected. Their presence in the foveal mosaic has been discussed as limiting aliasing image components with high spatial frequencies [22, 23, 24]. In the view of the current findings the patch-wise organization of the foveal mosaic is not accidental or directly linked to optimized image representation but is an obligatory feature of mosaic condensation. Lattice packing optimization requires midrange

Table 1. Substructuring along foveal cone elements

Section level	Discontinuity	Orientation	(Patch) Dimensions
Inner segments	hexag. iso-orientation patches	2D tangential	ca. 10 × 8 × 7 polygonal
ELM	discontinuous zonulae adherents	2D tangential	irregular
ONL	hexag. stacked arrays of cell bodies	3D radial/oblique	3–12 cells/series
Proximal axons	hexagonally bundled	2D radial/frontal	ca. 8 × 12 axons
Pedicles	orthogonal arrangement	2D tangential/ concentric	?

relaxation and axial reorientation whereas limitation of aliasing then arises as a positive side effect.

It has to be emphasized that the present data cannot establish a direct link between the grouping phenomena along the consecutive levels of foveal cone organizations (Table 1). Adequate marker experiments need to be combined with serial sectioning and reconstruction to definitely resolve these issues. Table 1 lists the modular elements including the pedicle lattice. Possibly the modular substructure of the macular cones is preserved down to the ganglion cells.

The bundling phenomena could possibly be a source for entoptic granular patterns attributed to "nerve fiber elements" [13]. Extensive discontinuities present in the external limiting membranes [11] may be also linked to the modular organization. Local lack of tight junctions may be indicative of borders between neighboring modules. If the gaps persist or increase during life they could be predisposed for retinoschisis in pathological or traumatic conditions.

Acknowledgements and support

The provision of tissue by the Cornea Transplant Lab, Eye Clinic, Med. University Vienna and J.E. Morgan, University Hospital of Wales, Heath Park, Cardiff, United Kingdom, is gratefully acknowledged. Supported by European Community Grant QLK6CT200100279.

References

1. Ahnelt PK (1998) The photoreceptor mosaic. Eye 12:531–40
2. Ahnelt PK, Pflug R (1986) Telodendrial contacts between foveolar cone pedicles in the human retina. Experientia 42:298–300
3. Ahnelt PK, Kolb H (2000) The mammalian photoreceptor mosaic-adaptive design. Prog Retin Eye Res 19:711–77
4. Ahnelt PK, Kolb H, Pflug R (1987) Identification of a subtype of cone photoreceptor, likely to be blue sensitive, in the human retina. J Comp Neurol 255:18–34
5. Curcio CA, Sloan KR (1992) Packing geometry of human cone photoreceptors: variation with eccentricity and evidence for local anisotropy. Vis Neurosci 9:169–80
6. Curcio CA, Sloan KR, Kalina RE, Hendrickson AE (1990) Human photoreceptor topography. J Comp Neurol 292:497–523
7. Fine BS, Yanoff (1988) Ocular histology, 2nd edn, Harper & Row, New York
8. Hendrickson AE, Yuodelis C (1984) The morphological development of the human fovea. Ophthalmology 91:603–12
9. Hirsch J, Curcio CA (1989) The spatial resolution capacity of human foveal retina. Vision Res 29:1095–101

10. Hoang QV, Linsenmeier RA, Chung CK, Curcio CA (2002) Photoreceptor inner segments in monkey and human retina: mitochondrial density, optics, and regional variation. Vis Neurosci 19:395–407

11. Krebs IP, Krebs W (1989) Discontinuities of the external limiting membrane in the fovea centralis of the primate retina. Exp Eye Res 48:295–301

12. Miller WH, Bernard GD (1983) Averaging over the foveal receptor aperture curtails aliasing. Vision Res 23:1365–9

13. Murillo Lopez F, Fukuhara J, Wisnicki HJ, Guyton DL (1994) Origin of the foveal granular pattern in entoptic viewing. Invest Ophthalmol Vis Sci 35:3319–24

14. Perry VH, Cowey A (1985) The ganglion cell and cone distributions in the monkey's retina: implications for central magnification factors. Vision Res 25:1795–810

15. Pöppe CH (1989) Graphische Darstellung komplex-analytischer Funktionen. Spektrum Wiss 8:8–13

16. Provis JM, Diaz CM, Dreher B (1998) Ontogeny of the primate fovea: a central issue in retinal development. Prog Neurobiol 54:549–80

17. Provis JM, van Driel D, Billson FA, Russell P (1985) Development of the human retina: patterns of cell distribution and redistribution in the ganglion cell layer. J Comp Neurol 233:429–51

18. Pum D, Ahnelt PK, Grasl M (1990) Iso-orientation areas in the foveal cone mosaic. Vis Neurosci 5:511–23

19. Schein SJ (1988) Anatomy of macaque fovea and spatial densities of neurons in foveal representation. J Comp Neurol 269:479–505

20. Sekiguchi N, Williams DR, Packer O (1991) Nonlinear distortion of gratings at the foveal resolution limit. Vision Res 31:815–31

21. Sjöstrand J, Popovic Z, Conradi N, Marshall J (1999) Morphometric study of the displacement of retinal ganglion cells subserving cones within the human fovea. Graefes Arch Clin Exp Ophthalmol 237:1014–23

22. Williams DR (1985) Aliasing in human foveal vision. Vision Res 25:195–205

23. Williams DR (1988) Topography of the foveal cone mosaic in the living human eye [see comments]. Vision Res 28:433–54

24. Yellott JI, Jr (1983) Spectral consequences of photoreceptor sampling in the rhesus retina. Science 221:382–5

Correspondence: a.Univ.Prof. Dr. Peter Ahnelt (e-mail: peter.ahnelt@univie.ac.at), Institut für Physiologie, Med. Universität Wien, Schwarzspanierstrasse 17, A-1090 Wien, Austria.

Macular pigment – its role in health and disease

M. Boulton

School of Optometry and Vision Sciences, Cardiff University,
Redwood Building, Cardiff, UK

Interest in macular pigment has increased over the last two decades with the realisation that it plays a major role in maintaining retinal homeostasis and that it may contribute to retinal pathologies [2, 15]. Macular pigment consists predominantly of two hydroxy carotenoids namely zeaxanthin and lutein (Fig. 1). However, a number of oxidised forms of lutein and zeaxanthin can also be identified in the retina of which meso-zeaxanthin (a product of oxidative modification of zeaxanthin) is the most common. Visually, macular pigment presents as a yellow colouration concentrated in the fovea. However, more objective methodologies such as spectrophotometry and HPLC have mapped the topographical distribution of macular pigment both across and within the layers of the retina. The absorption spectrum of macular pigment peaks in the blue light region of the visible spectrum (460 nm) but does not absorb in the green. By comparing the absorption of green and blue light in tissue sections through the fovea of adult primates it was demonstrated that macular pigment is concentrated in the foveola and avascular fovea regions [21]. Further analysis showed the macular pigment to be predominately located in the photoreceptor axons with significant but lesser amounts in the inner retinal neurons. Significantly lower levels are observed throughout the retina and macular pigment is often found in association with photoreceptor outer segments [18]. Biochemical analyses confirms that the macular carotenoids are assymetrically distributed throughout the retina but are concentrated in the macular and account for 36% of the total retinal carotenoids [4]. Carotenoid concentrations are estimated at 1.33 ng/mm^2 at the foveal centre, decreasing to 0.81 ng/mm^2 at eccentricity of 2.5 mm and decreasing significantly thereafter [4]. Interestingly the zeaxanthin : lutein ratio is dependent upon retinal location – zeaxanthin is the predominant carotenoid at the fovea while lutein is predominant in the peripheral retina [4, 22]. Snodderly and colleagues [22] have proposed lutein and zeaxanthin exhibit respectively a rod-cone specificity. The last decade has seen considerable emphasis placed on *in vivo* measures (e.g. heterochromic flicker photometry, fundus reflectometry) of macular pigment to obtain a better understanding of dietary and pathological conditions in the regulation of retinal carotenoid concentration. *In vivo* analysis of macular pigment optical density demonstrates that while there is considerable inter-individual variation in macular pigment levels within the UK population, there is a good correlation between macular pigment density between the left and right eyes of individuals [3]. The question of whether macular pigment density decreases with age is equivocal. Some authors report a highly significant decrease in carotenoids of the macular with increasing donor age and propose that those with the lowest macular pigment density may be at most risk of developing age-related macular degeneration (AMD) [3, 8]. However, this age-related decrease in macular pigment has not been observed in all studies and has not been confirmed by chemical analysis of retinas from different age groups [15]. It is important that in-depth studies are undertaken to clarify this issue and to confirm whether a deficit in retinal carotenoids contributes to macular disease.

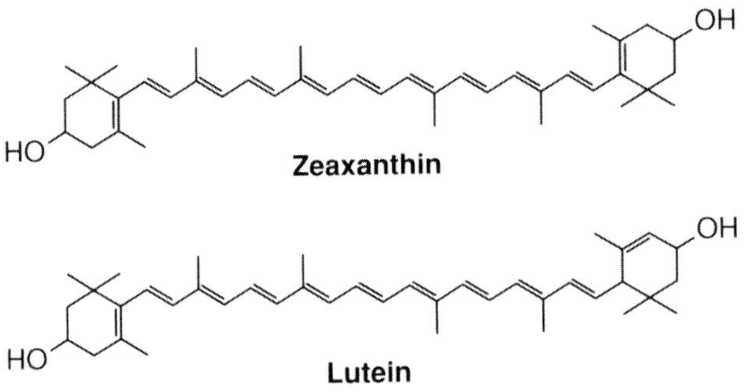

Fig. 1. Chemical structure of zeaxanthin and lutein

Physiological considerations

De novo synthesis of carotenoids does not occur in animals and thus the retinal carotenoids can only be obtained from the diet [2]. It has been previously demonstrated that monkeys fed a carotenoid-free diet have a total absence of macular pigment [16]. Furthermore, clinical trials have demonstrated that macular pigment can be elevated by dietary supplementation. In a study by Landrum et al. [14] individuals supplemented with lutein at 30 mg per day for 140 days showed no significant increase in macular pigment up to 14 days but thereafter a steady increase up to the point at which supplementation was ceased. Interestingly, this increase continued for at least 50 days following cessation of supplementation despite an obvious decrease in lutein serum levels. Thereafter, the macular pigment concentration remained elevated but constant for up to 400 days. This suggests a low turnover of carotenoids in the retina and that macular pigment levels reflect long-term carotenoid consumption. However, little is known of the process by which carotenoids reach the retina and how this may be affected in ageing and age-related disease and by gender differences (males are reported to have an average of 38% more macular pigment than females [9]).

The function of macular pigment

The precise role of macular pigment remains uncertain although there are an increasing number of reports that retinal carotenoids are related to visual performance in both normal subjects and those with ocular pathology. Three principal functions have been proposed; improved visual function, protection of the retina from potentially damaging blue light, and/or by acting directly as an antioxidant.

Visual function

It has been proposed that lutein and zeaxanthin can improve visual function through either increased visual acuity or improved visability (reviewed in Wooten and Hammond [25]). Based on theoretical modelling of the absorption of short wave length light by macular pigment Reading and Weale concluded that it was able to filter out the aberrant part of the visible spectrum and this reduced dramatic aberration to the lower threshold leading to improved visual acuity. However, it has also been proposed that macular pigment may improve visibility by preferentially absorbing blue haze.

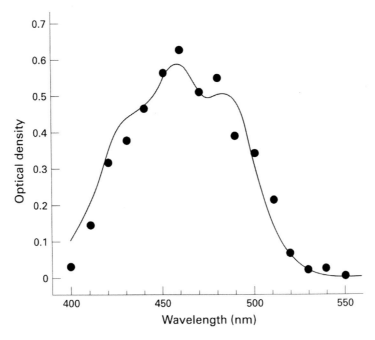

Fig. 2. Absorption spectrum of macular pigment as plotted by Wyszecki and Stiles (line) and Werner et al. (points). Reprinted from Werner et al. with permission from Elsevier Science [see 2]

Blue light filter

The absorption spectrum for macular pigment demonstrates absorbtion between 400–520 nm with peak absorbtion at 460 nm (Fig. 2). This makes macular pigment an excellent filter for blue light thus restricting the most energetic form of non-ionising radiation from reaching the retina where it has the potential for photochemical damage (reviewed in Boulton et al. [6]; [2]). This filtration is enhanced by the location of macular pigment in the retinal layers; a) macular carotenoids reach their highest levels in the receptor axon layer of the foveola with relatively high concentrations in the receptor axon and inner plexiform layers in the extra foveola macular, b) the macular pigment is distributed throughout the photoreceptor cell and thus each photoreceptor screens other photoreceptors as well as itself because of the lateral course of the axons and c) the orientation of the macular pigment within retinal cells enhances blue light absorption. Transmission studies have demonstrated that macular pigment can achieve sufficient density to prevent over 80% of 460 nm light from reaching the retina [10]. However, due to the considerable inter-individual variation in the macular pigment noted earlier those individuals with a low density of carotenoids may only screen about 10% of 460 nm light. The properties and location of macular pigment indicate that it will make a significant contribution towards protection of the retina against blue light-induced oxidative damage.

Antioxidant

Constant exposure to light, high oxygen levels and a readily oxidisable substrate in polyunsaturated fatty acids makes the retina an ideal tissue for the formation of potentially damaging reactive oxygen species (ROS). Numerous studies have demonstrated that the retina has evolved three mechanisms to protect against ROS [5]; a) repair systems

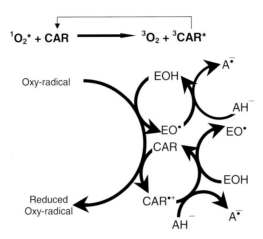

Fig. 3. A schematic representation of the co-operative antioxidant interactions of carotenoids (CAR), α tocopherol (E) and ascorbate (A). • radical; CAR* carotenoid radical

which replace damaged molecules, genes or proteins, b) enzymic antioxidants such as superoxide dismutase, catalase and glutathione peroxidase and c) non-enzymic antioxidants (e.g. vitamin C, vitamin E, glutathione and melanin). However, there is increasing evidence that the carotenoids also play a major role as scavengers of reactive oxygen species in the retina. Carotenoids are effective at neutralising both singlet oxygen and oxyradicals which itself results in a lower energy carotenoid radical that in turn requires neutralisation by other antioxidants such as α-tocopherol and ascorbate (Fig. 3) [5, 26]. Carotenoids are potent neutralising agents for oxyradicals and singlet oxygen with lycopene being the most potent followed by zeaxanthin and lutein.

The antioxidant properties of the retinal carotenoids include the ability to quench the triplet state of photosensitisers and singlet oxygen, reactivity with free radicals, and chain breaking antioxidant properties to retard the peroxidation of membrane phospholipids. Zeaxanthin is a particularly efficient singlet oxygen quencher with a biomolecular rate constant close to that controlled by diffusion, while lutein, having one less conjugated double bond, is half as effective in interactions with single oxygen. It has been shown that zeaxanthin is more efficient than betacarotene in inhibiting lipid peroxidation. Carotenoid radical cations, unless scavenged by other antioxidants such as vitamin E, vitamin C or melanin, may become damaging to biological molecules. However, antioxidants such as α-tocopherol and ascorbate also act synergistically with macular carotenoids in addition to neutralising carotenoid radicals. For example, recent studies in our laboratory (Rozanowska, Rozanowski, Boulton, unpublished observation) have compared the efficiency of individual antioxidants (e.g. lutein, α-tocopherol and ascorbate) and in combinations thereof in protecting human RPE cells against photooxidative damage. Our results show that a combination of a singlet oxygen quencher (e.g. carotenoid) and a free radical scavenger (e.g. ascorbate) offer better protection against photooxidative damage than increasing concentrations of individual antioxidants.

Macular pigments in aging and disease

The cumulative photochemical damage of the retina is reflected in the age-related morphological and functional changes that occur in the macular, e.g. a loss of rods in the perimacular region, a reduction in cone density and a loss of sensitivity of the short wavelength sensitive cones [7, 11, 24]. However, evidence for macular pigment providing protection against retinal photodamage, especially from the blue light component of the visible spectrum is at best circumstantial. Clinical observations and experiments on monkeys indicate a positive correlation between high macular pigment density and a reduced susceptibility to photodamage. There is also evidence that the outer fovea is more susceptible to photodamage than the foveola despite that in the foveola there is a higher density of cones which at other locations have been shown to be more susceptible to photodamage. Further evidence comes from the observation that the central macular is spared in a number of retinal pathologies for which light is a risk factor, e.g. age-related macular degeneration, chloroquine-induced retinopathy, pigmentary retinopathy [5]. In all these ocular conditions sparing of the central retina correlates with the region of the highest optical density of macular pigments.

Macular pigment and age related macular degeneration

It remains equivocal whether reductions in retinal carotenoid levels in the retina contribute to the aetiology of AMD and if they do whether they are cause or consequence of the condition. However, there is evidence from this and other laboratories that macular pigment is reduced in age-related macular degeneration [3, 13]. In our study macular pigment was significantly lower in high risk eyes (e.g. the fellow eye was already exhibiting AMD) compared to standard risk eyes in which there was no evidence of age-related macular degeneration in either eye [3]. It should be noted that, while macular pigment optical density was decreased in the majority of eyes with age-related macular degeneration, the overall optical density of pigment was highly variable between individuals. Furthermore, a limitation of this type of study is that at least 30% of standard risk eyes are likely to develop AMD later in life.

Carotenoid supplementation

Perhaps the simplest way to confirm a role for carotenoids in AMD is to see if dietary supplementation will prevent, slow or halt the progression of AMD. The idea of dietary supplementation with antioxidants has been extensively assessed but due to limitations in study design the efficacy of antioxidant therapy is not clearly proven. In the most recent ARED study, antioxidants plus zinc were able to reduce the rate of progression of AMD and reduce the loss of visual acuity compared to untreated controls [1]. However, while this was a significant effect it was not particularly large and required very high concentrations of antioxidants, suggesting that either the combination of antioxidants (vitamin C, vitamin E, beta-carotene and zinc oxide) was not optimal, other antioxidants (e.g. lutein and zeaxanthin) are necessary (an observation supported by our laboratory studies and discussed earlier in this review), or that there are other mechanisms involved in the progression of AMD. Dietary supplementation with the retinal carotenoids lutein and zeaxanthin is being strongly advocated by the commercial sector. Despite numerous studies the benefits of such supplementation remains inconclusive. The EDCC study in 1994 reported that a high dietary intake of carotenoids protected against AMD [20]. After adjusting for other risk factors, the highest quintile of carotenoid intake was associated with a 43% reduction in AMD. Of the carotenoids tested lutein and zeaxanthin were found to be the most protective. However in the subsequent BDES study no protective effect could be observed [17]. Perhaps the problem lies in our failure to realise that there is cooperation between antioxidants and that we have yet to supplement with the appropriate cocktail of antioxidants at the optimal concentration.

Conclusions

In summary, while macular pigment is considered to play an important role in macular physiology and disease this remains equivocal. Furthermore, while antioxidant supplementation is strongly advocated to ensure an adequate macular pigment density and to prevent or slow down the progression of retinal disease I leave you a recent quote from the National Eye Institute, July 2002: "Claims made about an association between lutein and eye health are speculative and should be viewed with caution. The possible benefits of lutein for the eye are uncertain." Despite these reservations, there is no objection to AMD sufferers or the population as a whole taking oral antioxidants, provided that they are at safe levels. However, perhaps the simplest way to ensure a healthy macular pigment density is to have a healthy diet containing egg yolk, maize, orange peppers, grapes, spinach and orange juice which are rich in lutein and zeaxanthin [23].

References

1. Age-Related Eye Disease Study Research Group (2001) A randomized, placebo-controlled, clinical trial of high-dose supplementation with vitamins C and E, beta carotene, and zinc for age-related macular degeneration and vision loss: AREDS report no. 8. Arch Ophthalmol 119:1417–36
2. Beatty S, Boulton M, Henson D, Koh H-H, Murray I (1999) Macular pigment and age-related macular degeneration. Br J Ophthalmol 83:867–77
3. Beatty S, Murray I, Henson D, Carden D, Koh H, Boulton M (2001) Macular pigment and risk for age-related macular degeneration in subjects from a Northern European population. Invest Ophthalmol Vis Sci 42:439–46
4. Bone R, Landrum J, Fernandez L, Tarsis L (1988) Analysis of the macular pigment by HPLC: retinal distribution and age study. Invest Ophthalmol Vis Sci 29:843–9
5. Boulton M, Dayhaw-Barker P (2001) The role of retinal pigment epithelium: topographical variation and ageing changes. Eye 15:384–9
6. Boulton M, Rózanowska M, Rózanowska B (2001) Retinal photodamage. J Photochem Photobiol B (biol) 64:144–61
7. Farber D, Flannery J, Lolley R, Bok D (1985) Distribution of patterns of photoreceptors, proteins and cyclic nucleotides in the human retina. Invest Ophthalmol Vis Sci 25:1558–68
8. Hammond B, Caruso-Avery M (2000) Macular pigment optical density in a Southwestern sample. Invest Ophthalmol Vis Sci 41:1492–7
9. Hammond B, Curran-Celentano J, Judd S, Fuld K, Krinsky NI, Wooten B, Snodderly D (1996) Sex differences in macular pigment optical density: relation to plasma carotenoid concentrations and dietary patterns. Vision Res 36:2001–12
10. Hammond B, Wooten B, Celentano J (2001) Carotenoids in the retina and lens: possible acute and chronic effects on visual performance. Arch Biochem Biophys 385:41–6
11. Jackson GR, Owsley C, Curcio CA (2002) Photoreceptor degeneration and dysfunction in aging and age-related maculopathy. Ageing Res Rev 1:381–96
12. Jaffe G, Wood I (1988) Retinal phototoxicity from the operating microscope: a protective effect by the fovea. Arch Ophthalmol 106:445–6
13. Landrum J, Bone R, Chen Y, Herrero C, Llerna C, Twarowska E (2000) Carotenoids in the human retina. Pure Appl Chem 71:2237–44
14. Landrum J, Bone R, Joa H, Kilburn M, Moore L, Sprauge K (1997) A one year study of the macular pigment: the effect of 140 days of a lutein supplement. Exp Eye Res 65:57–62
15. Landrum J, Bone R (2001) Lutein, zeaxanthin, and the macular pigment. Arch Biochem Biophys 385:28–40
16. Malinow M, Feeney-Burns L, Peterson L, Klein M, Neuringer M (1980) Diet-related macular anomalies in monkeys. Invest Ophthalmol Vis Sci 19:857–63
17. Marles-Perlman J, Klein R, Klein B, et al (1996) Association of zinc and antioxidant nutrients with age-related maculopathy. Arch Ophthalmol 114:991–7
18. Rapp L, Maple S, Choi J (2000) Lutein and zeaxanthin concentrations in rod outer segment membranes from perifoveal and peripheral human retina. Invest Ophthalmol Vis Sci 41:1200–9

19. Reading V, Weale R (1974) Macular pigment and chromatic aberration. J Am Optom Assoc 64:231–4

20. Seddon J, Ajani U, Spertudo R, et al (1994) Dietary carotenoids, Vitamins A, C, and E, and advanced age-related macular degeneration. Eye Disease case Control Study Group. JAMA 272:1413–20

21. Snodderly D, Auran J, Delori F (1984) The macular pigment. II. Spatial distribution in primate retinas. Invest Ophthalmol Vis Sci 25:674–85

22. Snodderly D, Handelman G, Adler J (1991) Distribution of individual macular pigment carotenoids in central retina of macaque and squirrel monkeys. Invest Ophthalmol Vis Sci 32:268–79

23. Sommerburg O, Keunen J, Bird A, van Kuijk F (1998) Fruits and vegetables which are sources for lutein and zeaxanthin: the macular pigment in human eyes. Br J Ophthalmol 82:907–10

24. Werner J, Steele V, Pfoff D (1989) Loss of human photoreceptor sensitivity associated with chronic exposure to ultraviolet radiation. Ophthalmol 96:1552–8

25. Wooten B, Hammond B (2002) Macular pigment: influences on visual acuity and visibility. Prog Retinal Eye Res 21:225–40

26. Young A, Lowe G (2001) Antioxidant and prooxidant properties of carotenoids. Arch Biochem Biophys 385:20–7

Correspondence: Mike Boulton (e-mail: BoultonM@cf.ac.uk), School of Optometry and Vision Sciences, Cardiff University, Redwood Building, King Edward VII Avenue, Cardiff CF10 3NB, UK.

The importance of maintaining the RPE phenotype in retinal transplantation

M. Boulton

School of Optometry and Vision Sciences, Cardiff University,
Redwood Building, Cardiff, UK

Retinal degeneration is a major cause of visual loss and is associated with a variety of conditions (e.g. age-related macular degeneration (AMD), retinitis pigmentosa, macular dystrophy). Morphologically, such degeneration can occur in the neural retina (e.g. retinitis pigmentosa) or retinal pigment epithelium (e.g. AMD). While a number of therapies have been proposed for the treatment of retinal degeneration, transplantation of cells or tissue has received considerable attention in the last decade [18, 20]. Of particular interest is retinal pigment epithelium (RPE) transplantation which has the advantage over neural retinal transplantation that it only involves one cell type, does not require neural networking and is a reasonably straightforward procedure, although not without complications as will be discussed later.

There are a number of requirements for a successful outcome in RPE transplantation.

- Replacement of diseased cells
- The transplanted cells *must* carry out the functions of the RPE
- The transplanted cells *must* establish themselves in the host eye and should at least maintain, if not improve, vision

To achieve this it is essential to have a source of donor cells, to be able to deliver the cells to the transplantation site and, once delivered, to minimise any inflammatory response in order to avoid the possibility of rejection and associated retinal degeneration. The transplanted cells, if they survive, should ideally acquire the normal *in vivo* RPE phenotype as well as establish and stabilise within the host in order to contribute towards the maintenance of retinal homeostasis. In the author's view, while we have overcome many of the problems associated with RPE transplantation, a major outstanding issue is ensuring that the transplanted cells exhibit a true *in vivo* RPE phenotype which will undertake the essential functions required of it. Unfortunately, despite claims that transplanted cells are functional in the host eye the tendency is to look only for a few major markers of activity (e.g. phagocytosis, attachment, polarisation) while ignoring a multitude of other markers critical for successful function and retinal homeostasis.

RPE physiology in the context of retinal transplantation

Before discussing further the limitations of RPE transplantation it is important to briefly review normal RPE structure and function [5, 9, 15]. The RPE is a continuous monolayer of hexano-cuboidal epithelial cells located between the photoreceptors and Bruch's membrane (Fig. 1). These cells do not normally divide in the adult except in cases of trauma or pathology. Two types of microvilli are present on the RPE apical surface: long thin microvilli 5–7 μm in length, which are believed to maximise the surface area of the plasma

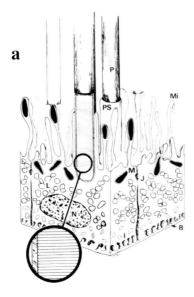
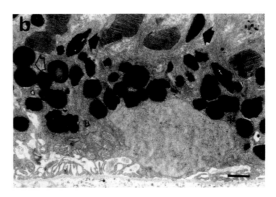

Fig. 1. a A schematic representation of the RPE/photoreceptor outer segment complex. J – Intercellular junctional complexes; Mi – microvilli; PS – photoreceptor sheath; P – photoreceptor outer segment; I – basal invaginations; B – Bruch's membrane; N – nucleus; M – melanosomes; L – lipofuscin granules. **b** Electron micrograph of *in situ* RPE from an 80 year old. Closed arrows – melanosomes; open arrows – lipofuscin; stars – melanolipofuscin complexes. The bar marker is 1 μm

membrane available for transepithelial transport and specialised microvilli which surround photoreceptor outer segment tips and are often referred to as photoreceptor sheaths. The basal surface of the RPE contains numerous infoldings which, like the apical surface, maximise surface area for the transfer of molecules. An outer blood-retinal barrier is established by the continuous belt of occluding junctions located between the lateral membranes of adjacent cells. Intracellular gap junctions are also present on the lateral membranes of RPE cells and ensure that the entire RPE layer is metabolically coupled. The RPE is rich in organelles which reflects its high metabolic rate. Abundant mitochondria are located towards the base of each cell while a rich provision of the smooth endoplasmic reticulum and lysosomes are distributed throughout the cell. In addition, melanin granules 2–3 μm in length are, for the most part, vertically orientated lying parallel to one another at the base of, or within the, apical processes presumably to maximise light absorption. It is quite evident that the RPE cell is a highly differentiated structure with clear morphological and metabolic compartmentalisation.

Most text books [14, 21] identify the critical functions of the RPE as:

- Provision of an outer blood-retinal barrier
- Transepithelial transport
- Transport and storage of retinoids
- Phagocytosis and degradation of photoreceptor outer segments
- Protection against light and oxidative damage
- Production of growth factors

Gases diffuse freely across the cell layer with high levels of oxygen moving from the choriocapillaris to the photoreceptors. However, in its role as the outer blood-retinal barrier, the RPE regulates the transepithelial transport of ions, fluid, metabolites and waste products via specialised transport proteins within the apical and/or basal plasma membranes. The asymmetric distribution and regulation of these proteins ensures that the RPE can control the micro environment bathing the photoreceptors.

The RPE is critical for the maintenance of the visual cycle due to its ability to transport, store and modify retinoids [12]. Retinol is present in the blood bound to a retinol binding protein (RBP) from which it is transferred into the cell via specific RBP binding sites localised to the basal and basolateral surfaces of RPE cells. Upon entering the cell all-*trans*-retinol immediately becomes esterified and provides a non-toxic substrate for isomerisation to the 11-*cis* conformation. Esterification of retinol also provides an intracellular store of retinoids. 11-*cis*-retinol is converted to 11-*cis* retinal and transported via interphotoreceptor matrix binding protein (IRBP) to the photoreceptors where it combines in rods with opsin to produce rhodopsin. In the photoreceptors, 11-*cis* retinal is converted to all-*trans*-retinal within picoseconds of absorbing a photon of light and transferred back to the RPE to be recycled either conjugated to IRBP (or as a function of the phagocytosis of outer segments).

The RPE is constantly ingesting the spent tips of photoreceptor outer segments throughout life. The recognition signals for outer segment binding and ingestion are poorly understood although a number of receptor molecules have been identified (e.g. the mannose receptor, αVβ3 integrin, CD38 and Mertk [5]). Once ingested the resultant phagosome fuses with a lysosome to form a secondary phagosome or phagolysosome in which the ingested outer segments are digested by a combination of over 40 lysosomal enzymes capable of degrading proteins, polysaccharides, lipids and nucleic acids. It is important to note that this degradation is incomplete and that this accounts for the age-related accumulation of lipofuscin within the RPE.

The RPE is in an ideal environment for the formation of reactive oxygen species with a potential to damage proteins, DNA and lipids in that it is constantly exposed to long periods of visible light and high local oxygen tensions, has a high metabolic activity and phagocytoses photoreceptor outer segments (a source of reactive oxygen species) on a daily basis [5, 8]. To limit oxidative damage the retina/RPE has evolved three lines of defence [3, 27]. First, the wavelength and intensity of light reaching the RPE can be attenuated by macular pigments which filter out potentially damaging reactive blue light and by melanin which will act as a neutral density filter and reduce light levels entering the RPE. Second, the RPE contains both enzymatic (e.g. superoxide dismutase, catalase and glutathione peroxidase) and non-enzymic (e.g. glutathione, ascorbate, α-tocopherol and carotenoids) antioxidants which neutralise reactive oxygen species before they can cause cellular damage. Third, some oxidative damage is inevitable and to overcome this, the RPE has evolved an efficient mechanism to repair oxidative damage up to a certain threshold.

The RPE can produce a wide variety of growth factors and cytokines (e.g. FGF, TGFβ, IGF-1, PDGF, VEGF, TNFα and members of the interleukin family) which are normally constitutively expressed at low levels but can become significantly upregulated in pathology [10]. The role of these growth factors remains unclear with some possibly acting as neuroprotective agents, some regulating synthesis and turnover of matrix, while others are controlling capillary permeability and maintaining vascular quiescence.

It is important to note that all the functions of the normal healthy RPE appear to operate above threshold levels of activity required for retinal homeostasis. This would indicate that there is considerable redundancy in the system and that the RPE is likely to be able to undergo considerable alteration before retinal function is compromised. Furthermore, it should also be realised that RPE structure and function varies with retinal location [5].

While the functional and metabolic activities highlighted above are critical for the maintenance of retinal homeostasis, it must be realised that a successful RPE phenotype, like most cell types, is dependent on a much greater number of physiological parameters which are finely tuned and interdependent on each other [13, 19]. Examples include:

- Polarity
- Adhesion and growth factor receptors
- Matrix synthesis and turnover
- Transport proteins (ion channels, glucose transporters)
- Pigmentation
- Protein targeting
- Compartmentalisation
- Environmental regulation

It is not sufficient simply to say that RPE cells have microvilli. To carry out their functions adequately, they must have the appropriate number and type that ensure the optimal transport characteristics of the RPE and allow for the ingestion of photoreceptor outer segments. Similarly, it is not sufficient to say that RPE cells are capable of phagocytosing photoreceptor outer segments; they must ingest them at the correct rate and they must dispose of them in the appropriate way.

What are the choices as a source of RPE cells?

Returning to the importance of RPE phenotype in retinal transplantation much is dependent on the source of the cells, how they are prepared, the method of transplantation and the status of the host eye. The source of RPE can be autologous cells, e.g. from the host eye, or non-autologous cells from donor eyes of human or non-human origin. Autologous cells are normally obtained from the peripheral retina with the disadvantage that they can only be obtained in relatively small numbers and that there will always be the possibility of consequent complications such as proliferative vitreoretinopathy. By contrast, non-autologous RPE cells from donor eyes can be obtained in large numbers and can be obtained from the central retina. However, the disadvantage of non-autologous cells is that they often provoke an immunogenic response which can ultimately result in rejection. Given the considerable differences in both morphology and metabolic capability between RPE cells from different retinal locations, it may well be very important to use central cells as opposed to peripheral cells to treat a central retinal pathology. Other considerations which are important are the post mortem time in the case of non-autologous cells, as the longer the post mortem time, the more likely the cells are going to have irretrievably lost some of their *in vivo* function. Another important issue relevant to non-autologous cells is whether to use foetal, young or old donor RPE cells. Foetal cells will provide a very morphologically differentiated cell type with some polarisation, but this does not appear to represent the adult phenotype. By comparison old cells have often lost many of their functional characteristics and are thus not the best donor cells for producing rejuvenation in a dysfunctional eye. For these reasons the best choice is tissue from young donors, but such eyes only rarely become available.

Should we transplant fresh or cultured cells?

There seems to be considerable differences in viewpoint on this issue with advocates and detractors for fresh and cultured cells (Fig. 2). The obvious advantage of freshly isolated cells is the retention of phenotype, but the disadvantage is that these cells will often be

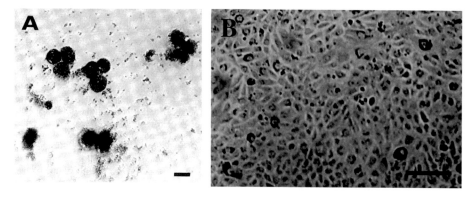

Fig. 2. A Freshly isolated RPE cells showing clumps of both intact and damaged cells. The bar marker is 20 μm. **B** A primary culture of human RPE cells. The bar marker is 150 μm

damaged by the recent procedure required to obtain them. Overt damage is commonly identified by Trypan blue staining. However, Trypan blue is a large molecular weight protein dye which will only enter cells that have large holes in their plasma membrane and will not identify more subtle but equally relevant damage such as shearing of integral membrane proteins, loss of adhesion receptors, and/or loss of apical microvilli, any of which will still result in a dysfunctional cell. Furthermore, fresh cells only provide a limited source of tissue as there is no means of amplification. This shortcoming can, in part, be overcome with the use of cultured cells in which it is possible to amplify small numbers of RPE cells (e.g. from chorioretinal biopsies [12]), to provide sufficient cell numbers to cover a large area of Bruch's membrane. However, the disadvantage of these cultured cells is that they lose many of their normal phenotypic characteristics. In addition, primary cell culture tends to select for cells with the greatest survival and proliferative capacities – the latter being hardly the ideal requirement for a retinal pigment epithelial cell once transplanted into the eye! If we look carefully at the loss of phenotypic characteristics in retinal pigment epithelial cells in culture, we can identify one or more of the following: reduction in surface area, reduction in the number of cell organelles, reduction in enzymic activity, loss of pigment, lower transepithelial resistance, often exposure to non-human proteins during culture (e.g. fetal calf serum), loss of polarity, loss of receptors, loss of compartmentalisation and increased contractility. From these observations, it must be concluded that we currently transplant "highly stressed" RPE cells, whether fresh or cultured, with reduced metabolic function into an adverse environment. Surprisingly, we then expect these cells to establish and perform their normal *in vivo* functions and are astonished when this does not happen!

Rejuvenation of phenotype

It is possible to recover, at least in part, the normal RPE in cultured retinal pigment epithelial cells by a number of additional manipulations [6, 7, 11]. Some examples of these procedures include: a) upregulating the number of apical microvilli and lysosomal enzymes by repeated feeding of cells with photoreceptor outer segments (Fig. 3), b) growing cells on a defined matrix which produces a better and more differentiated epithelial monolayer and c) maintaining the cells in a more appropriate oxygen environment (cells are routinely cultured under hyperoxic conditions). However, these additional manipulations are costly in terms of time and money, and as a result, may not represent a feasible approach if RPE transplantation is to become a routine procedure.

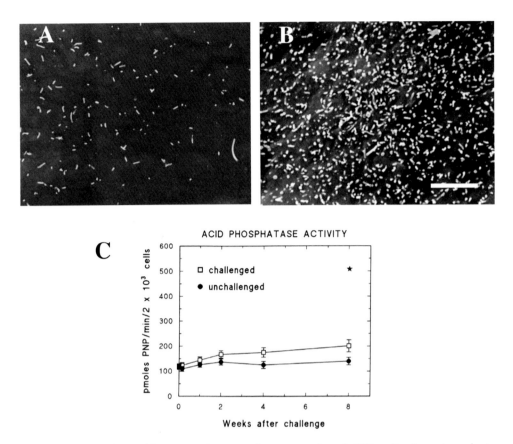

Fig. 3. Examples of possible approaches to rejuvenate cultured RPE cells. Scanning electron micrographs of the apical surface of subcultured human RPE cells. **A** shows unchallenged whilst **B** shows cells 24 hr after challenge with photoreceptor outer segments. The bar marker is 150 μm. The graph, **C**, shows a significant increase in acid phosphatase activity 8 weeks after daily challenge with rod outer segments. The asterisk shows lysosomal enzyme activity in the equivalent number of freshly isolated human RPE cells

Transplantation of RPE cells

Having obtained the RPE cells, either fresh or cultured, from autologous or non-autologous eyes, the next difficulty is how to present them to the diseased retina. Although RPE cells are relatively easy to deliver, there may be considerable trauma at dissociation whether using fresh or cultured cells, which may reduce their attachment ability. Ideally a single layer of transplanted RPE cells must attach to the basal substrate of Bruch's membrane in order to become established and function correctly. Histological analysis indicates that injection of cell suspensions often leads to multi-layering of retinal pigment epithelial cells. RPE cell sheets are particularly easy to produce in culture as they can be grown on a variety of biological and synthetic matrices (e.g. collagen, Bruch's membrane preparation, lens capsule, gelatine and other biodegradable substrates). There is reasonable quality control and no extreme trauma to the cells prior to transplantation. However, delivery of these sheets can be difficult resulting in the sheets, once at the transplant site, being wrinkled or the cell layer inverted. Once transplanted the overall clinical outcome in terms of restoring retinal function appears to be limited although this is often difficult to assess since transplants to date have largely been undertaken during the late stage of disease. However, the RPE cells are normally located appropriately between the photoreceptors and Bruch's membrane and demonstrate some limited functionality, e.g. they can phagocytose rod outer segments and demonstrate the presence of a retinoid system [20, 24]. Rejection associated with non-autologous cells can usually be avoided with immunosuppression. The efficacy of procedure is difficult to evaluate in humans, some improvement in vision has been reported although stabilisation is often considered a good end result [1, 4].

An additional manipulation is to modify the cells *ex vivo* before transplantation e.g. by inducing them to over express a required gene product. A number of studies have demonstrated that ex *vivo* gene therapy is feasible and that cultured human RPE cells can be transfected to over express a gene product when transplanted *in vivo* [16, 22]. Researchers are now investigating the possibilities of providing cells which over express brain-derived neurotrophic factor (BDNF) to promote retinal cell survival or over express pigment epithelial-derived growth factor to prevent aberrant angiogenesis such as occurs in sub-retinal neovascularisation [16]. Such phenotypic modification of transplanted retinal pigment epithelial cells offers the possibility that even a dysfunctional donor RPE cell can be restored to perform a required specific function in the retina which may in turn help prevent or slow down the degenerative process. Such an effect may also be beneficial even when RPE cells only offer some limited, short term establishment in the retina.

Future challenges

This review has concentrated on transplantation of human RPE cells, but it should be realised that there are a number of alternative transplant approaches which can be considered. Cells with a similar phenotype to the retinal pigment epithelial cell may be a realistic substitute. For example, researchers have shown that autologous iris pigment epithelium, which can be obtained in reasonably large numbers, can demonstrate some of the phenotypic characteristics of the RPE, both *in vivo* and *in vitro* [25, 26]. It is also possible to consider the transplantation of autologous cells with multipotential properties (e.g. stem cells [2]). However, it is likely that this procedure will not be effective since the differentiation of these primitive cells is dependent on the localised environment and that the adverse environment in the diseased eye is not likely to lead to the required form of differentiation. The final possibility is the use of genetically engineered tissue, such as porcine RPE which is designed to express human antigens [23].

Summary

In conclusion, while this review may appear to portray an overly pessimistic view of RPE transplantation, this is not the intention. Many of the limitations discussed can almost certainly be overcome with further research, leading to refinement of technique, *ex vivo* gene therapy, improved phenotype and new procedures for transplantation that will limit the damage associated with the dissociation process. The only aspect which is difficult to change following transplantation is the adverse local environment in the host eye. However, perhaps even this problem can be partly overcome by encasing the donor RPE cells in a "protective gel" which promotes their viability and phenotype during the first hours, days or weeks of their life in the host retina.

References

1. Algvere PV, Gouras P, Dafgard Kopp E (1999) Long-term outcome of RPE allografts in non-immunosuppressed patients with AMD. Eur J Ophthalmol 9:217–30

2. Arsenijevic Y, Taverney N, Kostic C, Tekaya M, Riva F, Zografos L, Schorderet D, Munier F (2003) Non-neural regions of the adult human eye: a potential source of neurons? Invest Ophthalmol Vis Sci 44:799–807

3. Beatty S, Koh H-H, Henson D, Boulton M (2000) The role of oxidative stress in the pathogenesis of age-related macular degeneration. Surv Ophthalmol 45:115–34

4. Binder S, Stolba U, Krebs I, Kellner L, Jahn C, Feichtinger H, Povelka M, Frohner U, Kruger A, Hilgers RD, Krugluger W (2002) Transplantation of autologous retinal pigment epithelium in eyes with foveal neovascularization resulting from age-related macular degeneration: a pilot study. Am J Ophthalmol 133:215–25

5. Boulton M, Dayhaw-Barker P (2001) The role of retinal pigment epithelium: topographical variation and ageing changes. Eye 15:384–9

6. Boulton M, Khaliq A, McLeod D, Moriarty P (1994) Effect of "hypoxia" on the proliferation of retinal microvascular cells in vitro. Exp Eye Res 59:243–6

7. Boulton M, Marshall J, Mellerio J (1984) Retinitis pigmentosa: a quantitative study of the apical membrane of normal and dystrophic human retinal pigment epithelial cells in tissue culture in relation to phagocytosis. Graefe's Arch Ophthalmol 221:214–29

8. Boulton M, Rózanowska M, Rózanowska B (2001) Retinal photodamage. J Photochem Photobiol B (biol) 64:144–61

9. Boulton ME (1991) Ageing of the retinal pigment epithelium. In: Osborne N, Charder G (eds) Progress in retinal research, vol 11. Oxford, New York: Pergamon Press, pp 125–51

10. Campochiaro P (1998) Growth factors in the retinal pigment epithelium and retina. In: Marmor M, Wolfensberger T (eds) The retinal pigment epithelium. New York, Oxford: Oxford University Press, pp 459–77

11. Campochiaro PA, Jerdan JA, Glaser BM (1986) The extracellular matrix of human retinal pigment epithelial cells in vivo and its synthesis in vitro. Invest Ophthalmol Vis Sci 27:1615–21

12. Chader G, Peppergerg D, Crouch R, Wiggert B (1998) Retinoids and the retinal pigment epithelium. In: Marmor M, Wolfensberger T (eds) The retinal pigment epithelium. New York, Oxford: Oxford University Press, pp 68–85

13. Cooper G (2000) The cell: a molecular approach. Washington: ASM Associates; Sunderland, Massachusetts: Sinauer Associates

14. Forrester J, Dick A, McMenamin P, Lee W (1999) The eye: basic science in practice. Edinburgh, London: WB Saunders

15. Hogan M, Alvarado J, Weddell J (1971) Histology of the human eye. Philadelphia: Saunders

16. Kanuga N, Winton HL, Beauchene L, Koman A, Zerbib A, Halford S, Couraud PO, Keegan D, Coffey P, Lund RD, Adamson P, Greenwood J (2002) Characterization of genetically modified human retinal pigment epithelial cells developed for in vitro and transplantation studies. Invest Ophthalmol Vis Sci 43(2):546–55

17. Lane C, Boulton M, Bird A, Marshall J (1988) Growth of pure cultures of retinal pigment epithelial cells using chorioretinal biopsies in the miniature pig. Exp Eye Res 46:813–7

18. Litchfield TM, Whiteley SJ, Lund RD (1997) Transplantation of retinal pigment epithelial, photoreceptor and other cells as treatment for retinal degeneration. Exp Eye Res 64:655–66

19. Lodish H, Berk A, Zipursky S, Matsudaira D, Darnell J (2001) Molecular cell biology. New York: WH Freeman

20. Lund RD, Kwan AS, Keegan DJ, Sauve Y, Coffey PJ, Lawrence JM (2001) Cell transplantation as a treatment for retinal disease. Prog Retin Eye Res 20:415–49

21. Marmor M, Wolfensberger T (1998) The retinal pigment epithelium. New York, Oxford: Oxford University Press

22. Murata T, Cui J, Taba KE, Oh JY, Spee C, Hinton DR, Ryan SJ (2000) The possibility of gene therapy for the treatment of choroidal neovascularization. Ophthalmol 107:1364–73

23. Niemann H (2001) Current status and perspectives for the generation of transgenic pigs for xenotransplantation. Ann Transplant 6:6–9

24. Sheng Y, Gouras P, Cao H, Berglin L, Kjeldbye H, Lopez R, Rosskothen H (1995) Patch transplants of human fetal retinal pigment epithelium in rabbit and monkey retina. Invest Ophthalmol Vis Sci 36:381–90

25. Thumann G, Aisenbrey S, Schraermeyer U, Lafaut B, Esser P, Walter P, Bartz-Schmidt KU (2000) Transplantation of autologous iris pigment epithelium after removal of choroidal neovascular membranes. Arch Ophthalmol 118:1350–5

26. Thumann G (2001) Development and cellular functions of the iris pigment epithelium. Surv Ophthalmol 45:345–54

27. Winkler B, Boulton ME, Gottsch J, Sternberg P (1999) Oxidative damage and age-related macular degeneration. Molecular Vision 5:32

Correspondence: Mike Boulton (e-mail: BoultonM@Cardiff.ac.uk), School of Optometry and Vision Sciences, Cardiff University, Redwood Building, King Edward VII Avenue, Cathays Park, Cardiff, CF10 3NB, UK.

What are the problems with retinal cell transplants?

P. Gouras

Columbia University, New York City, NY, USA

Introduction

Retinal cell transplantation offers the possibility of preserving and/or restoring function in a degenerating retina. This is a difficult but ultimately do-able project and the retina may be an ideal structure in which to pursue such central nervous system reconstruction. The retina is accessible, layered and the photoreceptor layer transmits signals in one direction in contrast to most neuronal circuits in the central nervous system. There are two areas to which this research has been directed. One involves the retinal epithelium and the second the neural retina, in particular the photoreceptors. Although some problems are similar in these two approaches, there are major differences requiring the topics to be considered separately.

Transplantation of retinal epithelium is inherently easier. The tissue can be cultured, dissociated, re-associated and manipulated in vitro. Its functional role, which is to metabolically support the highly specialized photoreceptor layer, requires only close apposition to the outer segments of the receptors. The technique has been proven successful in the Royal College Surgeons strain of rats, a model of a form of recessive retinitis pigmentosa [6, 11] and recently in a murine model of Leber's Congenital Amaurosis, the RPE65 –/– mouse [7]. In both models, photoreceptor degeneration can be stopped or delayed and photoreceptor function preserved or restored by retinal epithelial transplants. The major impediment found in both models has been evidence of rejection which appears to limit a long-term therapeutic success. Rejection has been even more of an impediment in attempts to use retinal epithelium transplants to treat age related macular degeneration, especially neovascularization. In human trials, rejection has been more rapid and aggressive than in the rodent models. I believe that this is related to breakdown of the blood retinal barrier caused by the transplantation surgery itself, which must be exacerbated in the case of neovascularization. I shall present evidence indicating that transient immunosuppression during and just after transplantation, may be able to avert rejection entirely.

Transplantation of photoreceptors is a different problem. Here rejection has been surprisingly minimal. Communication with the host retina is the major problem. No one has unequivocally demonstrated functional connectivity between transplant and host neurons. This is a major hurdle. I will present evidence that photoreceptors in such transplants can make membrane to membrane contact with host bipolars, which could allow ephatic communication between transplant and host. Synaptic contacts between transplant and host on the other hand have been difficult to find. I believe the solution to the problem of synaptic communication can come from using embryonic photoreceptors that have been liberated from their postsynaptic contacts. I shall show how it is possible to do this with the excimer laser.

Retinal epithelial transplants rescue function in the RPE65 –/– mice

We have been testing the effects of retinal epithelial transplants in the RPE65 –/– mouse. Here the defect is expressed in the epithelial layer, which prevents these mice from con-

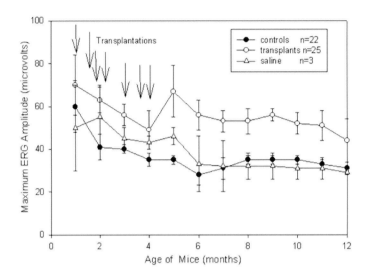

Fig. 1. Relationship between the average ERG responses in control and test eyes and the age of the mice in all seven litters. Three control subjects received an injection of saline. The other control eyes were untouched. Arrows age of the mice when mice received transplants. Vertical bars represent standard errors of the mean

verting all-trans to 11-cis retinol. This causes a large reduction in the photoreceptor response, monitored by the electroretinogram (ERG), and to a slow degeneration of the photoreceptor layer. By transplanting normal retinal epithelium into the subretinal space, photoreceptor function can be restored and anatomical degeneration slowed. Figure 1 illustrates the increase in ERG amplitude produced by transplantation at different ages in the life of the affected mice. The only disappointment has been that the functional recovery diminishes with time. We are not sure why. There is also a progressive reduction in the amount of transplanted cells found with time, indicating that they are not surviving. This is shown in Figs. 2 and 3 where multiple transplanted epithelial cells can be seen in the subretinal space at two weeks after transplantation (Fig. 2) versus only rare cells at 8 months after transplantation (Fig. 3). This may be the result of rejection although we have seen no evidence of inflammation, an invariable sign of rejection. Further research is necessary to clarify this. Several groups have reported that gene therapy can also rescue function in this model but the long-term results are still being determined.

Identifying rejection non-invasively

Rejection is a significant consideration with retinal epithelial allografts. We are now able to identify and follow rejection of retinal epithelium in vivo without having to sacrificing the animal. This is useful because it allows continuous monitoring, which can be done by ophthalmoscopy, in particular the scanning laser ophthalmoscope (SLO). There are several clues to rejection. These clues have become evident from the use of a reporter trans-gene expressible in the retinal epithelium and introduced into the epithelium by a lentiviral vector [5]. This jelly fish gene expresses a green fluorescent protein (GFP), which can be followed in single retinal epithelial cells by SLO. When GFP is expressed strongly, however, it leads to rejection within a few weeks. We have detected serum antibodies to GFP in these rabbits paralleling rejection, which provides strong evidence that GFP is the responsible antigen. By following GFP expression we have noticed several clues to rejection (Figs. 4 and 5). In Fig. 4 GFP expression is seen at 12 days after surgery. At 21 days

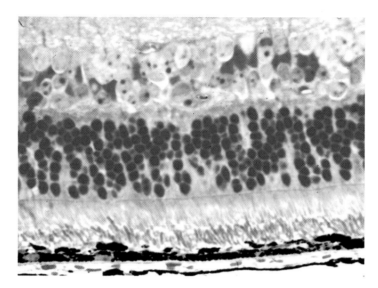

Fig. 2. Transplants in the subretinal space of a RPE65 –/– mouse at 2 weeks after surgery

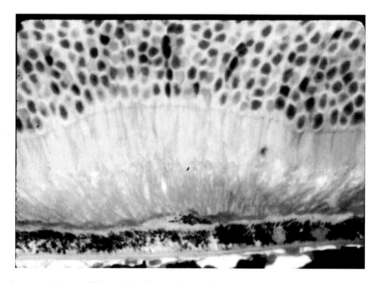

Fig. 3. A single transplant still found in the subretinal space at 8 months after surgery; such transplants are rarely found

after surgery, GFP fluorescence has been lost and the area of previous gene expression shows a "piebald" appearance due to disruption of this layer by the inflammatory response. Histology shows that the piebald appearance is due to piling up of the epithelium in some areas and migration and dilution of pigment in other areas [5]. Figure 5 shows how rapidly this rejection occurs and in addition another clue to rejection. At 14 days there is considerable GFP expression. At 17 days there is a blurring of the blue light image of the target area because of an edema. At this point there is only faint GFP expression visible. At 20 days all expression is lost and the target area shows the typical piebald appearance of rejection.

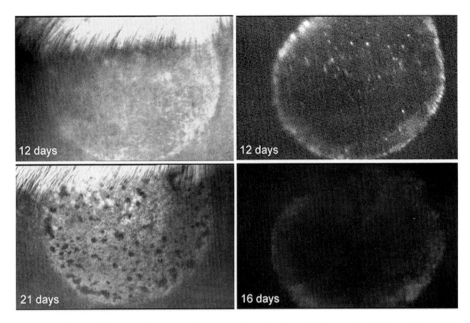

Fig. 4. Lentiviral transduction of GFP is shown in the retinal epithelium of rabbit at 12 and 21 days after surgery. On the left are blue SLO images; on the right are fluorescent images. At 12 days there is gene expression of GFP seen on the right; at 21 days there has been rejection

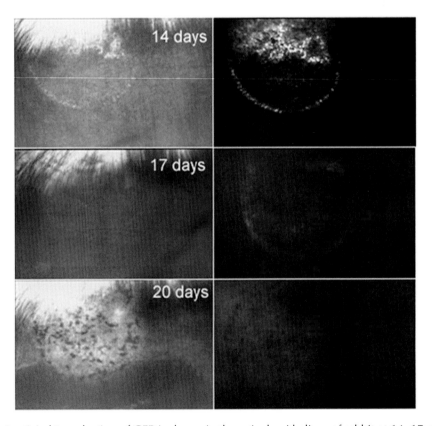

Fig. 5. Lentiviral transduction of GFP is shown in the retinal epithelium of rabbit at 14, 17 and 20 days after surgery. On the left are blue SLO images; on the right are fluorescent images. At 14 days there is gene expression of GFP seen on the right. At 17 days there is mild edema at the target area and GFP expression is almost lost. At 20 days the target area has a piebald appearance and all GFP fluorescence is lost

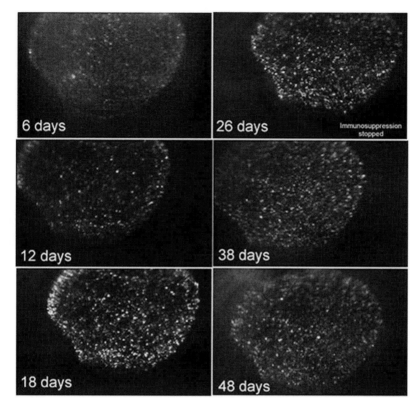

Fig. 6. Lentiviral transduction of GFP is shown in the retinal epithelium of rabbit that has been immunosuppressed at and for one month after surgery. Rejection does not occur for months after immunosuppression has ceased

Counteracting rejection

This is a summary of an on-going research project being carried out by Ken Doi, Jian Kong, Janos Hargitai, Steve Goff and myself on lentiviral transduction of rabbit and mouse retina. I present it here because it is relevant to the problem of rejection of retinal epithelium in general. If you immunosuppress a rabbit using cyclosporine, aza-thioprine and prednisolone administered daily starting on the day before surgery for viral transfection, you can prevent rejection. If you stop the immunosuppression after one month, rejection never occurs again. Figure 6 shows an example of lentiviral induced expression of GFP in rabbit retina for 6 months with no indication of rejection. There is continuous and strong expression of GFP throughout the transduced area. This has been seen repeatedly and it occurs without the appearance of any serum antibodies to GFP. If, however, a viral injection is placed in the contralateral eye and immunosup-pression is not instituted, both areas of GFP expression will be rejected. Rejection appears to depend on the initial phases of the subretinal surgery. If immunosuppression can be maintained for this period which at present involves at least a month's time, tolerance can be produced indefinitely. The detection of the foreign antigen or antigens must be facilitated by factors occurring contemporaneously with the subretinal surgery. Once these factors have disappeared or dissipated, the immune system can no longer detect the foreign material. This approach should be carefully explored with retinal epithelial transplants.

Another strategy to counteract rejection is to use homografts of iris retinal epithelium from the subject requiring retinal epithelium transplantation. This completely eliminates rejection but has several other problems. One is that the iris epithelium does not have all the enzymatic machinery to handle the outer segment but it is possible that it could modify its behavior when confronting the photoreceptor. In addition, the movement of lipophyllic molecules, such as vitamin A, needed for phototransduction might be able to move from membrane to membrane across considerable distances. Clinical trials on this strategy are underway.

Another approach has been used by Susan Binder in which retinal epithelium from elsewhere in the retina has been used to cover the area that must be covered in the macula [4]. This has the problem that you are using aged and probably somewhat defective epithelium and there is a chance that the removal technique damages a significant and unknown number of cells.

Stem cells are perhaps another possibility but they have the problem that one doesn't know where to find them especially in older subjects needing the transplant repair and secondly the stem cells have to differentiate into retinal epithelium which has not yet been demonstrated.

A very intriguing way of creating healthy, young or embryonic retinal epithelium from the same donor is to clone this individual to the fetal stage and then sacrifice the fetus in order to obtain the retinal epithelium. This has serious ethical considerations. Its success has recently been demonstrated in the mouse [12].

Transplantation of neural retina

One of the most intriguing concepts in treating blindness is to try to restore photoreceptor function in a blind retina. This area of research has been evolving slowly over more than a decade. The most extraordinary result so far is the fact that when photoreceptors, especially embryonic ones, are placed in the subretinal space they survive extremely well and will develop normal appearing outer segments when these photoreceptors are properly oriented toward the retinal epithelium. There is also unequivocal evidence that these transplanted photoreceptors respond to light [1, 14]. There is little indication of rejection of such neural transplants. The major problem, however, in this research in the communication of these photoreceptor transplants is a failure of any evidence that they can communicate with the host retina. This is a major impasse.

We have attempted to use small microaggregates of embryonic murine retina to determine how well they integrate with the retina of the adult dystrophic rd mouse. One of the advantages of our method is that we have labeled both the donor rods and the host rod bipolars. We have produced an rd mouse with such LacZ labeled bipolars [8, 9]. In Fig. 7, the transplant on the right is oriented appropriately toward the epithelium and well developed outer segments, stained blue, are visible in the subretinal space of the adult rd mouse. Electron micrographs of labeled rod transplants show them to be contacting the retinal epithelial layer of adult rd mice (Figs. 8, 9). The rods of the normal donor mice are labeled with the LacZ reporter gene and the rod bipolars of the rd host retina is also labeled with the same reporter gene. This has allowed us to trace the neural structures of transplanted rods and those of donor rod bipolars with considerable precision. What we have found is that there is a partial barrier to communication between donor and host tissue formed by the Muller cells of the host. There are however, breaks in this glial barrier which allow close contacts to form between donor and host neurons. At these points, we have found evidence that donor rod cell bodies make membrane to membrane contacts with host rod bipolars. Figure 10 shows a typical example of such membrane to membrane contacts between these donor and host neurons. This provides a way for ionic

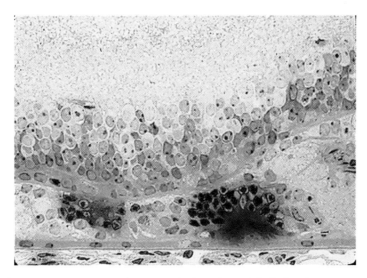

Fig. 7. Retinal microaggregate transplants in which rods are labeled with LacZ reporter gene are shown in the subretinal space of rd mice in which rod bipolars are labeled with the same reporter gene. The transplants on the right are appropriately oriented toward the retinal epithelium

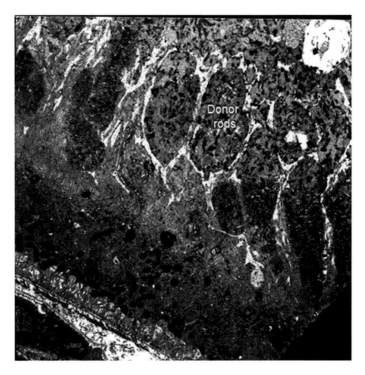

Fig. 8. Electron micrograph showing labeled rods in the subretinal space of an rd mouse, months after transplantation

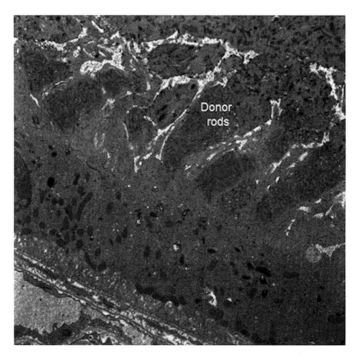

Fig. 9. Electron micrograph showing labeled rods in the subretinal space of an rd mouse, months after transplantation

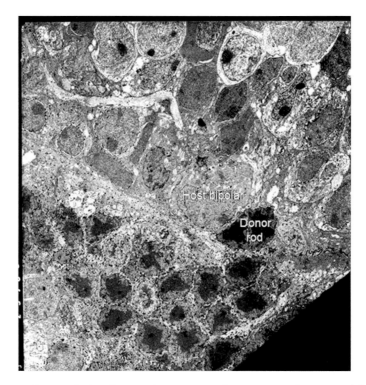

Fig. 10. Electron micrograph showing membrane to membrane contact between a labeled host rod bipolar and a labeled donor rod. Such contacts can be the site of ionic communication between transplant and host neurons

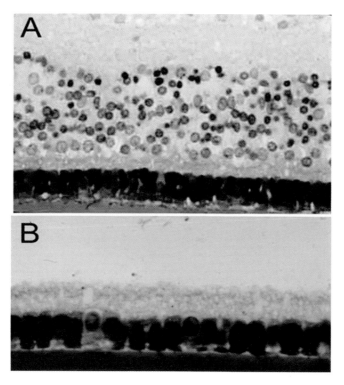

Fig. 11. Light micrograph shows in **A**. the normal 20 week old human fetal retina in the macular area and in **B**. how the inner layers have been selectively removed by the excimer laser

communication between these two systems. This communication is known as ephaptic communication in contrast to synaptic communication. It is certainly un-physiological but provides some explanation for recent evidence that such transplants are able to weakly influence the ganglion cells of the host retina. What we have not been able to detect is strong evidence for any synaptic communication between these two systems. Very occasionally we do find processes of rods entering the territory of the host making contacts with postsynaptic structures labeled as host rod bipolars. Because there are reasons to worry about artifacts leading to such rare events, we are reluctant to accept this as unequivocal.

It is our impression that the best strategy to use to improve this approach is to free up the donor photoreceptors from their second order postsynaptic structures before transplantation. We have found a good way to do this, using embryonic human retina. What is remarkable about the developing human or primate retina in general is that the foveal area develops relatively early in embryonic life and is separated from the inner nuclear layer by a distinct outer plexiform layer. This separation between outer and inner nuclear layers does not exist in non-foveal areas of the retina. The separation allows the excimer laser to destroy all the inner layers of the retina and leave the primordial foveal cone layer relatively undisturbed. This is not possible elsewhere in this developing retina. Figure 11A illustrates this separation of the foveal cone photoreceptor layer, primarily cones, from the inner nuclear layer. Figure 11B shows how the excimer laser has completely removed all the inner layers of this embryonic retina except the photoreceptor layer. Figure 12 shows electron micrographs of such an isolated layer of cones with the synaptic terminals of these cones altered but sealed by a complete plasma membrane. Proof that these cells are alive comes from the fact that they survive quite well when cultured in this state.

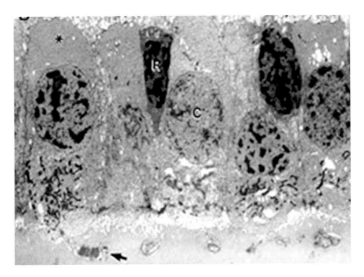

Fig. 12. Electron micrograph showing the survival of a monolayer of fetal human foveal cones and a few rods in tissue culture after the inner layers of the retina have been removed by the excimer laser

Therefore it is possible to isolate pure cones and some rods separated from their second order contacts. We believe that this approach could allow a better opportunity for transplanted photoreceptors and cones in particular to form synaptic contacts with second order host neurons. Of course this is only a small step in establishing such contacts. There are many other obstacles involved in addition to the Muller cell gliosis.

Summary

I have attempted to summarize the research we have recently performed and which we and others are planning in the future. Retinal cell transplantation is a difficult area of research but it is not in my opinion a blind end unworthy of support. It can work in animals and therefore it should also be able to work in humans with retinal degeneration. It is a more biological approach than the electronic chip which also has great obstacles to success. The fact that one is forced to work with the cells that are at the root of the problem of retinal blindness, the retinal epithelium and the photoreceptors, is one of the most appealing aspects of this research. If it were possible to replace degenerating cells with healthy ones, this would most certainly lead to a revolutionary means of restoring function and vision to the retina and macula in particular. Careful and imaginative atention to the factors that can improve manipulating cells in microscopic ways in the subretinal space hold the roots of success in this endeavor.

References

1. Adolph AR, Zucker CL, Ehinger B, Bergstrom A (1994) Function and structure in retinal transplants. J Neural Transplant 5:147–62
2. Algvere P, Gouras P, Kopp ED (1999) Long term outcome of RPE allografts in non-immunosuppressed patients with age related macular degeneration (AMD). Eur J Ophthalmol 97:23–31

3. Aramant RB, Seiler MJ (1995) Fiber and synaptic connections between embryonic retinal transplants and host retina. Exper Neurol 133:244–55

4. Binder S, Stolba U, Krebs I, Kellner L, Jahn C, Feichtinger H, Povelka M, Kruger A, Hilgers RC, Krugluger W (2002) Transplantation of autologous retinal pigment epithelium in eyes with foveal neovascularizaton resulting from age related macular degeneration: a pilot study. Am J Ophthalmol 133:215–25

5. Doi K, Hargitai J, Kong J, Tsang SH, Wheatley M, Chang S, Goff S, Gouras P (2002) Lentiviral transduction of green fluorescent protein in retinal epithelium: evidence of rejection. Vision Res 42:551–8

6. Gouras P (1998) Transplantation of retinal pigment epithelium. In: Marmor M, Wolfensberger TJ (eds) The retinal pigment epithelium, function and disease. New York, Oxford: Oxford University Press, pp 492–507

7. Gouras P, Kong, J, Tsang SH (2002) Retinal degeneration and RPE transplantation in Rpe65 –/– mice. Invest Ophthalmol Vis Sci 43:3307–11

8. Gouras P, Tanabe T (2003a) Survival and integration of neural retinal transplants in rd mice. Graefes Arch Clin Exp Ophthalmol (in press)

9. Gouras P, Tanabe T (2003b) Ultrastructure of adult rd mouse retina. Graefes Arch Clin Exp Ophthalmol (in press)

10. Lai C, Gouras P, Doi K, Lu F, Keldbye H, Goff SP, Pawliuk R, Leboulch, P, Tsang SH (1990) Tracking RPE transplants labeled by retroviral gene transfer with green fluorescent protein. Invest Ophthalmol Vis Sci 40:2141–6

11. Lund RD, Kwan ASL, Keegan DJ, Sauve Y, Coffey PJ, Lawrence JM (2001) Cell transplantation as a treatment for retinal disease. Progress in Retinal & Eye Res 20:415–49

12. Rideout WM, Hochedlinger K, Kyba M, Daley GQ, Jaenisch R (2002) Correction of a genetic defect by nuclear transplantation and combined cell and gene therapy. Cell 109:17–27

13. Salchow DJ, Trokel SL, Kjeldbye H, Dudley T, Gouras P (2001) Isolation of human fetal cones. Curr Eye Res 22:85–9

14. Seiler MJ, Aramant RB, Ball SL (1999) Photoreceptor function of retinal transplants as indicated by light-dark shift of S-antigen and rod transducin. Vision Res 39:2589–96

15. Woch G, Aramant RB, Seiler MJ, Sagdullaev BT, McCall MA (2001) Retinal transplants restore visually evoked responses in rats with photoreceptor degeneration. Invest Ophthalmol Vis Sci 42:1669–76

Correspondence: Peter Gouras M.D., Columbia University, 630 West 168th Street, New York City, NY, 10032, USA.

Experimental transplantation of IPE to the subretinal space-morphology and photoreceptor survival

S. Crafoord

Department of Ophthalmology, University Hospital Örebro, Sweden

Abstract

Background: Age-related macular degeneration (AMD) is associated with degeneration and subsequent loss of the retinal pigment epithelium (RPE). Transplantation of allogeneic RPE cells seems to induce graft rejection. Therefore, autotransplantation was suggested. Iris pigment epithelial cells (IPE) are embryologically similar to RPE.

Methods: Suspensions of freshly harvested autologous IPE cells (without culturing) were transplanted to the subretinal space of 37 rabbits. The eyes were examined with light and electron microscopy after 1, 2, 3 and 6 months, respectively.

Results: On histological examination, the photoreceptor cells were preserved in grafted areas at 1–3 months and the transplanted IPE formed one or more contiguous layers on top of native RPE. There was no inflammatory response in the choroid and the choriocapillaris remained patent.

The grafted area retained the same configuration over 6 months but then appeared less pigmented and the photoreceptors disclosed a normal appearance. Only in circumscribed locations with multilayers of cells was there a focal photoreceptor damage.

Conclusion: When grafting freshly harvested autologous IPE cells to the subretinal space the photoreceptors generally survive for at least 6 months overlying the transplanted areas. Our observations suggest a scenario of remodeling of the cellular layers in the subretinal space over time where grafted IPE cells form a compound layer with the native RPE. Autologous IPE cells seem to have a potential of supporting photoreceptors, maybe also in diseases with RPE degeneration.

Introduction

Transplantation of RPE allograft has been performed both experimentally in animals and clinically in humans. A graft rejection is described. Therefore transplantation of *autologous* cells, such as iris pigment epithelial cells, allows us to exclude immunogenic cellular responses and immunogenic graft rejection.

Also graft failure of non-immunogenic causes, if present, can then be studied.

In vitro experiments have indicated that IPE cells acquire the ability to *phagocytose* photoreceptor outer segments.

IPE cells in culture did not show any retinoid metabolism but the presence of mRNA for cellular retinaldehyde binding protein (CRALBP) and for some related substances suggests the possibility that IPE cells may be able to *metabolize retinol* in a proper microenvironment. The *transdifferentiation* ability of IPE cells was previously reported showing lens-forming potency and recently also documented in chicken.

IPE cells in tissue culture also demonstrate a functional barrier against macromolecules similar to RPE and may subsequently be able to maintain *blood-retina barrier* in vivo.

In this study we present the results of IPE transplantation to the subretinal space of rabbit.

Methods

Autologous IPE cells were obtained from iridectomy specimens (Dutch belted rabbits).

The iridectomy specimen was treated with trypsin (0.25%) – EDTA (0.02%) solution for 10 min and the IPE cells gently brushed off the posterior iris surface using a Lewis–Tano instrument.

The fresh IPE cells were mixed with balanced salt solution to make a cellsuspension.

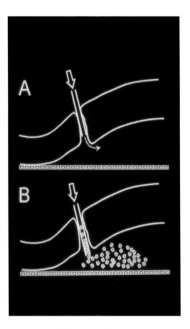

Fig. 1. A core vitrectomy was performed followed by an injection of a stream of BSS from a glass micropipette, connected to a silicone tube, which produced a small retinotomy and a subretinal bleb at the inferior part of the medullary ray (**A**). About 20–25 µl of the IPE cell suspension (approximately $2–4 \times 10^4$ cells) was injected through the retinotomy into the subretinal space with the same micropipette (**B**)

The grafts were monitored by ophthalmoscopy, fluorescein angiography and colour fundus photography. Rabbits were sacrificed at 1, 2, 3 and 6 months, respectively, and the eyes examined with light and electron microscopy, TUNEL-dye and immunohistochemistry.

Results and Conclusions

Following IPE cell transplantation the photoreceptors generally survive for six months. Transplanting fresh autologous IPE cells without culturing does not seem to be harmful on adjacent photoreceptors.

Shortcomings in the described method/study.

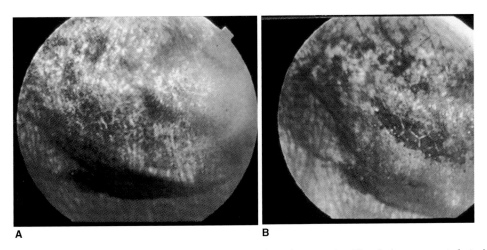

Fig. 2. Fundus photographs of live rabbit at 1 month and 6 months. The dark crescent inferiorly display the transplanted area

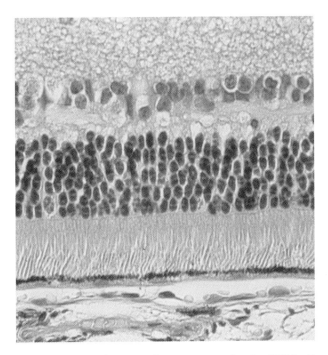

Fig. 3. This picture depicts the normal appearance of native RPE in Dutch rabbit

- It remains to be determined to what extent grafted IPE cells are capable of supporting photoreceptors and maintaining the normal physiological function.
- Identification of grafted cells.

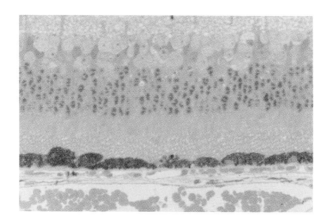

Fig. 4. Transplanted IPE cells appear heavily pigmented on top of the native RPE at one month

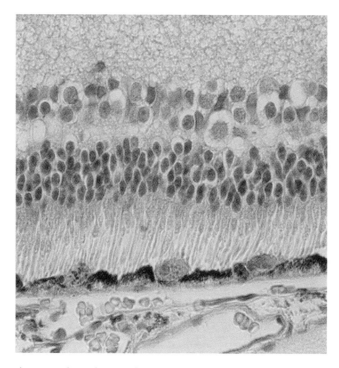

Fig. 5. At six months, transplanted IPE cells were seen to integrate into a compound layer with the RPE

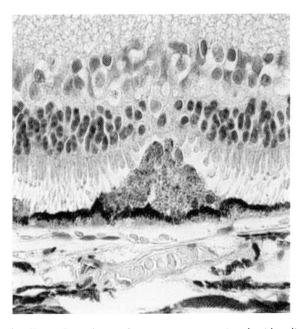

Fig. 6. Multilayers of cells in the subretinal space were associated with adjacent photoreceptor damage. In addition to transplanted IPE cells, the cellular multilayers disclosed native RPE and macrophages

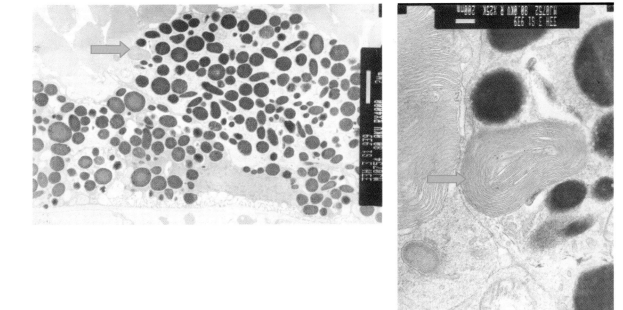

Fig. 7. Presumed IPE cell in close contact with native RPE and photoreceptor outer segments. Arrows show intracellular phagosom

Some questions remains to be answered in experimental transplantation.

1. Should we denude the original RPE before grafting?
2. How do we mark the transplanted cells?
3. Should we use fresh transplants or cultivated?
4. Basal lamina. Should that be included?
5. How does the transplanted area function?
6. Do vitamin A metabolism take place?

Correspondence: Sven Crafoord, M.D. PhD., Department of Ophthalmology, University Hospital Örebro, SE-701 85 Örebro, Sweden, E-mail: sven.crafoord@orebroll.se

Harvesting efficacy and viability of retinal pigment epithelial cells in aspirates from posterior retinal areas – a study on human eyes

A. Assadoullina[1], S. Binder[1], B. Stanzel[1], A. Abri[1],
W. Krugluger[2], S. Scholz[3], and H. Feichtinger[4]

[1] The Ludwig Boltzmann Institute of Retinology and Biomicroscopic Laser Surgery,
Department of Ophthalmology (Chairman: Prof. Dr. Susanne Binder),
Rudolf Foundation Clinic, Vienna, Austria
[2] Institute of Clinical Chemistry (Chairman: Prof. Dr. Pierre Hopmeier),
Rudolf Foundation Clinic, Vienna, Austria
[3] Department of Medical Statistic (Chairman: Prof. Dr. Peter Bauer),
University of Vienna, Austria
[4] Institute of Pathology and Bacteriology (Chairman: Prof. Dr.
Hans Feichtinger), Rudolf Foundation Clinic, Vienna, Austria

Abstract

A reproducible cell amount in the inoculate and its high viability are critical factors in autologous RPE transplantation. We therefore applied a technique of gentle mobilization and aspiration of RPE-s from the nasal area of the retina to 14 cadaver human eyes. The outcome was systematically evaluated for RPE cell amounts and their viability. Briefly, after retinotomy the retina was locally detached nasally of the optic disc with a subretinal injection of Ringer's solution. RPE cells were then gently mobilized over an area of 2–4 disc diameters, aspirated, stained with Trypan blue, and the dye exclusion immediately assessed. Total cell numbers ranged from 11.000 to 29.200 (19.976 ± 6.016), however, the harvesting efficacy (nr. of cells/disc area) was remarkably constant (6.165 ± 746). Cell viability was high (82,0 ± 6,9%). We conclude that reasonable cell numbers of high viability suitable for autologous RPE transplantation can be efficiently harvested even from small retinal areas.

Introduction

Surgical membrane excision and consecutive autologous RPE-transplantation in patients with subretinal neovascular membranes due to AMD performed within one operative session requires an optimal mobilization and harvest of RPE-s [1]. Beside other factors, the success of the procedure should be assessed in cell amount as well as their viability in the RPE suspension transplant [2]. Here we describe the application of a new microsurgical technique for RPE cell aspiration using human cadaver eyes as a model system to determine the aforementioned two parameters. The cells were collected from the nasal paracentral area of the retina.

The harvesting efficacy was determined as the number of cells per mobilization area for each single experiment.

We demonstrate that a gentle mobilization and aspiration of RPE cells within a circumscribed nasal area of the retina yields reasonable numbers of viable cells with a constant harvesting efficacy.

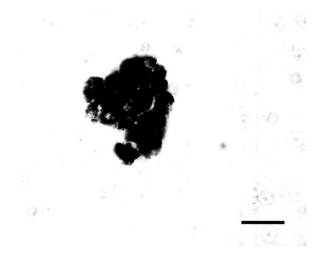

Fig. 1. Microscopic preparation of a RPE-Aspirate: RPE-cell complex in Fuchs-Rosenthal counting chamber. Calibration mark −20 μm

Materials and methods

We examined 14 human donor eyes (1 sample per eye) from 7 individuals (3 females, 4 males). The death-to-harvesting time ranged from 9 to 42 hours (mean, 21,1 ± 11,2).

The median age was 79 years (range 69 to 90 years). Eyes with signs of visible ocular surgery, ocular inflammation or retinal disease were excluded from the study.

After removal of the anterior segment a retinotomy was performed nasally from the optic disc with a subretinal pick. Retinal detachment was created by a subretinal injection of Ringer's solution. RPE cells were gently mobilised with a bent blunt 39-gauge subretinal cannula (BD Ophthalmic systems) over an area of 2–4 optic disc diameter. This cell suspension was then aspirated either manually with a tube connected to a tuberculin syringe (10 cases) or by using an oil hydraulic microinjection pump (Oil-Trans Injector/ Eppendorf) (4 cases). Cells were stained with trypan-blue and immediately counted in blood counting chambers (Bürker-Türk or Fuchs-Rosental) to assess their viability. The counts were carried out by 2 independent examiners. Harvesting efficacy was calculated in terms of cell number per optic disc surface area (1 da). To test the significance of differences, the Mann-Whitney-Wilcoxon and Student's – tests were applied. The Pearson Correlation was used to identify associations between variables.

Results

RPE cell yield in individual experiments ranged from 11.000–29.200 (19.976 ± 6.016 cells, /mean ± S.D.) (Table 1). Viability rate by trypan-blue staining was 82,0 ± 6,9%. Harvesting efficacy of samples was 6.165 ± 746 cells/1 disc area corresponding to 2.371 ± 297 cells/mm^2.

Mean harvesting efficacy and mean cell viability by using the syringe technique were 6.172 ± 813,4 and 81,8 ± 5,7, respectively. Similar numbers were achieved using the pump aspiration technique (6.147,7 ± 651,8 and 82,5 ± 10,4, respectively).

The amount of contaminating cells like erythrocytes, photoreceptors fragments and other debris in the RPE cell aspirates was not determined in our study.

Table 1. Cell count and viability rates in 14 aspirates

Aspirat nr.	Patient/ Sex	Age (years)	DHT (hours)	Aspiration technique	cell count	Area (da)	Harvesting efficacy (cells)	viability (%)*
1	1/f	90	15	syringe	11.200	2	5600	83
2	1/f	90	14	syringe	12.000	2	6000	87
3	2/m	69	33	syringe	16.320	3	5440	77
4	2/m	69	32	syringe	22.600	3	7533	76
5	3/f	88	42	pump	20.000	3	6666	67
6	3/f	88	41	syringe	24.000	4	6000	70
7	4/f	79	9	pump	27.000	4	6750	89
8	4/f	79	10	syringe	29.200	4	7300	87
9	5/m	77	13	pump	22.700	4	5675	88
10	5/m	77	14	syringe	19.000	3	6333	85
11	6/m	82	16	syringe	27.400	4	6850	86
12	6/m	82	17	syringe	16.250	3	5416	85
13	7/m	75	20	syringe	21.000	4	5250	82
14	7/m	75	19	pump	11.000	2	5500	86
Mean		$80,0 \pm 7,1$	$21,07 \pm 11,2$		19.976 ± 6.016		6.165 ± 746	$82,0 \pm 6,9$

DHT death-to-harvest time
da disc area
* using trypan blue staining

Discussion

The microsurgical technique of RPE cell aspiration applied in our study is a relatively simple method for harvesting cells for autologous transplantation [1]. We have chosen the nasal paracentral area of the retina mainly for two reasons. First, it represents a clearly visible zone optimal for intraoperative manipulations and the retinotomy in this area can be easily closed either with a gas tamponade or the defect closes even on its own because of the posterior location. Second, this region exhibits a high density of RPE cells [3, 4].

An important feature of this technique was the high reproducibility of RPE cell acquisition. Although an individual variation in average RPE cell density, especially in the older retina, is well known [3, 4] very similar cell numbers per one disc area could be harvested. We ascribed it the "harvesting-efficacy ratio". Its values have been remarkably constant in the present experimental setting (Table 1).

Corresponding to mobilization areas of 2 to 4 optic disc diameters the total number of aspirated RPE cells ranged from 11.000 to 29.200. We have chosen the parameter of the optic disc diameter intentionally, because it is a coined term used to determine the size of retinal structures in case of pathological changes and, furthermore, because of its usefulness for an intraoperative estimation of the RPE mobilization area. When transformed into the number of cells isolated per mm^2, our data (2019 to 2898 cells/mm^2) are fairly consistent with those from reports of different authors about RPE cell densities in the mid-peripheral nasal quadrant (about 3.200 cells/mm^2) [3, 4], if a certain degree of cell loss due to the procedure is considered. It is also important to note that this cell yield seems sufficient for transplantation, as even lower numbers of aspirated RPE cells have been shown sufficient to establish a confluent monolayer in an area of approximately 2,6–6 mm in diameter under optimal in vitro conditions [5, 6, 7]. However, it should also be mentioned, that RPE cell mobilization and acquisition is somewhat less crucial in the cadaver eye due to a progressive post-mortem decrease in Bruch's membrane adhesion. Intraoperatively in living patients, stronger adhesion could result in lower cell numbers in the inoculates used for transplantation.

The viability of RPE cells was high (82,0 ± 6,9%; range, 67% to 89%) and is in accordance with published data reporting RPE cell viabilities of 82% [8] and between 30–80% [6] in cadaver eyes within 48h after death, respectively. Dead-to-harvesting time (DHT) on the one hand and total cell number, harvesting efficacy and cell viability on the other hand showed a significant correlation only between DHT and viability ($r = -0,97$; $p \leq 0.001$, bonferroni adjusted). Neither general cell numbers, nor the level of harvesting efficacy seemed to be significantly associated with DHT duration.

Although only used in a small number of cases, two different techniques of aspiration – manual with syringe vs. microinjection pump – yielded similar amounts of RPE cells with similar viability rates. The oil hydraulic microinjection device has been successfully used in animal studies with the aim to minimize the traumatic effects on the transplantable cells and the recipient tissue [9]. A comparison of these two aspiration techniques by the Student's T-Test and the Mann–Whitney–Wilcoxon – Test yielded no striking difference in this small sample.

Conclusion

In conclusion, our procedure of mobilizing and harvesting of RPE cells from the nasal paracentral region of the retina represents a feasible technique to be used efficiently for therapeutic applications in patients, since even from relatively small retinal areas a reproducibly high number of viable RPE cells can be harvested for further use.

Acknowledgements

The authors would like to thank Monika Valtink, Judith Weichel, Katrin Engelmann and the team of the Cornea Bank of the Department of Ophthalmology, University of Hamburg, Germany for their help and advice in the experiments.

References

1. Binder S, Stolba U, Krebs I, Kellner L, Jahn Ch, Feichtinger H, Pavelka M, Frohner U, Kruger A, Hilgers RD, Krugluger W (2002) Transplantation of autologous retinal pigment epithelium in eyes with foveal neovascularization resulting from age-related macular degeneration: a pilot study. Am J Ophthalmol 133:215–25
2. Tsukahara I, Ninomiya S, Castellarin A, Yagi F, Sugino IK, Zarbin MA (2002) Early attachment of uncultured retinal pigment epithelium from aged donors onto Bruch's membrane explants. Exp Eye Res 74:255–6
3. Harman AM, Fleming PA, Hoskins RV, More SR (1997) Development and aging of cell topography in the human retinal pigment epithelium. Invest Ophthalmol Vis Sci 38:2016–26
4. Panda-Jonas S, Jonas JB, Jakobczyk-Zmija (1996) Retinal pigment epithelial cell count, distribution, and correlations in normal human eyes. Am J Ophthalmol 121:181–9
5. Kim KS, Tezel TH, Del Priore LV (1998) Minimum number of adult human retinal pigment epithelial cells required to establish a confluent monolayer in vitro. Curr Eye Res 17(10):262–9
6. Ishida M, Lui GM, Yamani A, Sugino IK, Zarbin MA (1998) Culture of human retinal pigment epithelial cells from peripheral scleral flap biopsies. Curr Eye Res 17:392–402
7. Stanzel BV, Huemer K-H, Ahnelt PK, Feichtinger H, Binder S (2002) Minimal plating density required for confluency of adult human RPE cells using a Ca^{++} adjusted DMEM/F12 culture medium. Invest Ophthalmol Vis Sci 43(4):3437 (B421)
8. Tezel TH, Del Priore LV, Kaplan HJ (1997) Harvest and storage of adult human retinal pigment epithelial sheets. Curr Eye Res 16:802–9

9. Weichel J, Valtink M, Richard G, Engelmann K (1999) Optimization of a surgical approach for transplanting adult human retinal pigment epithelial cells into the subretinal space of RCS rats. Invest Ophthalmol Vis Sci 40(4):S727

Correspondence: Adele Assadoullina, MD, The Ludwig Boltzmann Institute of Retinology and Bio-microscopic Laser Surgery, Department of Ophthalmology, Rudolf Foundation Clinic, Juchgasse 25, A-1030 Vienna, Austria, E-mail: adele.assadoullina@kar.magwien.gv.at

Iris pigment epithelium transplantation – experimental and clinical results

G. Thumann[1], S. Aisenbrey[2], and K. U. Bartz-Schmidt[3]

[1] Department of Ophthalmology, University of Cologne, Germany
[2] Department of Neuroscience, Tufts University, Boston, MA, USA
[3] University of Tübingen, Tübingen, Germany

Abstract

It has been hypothesized that transplantation of iris pigment epithelial (IPE) cells to the subretinal space may be useful in the treatment of exudative age-related macular degeneration following surgical removal of the neovascular complex. In practice, the success of IPE transplantation depends on (a) the transplantation of a sufficient number of IPE cells, (b) the ability of the transplanted IPE cells to form a monolayer that will cover the exposed photoreceptor outer segments, and (c) the acquisition of RPE cell characteristics and functions by the transplanted IPE cells.

We have transplanted autologous IPE cells as a single cell suspension to the subretinal space in 20 patients; during the three years of follow-up the cells survived and did not adversely affect photoreceptors function. Stabilization of visual acuity was achieved in the majority of patients after IPE transplantation, and by fluorescein angiography none of the twenty patients showed any sign of recurrent vascular disease. The transplanted cells appeared to have remained at the site of transplantation, however it was not possible to ascertain whether they had spread and formed a monolayer. Since the formation of a monolayer of cells is critical to the successful visual outcome of IPE transplantation, we have begun a series of experiments to optimize the culture of IPE and RPE cells and explore the feasibility of transplanting preformed monolayers of autologous IPE cells cultured on biodegradable substrates.

Introduction

Surgical extraction of subfoveal neovascular membranes in choroidal neovascularization is not particularly helpful since the underlying RPE is invariably removed resulting in poor visual outcome. Furthermore, several studies have shown progression of atrophy after membrane extraction and recurrence of the CNV in 30 to 40% of patients [4, 5, 8, 11, 16]. Transplantation of retinal pigment epithelial (RPE) cells to the subretinal space has been examined in a number of experimental and clinical studies as a means of restoring normal subretinal conditions. However, the transplantation of homologous adult as well as fetal RPE cells in human subjects has resulted in immunological rejection due to slow host-graft response. To prevent rejection it would be necessary to transplant autologous RPE cells, which is being actively investigated by Binder and co-workers [6, 17].

Since autologous human RPE cells are difficult to obtain, whereas iris pigment epithelial (IPE) cells are easily obtained, it has been suggested that IPE cells be used to transplant to the subretinal space as a substitute for RPE cells. A number of investigators have demonstrated that RPE and IPE cells have in common many critical properties, such as pigmentation, cellular morphology, and formation of tight junctions [9, 10, 15, 20]. In addition, it has been shown that in vitro human, porcine and rat IPE cells acquire the ability to phagocytize photoreceptor outer segments (ROS) and express proteins involved in retinol metabolism, which are specific properties of RPE cells in situ [20, 22]. It also has been shown that in rabbits a cell suspension of autologous IPE cells can be transplanted to the subretinal space, where they form a monolayer on top of the original RPE, phagocytize ROS, develop microvilli, establish contact with the photoreceptor outer segments, and show no evidence of rejection during a 20-week follow-up [7, 21]. Since adult IPE as well as RPE cells retain the ability to transdifferentiate into other cell types such as lens epithelial cells and neural retinal cells [12, 13, 24], it can be assumed that IPE cells transplanted into the subretinal space will transdifferentiate into RPE cells.

In practice, the success of IPE transplantation depends on three factors, namely (a) the transplantation of a sufficient number of IPE cells, (b) the ability of the transplanted IPE cells to form a monolayer that will cover the exposed photoreceptor outer segments, and (c) on the acquisition by the transplanted IPE cells of characteristics and functions of RPE cell. Since to prevent rejections, the cells to be transplanted should be from the same patient it may not be possible to obtain enough cells in all cases, and it may be necessary to culture cells. However, even the transplantation of an optimal number of cells will not insure that the cells will form a monolayer. Therefore, it may be necessary to transplant monolayers pre-formed by cells cultured on biodegradable membranes. However, since in culture with passage IPE as well as RPE cells loose many differentiated characteristics, it would be best to use primary cell cultures. Therefore, a method capable of yielding large numbers of primary IPE as well as RPE cells would be of great value for transplantation of these cells to the subretinal space.

Since freshly isolated primary IPE and RPE cells grow rather slowly when they are initially placed in culture, we have begun studies to optimize the culture of freshly isolated cells as well as studies to culture cells on biodegradable membranes, which can be easily manipulated and transplanted to the subretinal space.

Material and methods

Subretinal transplantation of IPE cells suspensions in CNV patients

Patients

Between June and November 1998, 20 patients (15 women and 5 men; age 33 to 85 years) with exudative maculopathy underwent surgery for removal of subretinal neovascular membranes followed by transplantation of IPE cells to the subretinal space. Criteria of inclusion consisted of (1) CNV that involved the geometric center of the foveal avascular zone, (2) best-corrected visual acuity of 20/50 or less in the eligible eye, and (3) decreased visual acuity within the last 3 months. All patients underwent a comprehensive ophthalmologic examination preoperatively, which included anterior segment biomicroscopy, intraocular pressure measurement, fundus examination, fluorescein and an indocyanin green angiography, and microperimetry. Best-corrected distance visual acuity was measured by a certified visual examiner with the use of the Early Treatment Diabetic Retinopathy Study (ETDRS) chart according to a fixed protocol.

Preparation of IPE cell suspension

IPE cells were isolated from iridectomy tissue obtained from the eye undergoing vitrectomy. The IPE cells were mechanically isolated from the underlying stroma without the use of enzymes to avoid damage and alteration of the cells. For each patient cells were prepared for injection into the subretinal space by suspending them in 20 µl of BSS. The cell suspension was drawn into a Hamilton syringe fitted with a glass pipette tip, which had previously been coated with autologous serum.

Injection of IPE cells into the subretinal space

In all patients a 3-port pars plana vitrectomy was performed. A small retinotomy was made superior or temporal to the fovea; the fibrovascular membrane was seized with a forceps and extracted slowly through the retinotomy. The Hamilton syringe containing the cells was introduced and positioned just over the retinotomy and the cells injected slowly. After the cells were injected, a fluid-air or a fluid-gas exchange was performed. In one case, cataract surgery was performed prior to iridectomy and vitrectomy. All patients were scheduled for examination at 3 weeks, 3, 6, 12 and 36 months. The three-year follow-up was completed in 17 patients.

Results

Cell transplantation

Submacular surgery with CNV extraction was performed in 20 eyes of 20 patients and autologous, freshly isolated IPE cells were successfully transplanted to the subretinal space in 19 out of the 20 patients. In these patients preoperative best-corrected visual acuity ranged from 20/1000 (logMAR 1.7) to 20/125 (logMAR 0.8), with a mean 20/320 (logMAR, 1.2). Preoperative fluorescein angiography showed classic subfoveal CNV due to AMD in 9 eyes, occult subfoveal CNV in 7 eyes, and either idiopathic CNV or CNV associated with dominant drusen or pathologic myopia in four eyes.

Three years after IPE transplantation, best-corrected visual acuity ranged from hand movements (logMAR, 2.0) to 20/100 (logMAR, 0.7), with a mean of 20/320 (logMAR, 1.2). Compared to preoperative visual acuity, one patient showed improvement of 3 lines or more on the ETDRS chart, 13 patients retained stable visual acuity with a change of less than 3 lines, and 3 patients showed decreased visual acuity of 3 lines or more. Of the 3 patients that showed decreased visual acuity, one patient had suffered from proliferative vitreoretinopathy (PVR) and had undergone 2 revisional vitrectomies.

In fundus photographs transplanted cells appeared as dark spots in the area of the transplant, which appeared to remain stable in size and shape throughout the observation period. Throughout the 36 to 44 months follow-up period, the retina appeared healthy with no evidence of immunologic rejection, e.g. macular edema. In postoperative angiograms, we did not observe any recurrence of CNV during the three-year follow-up period in any of the patients. By macular perimetry, none of the patients showed central fixation or responses over the transplanted areas three years after submacular surgery.

All 19 phakic patients developed a cataract and underwent cataract surgery; in one case, phakoemulsification was combined with the initial vitrectomy and IPE translocation. During the first two months postoperatively two of the 19 patients successfully injected with IPE cells experienced significant complications, namely retinal detachment and proliferative vitreoretinopathy (PVR), and underwent revision vitrectomy with silicone oil endotamponade at 3 months.

Discussion

The development of neovascularization leads to irreversible damage to the RPE and photoreceptors, and surgical excision of the membranes is associated with the traumatic loss of the RPE cell layer and damage to Bruch's membrane, which prevents restoration of vision. Therefore, membrane extraction should be accompanied by the restoration of the

Bruch's membrane-RPE complex. A number of investigators have attempted to repair the damaged RPE-Bruch's membrane complex by transplanting homologous RPE cells or fetal RPE cells to the subretinal space. However, these cells were rejected [1–3]. To prevent rejection it would be necessary to transplant autologous RPE cells. Even though possible, autologous RPE cells are difficult to obtain routinely, therefore, we have transplanted autologous IPE cells. The transplantation of IPE cells as a substitute for RPE cells is based on the hypothesis that IPE cells have the ability to transdifferentiate into RPE cells in the subretinal space environment. This hypothesis is supported by evidence that IPE cells are "plastic" and are able to transdifferentiate into lens cells and into neural retinal cells, etc. when given the appropriate environmental stimuli [12, 13, 24]. In vitro IPE cells have the ability to phagocytize ROS and express the appropriate enzymes to metabolize retinol [22, 23]. In addition, the hypothesis that IPE cells may acquire RPE functions in the subretinal space is supported by experiments in which single cell suspensions of IPE cells transplanted to the subretinal space of rabbits acquired morphological characteristics of RPE cells, phagocityzed rod outer segments and formed a monolayer [7, 21].

In the clinical study presented here, the majority of patients who were examined 3 years after autologous IPE transplantation showed improvement or stabilization of visual acuity, a visual outcome at least as good as those reported after classic membrane extraction. In addition, during the follow-up period (36 months or longer) there was no recurrence of neovascularization in any of the patients, suggesting that the transplanted IPE cells in the subretinal space synthesize anti-angiogenic substances and could be considered a treatment option for patients with exudative maculopathy in combination with surgical excision of the neovascular membranes.

In our series of patients, we observed that the transplanted IPE cells remained funduscopically unchanged at the site of transplantation, possibly as a clump, suggesting that they were not able to spread or migrate or divide. The cells must have remained alive, or after three years we would have expected to see only dispersed pigmented debris. However, clinical examination by funduscopy or other means can only suggest but does not allow the determination of cell morphology, location and fate of the transplanted cells. Determination of cell morphology and cell fate will require the development of an animal model, which develops choroidal neovascular membranes, which can be excised prior to cell transplantation.

In our study, IPE cells were successfully transplanted to the subretinal space of patients following excision of neovascular membranes and these cells may have contributed to the prevention of neovascularization recurrence and to the stabilization of visual acuity. However, the ultimate goal of improvement or restoration of vision was not achieved. There are a number of considerations for the lack of a better visual outcome in these patients, namely the cells did not differentiate functionally, the cells did not acquire the proper morphological position vis-à-vis the neural retina, or the cells did not spread and form a monolayer as the result of an altered or damaged Bruch's membrane. One obvious solution to reduce these problems would be the transplantation of IPE cells as a sheet of cells with apical and basal domains already established. Transplantation of a sheet of cells with the appropriate morphology requires an efficient cell culture system and an appropriate biodegradable substrate, which allows for efficient cell attachment and growth and that can be handled without severe damage to it or to the cells attached to it. In addition, a suitable instrument to handle such cell sheets must be developed.

We have begun a series of studies to develop a culture system that allows RPE and IPE cells to grow efficiently, to acquire and maintain epithelial morphology. A culture system of IPE and RPE cells that allows for efficient cell proliferation, while maintaining morphological and functional characteristics would be invaluable for studies of transplantation, differentiation, and gene transfer directed at the Bruch's membrane-retina complex [18]. In addition, we have begun studies to culture cells on biodegradable membranes, which allow for the growth and acquisition of proper morphological and functional characteristics. Our preliminary results indicate that these membranes with attached cells are durable enough to be manipulated and transplanted to the subretinal space. These studies are still at an early stage and it is difficult to assess whether transplantation of cell sheets in AMD patients will result in a better visual outcome than the transplantation of cell suspensions. We are also experimenting with different types of biodegradable membranes to define the most biologically appropriate membrane.

References

1. Algvere PV, Berglin L, Gouras P, Sheng Y (1995) Transplantation of fetal retinal pigment epithelium in age-related macular degeneration with subfoveal neovascularization. Graefe's Arch Clin Exp Ophthalmol 232:707–16
2. Algvere PV, Berglin L, Gouras P, Sheng Y, Dafgard Kopp E (1997) Transplantation of RPE in age-related macular degeneration: observations in disciform lesions and dry RPE atrophy. Graefe's Arch Clin Exp Ophthalmol 235:149–58
3. Algvere PV, Gouras P, Dafgard Kopp E (1999) Long-term outcome of RPE allografts in non-immunosuppressed patients with AMD. Eur J Ophthalmol 9:217–30
4. Benson MT, Callear A, Tsaloumas M, China J, Beatty S (1998) Surgical excision of subfoveal neovascular membranes. Eye 12:768–74
5. Berglin L, Algvere P, Olivestedt G, Crafoord S, Stenkula S, Hansson LJ, Tomic Z, Kvanta A, Seregard S (2001) The Swedish national survey of surgical excision for submacular choroidal neovascularization (CNV). Acta Ophthalmol Scand 79:580–4
6. Binder S, Stolba U, Krebs I, Kellner L, Jahn C, Feichtinger H, Povelka M, Frohner U, Kruger A, Hilgers RD, Krugluger W (2002) Transplantation of autologues retinal pigment epithelium in eyes with foveal neovascularization resulting from age-related macular degeneration: A pilot study. Am J Ophthalmol 133:215–24
7. Crafoord S, Geng L, Seregard S, Algvere PV (2001) Experimental transplantation of autologous iris pigment epithelial cells to the subretinal space. Acta Ophthalmol Scand 79:509–14
8. Eckardt C (1996) Surgical removal of submacular neovascularization membranes. Ophthalmologe 93:688–93
9. Hu DN, Ritch R, McCormick SA, Pelton-Henrion K (1992) Isolation and cultivation of human iris pigment epithelium. Invest Ophthalmol Vis Sci 33:2443–53
10. Hu DN, McCormick SA, Ritch R (1997) Isolation and culture of iris pigment epithelium from iridectomy specimens of eyes with and without exfoliation syndrome. Arch Ophthalmol 115:89–94
11. Merrill PT, LoRusso FJ, Lomeo MD, Saxe SJ, Khan MM, Lambert HM (1999) Surgical removal of subfoveal choroidal neovascularization in age-related macular degeneration. Ophthalmology 106:782–9
12. Okada TS (1980) Cellular metaplasia or transdifferentiation as a model for retinal cell differentiation. Curr Top Dev Biol 16:349–80
13. Okada TS, Yasuda K, Araki M, Eguchi G (1979) Possible demonstration of multipotential nature of embryonic neural retina by clonal cell culture. Dev Biol 68:600–17
14. Rezai KA, Lappas A, Farrokh-Siar L, Kohen L, Wiedemann P, Heimann K (1997) Iris pigment epithelial cells of Long Evans Rats demonstrate phagocytic activity. Exp Eye Res 65:23–9
15. Rezai KA, Lappas A, Kohen L, Wiedemann P, Heimann K (1997) Comparison of tight junction permeability for albumin in iris pigment epithelium and retinal pigment epithelium in vitro. Graefe's Arch Clin Exp Ophthalmol 235:48–55
16. Scheider A, Gündisch O, Kampik A (1999) Surgical extraction of subfoveal choroidal new vessels and submacular hemorrhage in age-related macular degeneration: results of a prospective study. Graefe's Arch Clin Exp Ophthalmol 237:10–15
17. Stanga PE, Kychenthal A, Fitzke FW, Halfyard AS, Chan R, Bird AC, Aylward GW (2002) Retinal pigment epithelium transplantation after choroidal neovascular membrane removal in age-related macular degeneration. Ophthalmology 109:1492–8
18. Thumann G (2002) Potential of pigment epithelium transplantation in the treatment of AMD. Graefe's Arch Clin Exp Ophthalmol 240:695–697

19. Thumann G, Aisenbrey S, Schraermeyer U, et al (2000) Transplantation of autologous iris pigment epithelium after removal of choroidal neovascular membranes. Arch Ophthalmol 118:1350–5
20. Thumann G, Bartz-Schmidt KU, Schraermeyer U, Heimann K (1997) Descemets membrane as autologous membranous support in RPE/IPE transplantation. Curr Eye Res 16:1236–8
21. Thumann G, Bartz-Schmidt KU, El Bakri H, Schraermeyer U, Spee C, Cui J, Hinton DR, Ryan SJ, Heimann K (1999) Transplantation of autologous iris pigment epithelium to the subretinal space in rabbits. Transplantation 68:195–201
22. Thumann G, Bartz-Schmidt KU, Heimann K, Schraermeyer U (1998) Phagocytosis of rod outer segments by human iris pigment epithelial cells in vitro. Graefe's Arch Clin Exp Ophthalmol 236:753–7
23. Thumann G, Kociok N, Bartz-Schmidt KU, Esser P, Schraermeyer U, Heimann K (1999) Detection of mRNA for proteins involved in retinol metabolism in iris pigment epithelium. Graefes Arch Clin Exp Ophthalmol 237:1046–51
24. Zhao S, Rizzolo LJ, Barnstable CJ (1997) Differentiation and transdifferentiation of the retinal pigment epithelium. Int Rev Cytol 171:225–66

Correspondence: Gabriele Thumann, M.D., Universitäts-Augenklinik, Joseph-Stelzmann-Strasse 9, D-50931 Köln, Germany, E-mail: G. Thumann@uni-koeln.de

Translocation of iris pigment epithelium in patients with exudative age-related macular degeneration – long term results

A. Lappas[1], A. M. H. Foerster[2], A. W. A. Weinberger[1],
S. Coburger[3], N. Schrage[1], and B. Kirchhof[2]

[1] University of Aachen, Department of Ophthalmology, Aachen, Germany
[2] University of Cologne, Department of Ophthalmology, Cologne, Germany
[3] University of Cologne, Department of Medical Statistics,
Informatics and Epidemiology, Cologne, Germany

Abstract

Objectives: To report practicability and efficacy of autologous iris pigment epithelium (IPE) translocation in exudative age-related macular degeneration (ARMD) over one year.
Methods: The consecutive interventional case series included 56 patients with exudative ARMD. During vitrectomy the submacular neovascular membrane (CNV) was removed and IPE cells, harvested from a peripheral iridectomy, were injected into the submacular space. Included were patients with subfoveal occult CNV (11 eyes), classic CNV (10 eyes), mixed CNV (18 eyes), CNV with a pigment epithelial detachment (13 eyes) or with a hemorrhage (5 eyes). Outcome measures were visual acuity, foveal fixation, size of CNV and rate of recurrence based on fluorescence angiographic imaging.

Results: All patients underwent successful surgical removal of the CNV with consecutive subretinal IPE injection. Mean preoperative visual acuity (1.0 +/– 0.3 logMAR units) did not change significantly after one year (1.0 +/– 0.3 logMAR units). Ten eyes (17.8%) developed a recurrence. Fixation within the surgically denuded area could be demonstrated in 25 eyes (45%).

Conclusions: Autologous IPE translocation for ARMD over one year can preserve foveal function on a low level, but cannot improve visual acuity. IPE translocation is technically feasible with a low rate of complication. Continued research seems justified to improve functional outcome.

Introduction

Age-related macular degeneration (ARMD) is characterized by diseased retinal pigment epithelium (RPE), Bruch's membrane and choriocapillaris followed by insufficiency of photoreceptor cells and visual loss. In exudative ARMD neovascular choroidal vessels grow through Bruch´s membrane underneath the retina or the RPE, accelerating photoreceptor cell loss. Selective removal of classic CNV [11] was found to be more beneficial in young patients with presumed ocular histoplasmosis syndrome (POHS) or myopia [17] than in patients with ARMD [8]. So far, CNV removal in ARMD has been unable to maintain or revive subfoveal RPE. As RPE cells are considered crucial for maintenance and function of photoreceptors, restoration of RPE cell function is under investigation either by translocation of the macula to neighbouring intact RPE [10] or by transplantation/translocation of pigmented cells. Autologous translocation of RPE cells has been reported [12]. Homologous RPE transplantation failed due to macular oedema, probably as a result of immunologic graft rejection [1]. Lately, IPE cells have been suggested as RPE-substitute [13]. IPE cells can easily be isolated from an iridectomy and be injected subretinally. IPE translocation was performed in patients with ARMD and followed for 6–8 months [9, 18]. Stable visual acuity was reported for up to 6 months. We now report the follow-up results one year after autologous IPE translocation in patients with exudative ARMD.

Method

A consecutive interventional case series was performed on patients with exudative ARMD recruited between 1998 and 2000 in Aachen (Germany). The prospective pilot study was set up on 56 consecutive patients (56 eyes), 38 women and 18 men.

Inclusion criteria were: Exudative ARMD, fluorescein angiographic evidence of classic, occult or a mixed subfoveal neovascularisation according to the MPS (Macular Photocoagulation Study Group) classification. Classic CNV size needed to be more than 2 disc areas, a size that was found not to be beneficial according to the MPS study [Macular Photocoagulation Study Group, 1991 #4]. Photodynamic therapy was not yet approved in Germany at the time of the study. Inclusion into the study also required a visual acuity below 20/63 and above light projection, that the patient had experienced a recent, subjectively relevant visual loss and willingness to participate in the trial and to attend all follow-up examinations after informed consent. Exclusion criteria were: prior macular laser photocoagulation, radiation therapy or submacular surgery; severe systemic or additional ophthalmic disease; participation in any other study.

Intervention

IPE translocation was done as reported in a previous study [9] with minor modifications. Briefly, isolation of IPE cells from 2 peripheral iridectomies was followed by a complete pars plana vitrectomy including a delamination of the posterior vitreous. According to the fluorescein angiographic images the edges of the neovascular membrane were evaluated and the retinotomy site determined. Usually, the retinotomy was positioned temporal to the fovea at the margin of the membrane. A retinal bleb was created by a slow subretinal injection of BSS with a 20 µl glass micropipette that was connected by a flexible tube to a 2.0 cc syringe. An angled subretinal pick was used to free the CNV from the surrounding tissue. Then the membrane was grasped and removed with a horizontally opening subretinal forceps (Dutch Ophthalmic Research Center, Int., b.v., Netherlands) through the same retinotomy. If necessary, additional BSS was injected into the retinal bleb to achieve a tight wall. A fluid air exchange was performed and any remaining fluid was removed from the posterior pole via flute needle. The isolated IPE cells were injected with the glass micropipette through the peak of the retinal bleb into the subretinal space. Patients were postured supine at the day of surgery to support adhesion of the injected cells until the subretinal bleb was absorbed. All treatments were given in accordance with the guidelines of national legislation and the declaration of Helsinki.

Main outcome measures

The size of the CNV was expressed in correlation to disc areas. The area of the CNV and the optic disc were measured using Heidelberg Eye Explorer software (Heidelberg,

Germany). The size of classic CNVs was determined during the early phase of fluorescein angiography including the area of hyperfluorescence and the surrounding hypofluorescent rim. The borders of occult CNVs were estimated by early leakage during the late phase of fluorescein angiography. The area of pigment epithelial detachments was assessed by early leakage in fluorescein angiography. The size of occult CNVs associated with submacular hemorrhage was estimated with fluorescein and indocyanin angiography including the dimensions of the CNV (late hyperfluorescence) and blocked fluorescence due to subretinal blood. Submacular bleeding was classified as hemorrhage when it covered an area over 6 disc areas.

Follow up examinations were performed 6 weeks, 3 months, 6 months and 1 year postoperatively. The size of the postoperative surgically denuded area was determined on the basis of the early hyperfluorescent area in fluorescence angiography. Pre- and postoperative examinations included best corrected visual acuity based on the Early Treatment Diabetic Retinopathy Study (ETDRS) chart. Means were calculated with LogMAR values. Hand movements were set to 2.0 logMAR units. Slit lamp examination, colour fundus photography, fluorescein and indocyanin angiography were performed at each follow up examination.

Macular fixation was determined using the Rodenstock scanning laser ophthalmoscope (SLO; Rodenstock, Germany) with refined software for microperimetry (Software Aachen) [19]. The size of the fixation cross was 10×10 to 20×20 pixels. Each fixation test involved an adaptation of the retinal image to the presented fixation cross with a retinal landmark. The microperimetrically determined fixation site was transferred to the fundus photographs and to the angiograms to relate it to the estimated fovea and the post-surgical RPE defect.

Subgroup analysis

As potential predictors for a significant change in visual acuity pre-, intra- and postoperative observations were considered. As preoperative factors age, gender, diagnosis, visual acuity and the size of the CNV were examined. As an intraoperative factor choroidal hemorrhage was included. As postoperative observations size of the surgically denuded area, change of fixation, recurrences and complications were taken into consideration. The influence of cataract surgery was also examined.

Patients were subdivided into groups within each factor and their P values were compared to determine a significant decrease in visual acuity using chi squared test or Fisher's exact test. The decision between chi square test and Fisher's exact test was made by expected cell frequencies. Logistic regression was used to evaluate the relationship between a significant decrease in visual acuity and the variables showing a distinct interdependency with the decrease of visual acuity of at least 3 lines.

Results

Of the 56 patients with subfoveal CNV 11 eyes (19.6%) showed an occult type, 10 eyes (17.9%) showed a classic type and 17 eyes (30.4%) showed a mixed type of CNV, 13 eyes (23.2%) had a PED and 5 eyes (8.9%) presented with submacular hemorrhage. Twenty-two patients (39.3%) were phakic when they entered the study; the remaining were pseudophakic (28 cases, 50%) or underwent cataract surgery with implantation of an intraocular lens during submacular surgery (6 cases, 10.7%).

Mean preoperative visual acuity was 20/200 (1.0 +/− 0.3 logMAR). The average time between IPE-translocation and drop of visual acuity was 17.4 (+/−12.9) weeks. One year after surgery mean visual acuity was 20/200 (1.0 +/− 0.3 logMAR).

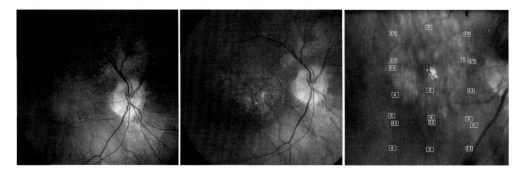

Fig. 1. Left, Preoperative photograph of a 67 year old, male patient with an occult CNV and a visual acuity of 20/1000. **Center**, The postoperative fundus photograph shows a surgically denuded area with pigmented material, visual acuity improved significantly to 20/320. **Right**, SLO microperimetric image demonstrating fixation within the surgically denuded area

Preoperatively 7 patients (12.5%) were found with a visual acuity better than 20/100, 12 (21.4%) had a visual acuity between 20/100 and 20/160, 26 (46.4%) between 20/200 and 20/320 and 11 (19.6%) had a visual acuity less than 20/320. Postoperatively 4 (7.1%) patients showed a visual acuity better than 20/100, 14 (25%) had a visual acuity between 20/100 to 20/160, 30 (53.6%) between 20/200 and 20/320 and 8 (14.3%) had a visual acuity less than 20/320.

A significant change in visual acuity was defined as a change of at least 3 ETDRS lines. According to this classification visual acuity improved significantly in 13 (23.2%) cases, decreased in 13 (23.2%) cases and remained unchanged in 30 (53.6%) cases.

With respect to preoperative visual acuity a significant improvement in visual acuity was observed in 9 out of 11 patients (81.9%) with a preoperative visual acuity lower than 20/320. A significant decrease was found in 5 out of 7 (71.4%) patients with a preoperative visual acuity better than 20/100. Most patients had a preoperative visual acuity between 20/100 and 20/320 (38 cases, 67.9%), only 21% (8 patients) of those developed a significant decrease in visual acuity. No patient with a low visual acuity (<20/320) showed a significant decrease in visual acuity.

There was no significant change in visual acuity with respect to type of CNV. Preoperative fixation was foveal in 43 (76.8%) patients and extrafoveal in 13 (23.2%) patients. Postoperatively, fixation crosses were related to the surgically denuded area that was left after removal of the CNV and could be identified with SLO perimetry as a bright area. In 25 (44.6%) patients fixation occurred within the surgically denuded area (Fig. 1). In 18 (32.1%) patients fixation occurred outside the surgically denuded area. These patients lost foveal fixation after surgery. In 13 (23.2%) eyes preoperatively, extrafoveal fixation was retained after surgery at an extrafoveal location at the margin or outside the surgically denuded area. In some patients pigmented areas could be detected as dark spots within the RPE defect.

Preservation of fixation within the RPE defect was not related to size of the RPE-defect. Preoperative foveal fixations were found in small as well as in large CNVs (71.4%–90% patients with foveal fixation) and could be found within small to large surgically denuded areas (39.1%–56.3% patients with fixation within the surgically denuded area, 1). Moreover, postoperative fixation within the RPE defect was not related to the type of CNV. Fixation within the RPE defect could be found in 36.4% (4 cases) of occult CNVs, 46.2% (6 cases) of pigment epithelial detachments (PED), 47.1% (8 cases) of mixed CNVs, 40% (4 cases) of classic CNVs and in 60% (3 cases) of patients with a submacular hemorrhage.

However, mean preoperative visual acuity, was significantly lower in patients with preoperative extrafoveal fixation (20/400, 1.3 +/– 0.3 logMAR) than in those with foveal fixation (20/200, 1.0 +/– 0.3 logMAR). Postoperatively, mean visual acuity did not differ significantly in patients with fixation within the surgically denuded area (20/200, 1.0 +/– 0.3 logMAR) compared to patients who lost foveal fixation or maintained extrafoveal fixation (20/200, 1.0 +/– 0.3 logMAR). Among the patients with a preoperative foveal fixation (43 patients, 76.8%) only 13 (30.2%) and none of those with a preoperative extrafoveal fixation experienced a significant decrease in visual acuity.

Postoperative fluorescein angiography revealed hyperfluorescence in the surgically denuded area without late leakage in most cases indicating that the choroidal neovascular membrane was removed successfully and did not recur. The mean preoperative size of the choroidal neovascular membranes was 6.5 +/– 6.0 disc areas (range 2–35 disc areas). Postoperatively, the mean size of the surgically denuded area was 9.5 +/– 6.8 disc areas (range 2–45 disc areas). Mean visual acuity did not differ significantly in small to large membranes both pre- and postoperatively.

In 10 patients (17.8%) we observed a recurrence or persistence of the CNV. Seven patients (12.5%) showed late hyperfluorescence as early as 6 weeks after surgery developing into a recurrence during the later follow up. In 3 cases (5.4%) late hyperfluorescence was found 3 months postoperatively. This suggests that in most cases a persistence could be the reason for a recurrent CNV. In 3 cases (5.4%) the recurrence was treated by argon laser photocoagulation as it showed well demarcated borders and was located extrafoveally.

Further postoperative complications were retinal detachment with PVR that was treated by pars plana vitrectomy and injection of silicone oil (1 eye). One patient developed a macular pucker and another patient showed subretinal bleeding and vitreous hemorrhage. Both underwent pars plana re-vitrectomy. Postoperative complications resulted in a decrease in visual acuity (mean preoperative visual acuity 1.0 +/– 0.2 logMAR units, mean postoperative visual acuity 1.4 +/– 0.4 logMAR units) whereas mean visual acuity in patients without complications remained unchanged (mean preoperative visual acuity 1.1 +/– 0.3 logMAR units, mean postoperative visual acuity 1.0 +/– 0.4 logMAR units).

Intraoperative bleeding during removal of the subfoveal membrane was observed in 5 cases (9%). Subretinal injections with balanced salt solution were performed to remove the hemorrhage until no further blood was left. Intraoperative bleeding resulted in a significant decrease in visual acuity in 4 out of 5 cases (80%; mean preoperative visual acuity 1.0 +/– 0.3 logMAR units, mean postoperative visual acuity 1.4 +/– 0.3 logMAR units).

Further surgical procedures included implantation of an intraocular lens in 11 cases (19.6%). Twenty-eight patients (50%) were pseudophakic preoperatively or an intraocular lens was implanted at the time of IPE translocation (6 cases, 10.7%). The remaining 11 patients (19.6%) were still phakic at the end of the follow up.

Discussion

We investigated the long-term results after removal of choroidal neovascular membranes and IPE translocation in patients with advanced exudative ARMD. After 12 months follow up mean visual acuity did not change significantly. In contrast to allogenic transplantation of fetal RPE no morphologic sign of rejection of the translocated cells could be found.

Only 13 patients (23%) experienced a significant decrease in visual acuity of at least 3 lines. According to the MPS, all patients with subfoveal classic membranes larger than 2 disc areas with or without laser treatment showed a mean decrease of 3 lines after 1 year. In our study mean visual acuity in classic CNVs remained unchanged. In the MPS study patients were not included if visual acuity was worse than 20/320 and the membrane was larger than 3.5 disc areas. In this study the mean CNV-size ranged from 2–35 disc areas (mean 6.6), and 11 patients (19.6%) had a preoperative visual acuity of less than 20/320.

In the Photodynamic Study Group (TAP) report, 58% of patients with mixed CNV were reported to loose at least 15 letters (3 lines) without treatment whereas only 40% of patients lost at least 3 lines with treatment. After IPE translocation a decrease of at least 3 lines was found in only 29% of patients with mixed CNV. However, in the PDT study 20/200 was the lower limit for visual acuity, the CNV size was not larger than 5400 μm (approximately 3.5 disc areas) and at least 50% of the CNV had to be classic.

In patients with occult CNV, a moderate to severe loss of vision of at least 3 lines can be expected without treatment in 66% of eyes after twelve months [3]. In this study, we observed a significant decrease (a decrease of at least 3 ETDRS lines) in 9% of patients with occult CNV and in 31% of patients with PED. In patients with subretinal haemorrhage and lesion sizes larger than 6 disc areas, a final visual acuity less than 20/200 can be expected in 71% of all cases [2].

In the Submacular Surgery Trial (SST), CNV removal was performed in patients with recurrent CNV after laser treatment of juxta- or extrafoveal lesions. A decrease of at least 2 lines was observed in 45% of all cases, compared to a decrease of 23% of at least 3 lines in this study. Again, comparability is limited as the size of the CNV was limited to 9 disc areas including the laser scar in the SST study. Considering that the subfoveal portion was a recurrence of juxta- or extrafoveal CNV the final shortest distance of the recurrent CNV between its outer margin to the fovea might have been smaller than with IPE translocation suggesting a better visual prognosis.

A retrospective study of patients who received subfoveal CNV-removal accompanied by subretinal injection of recombinant tissue plasminogen activator showed that 28% of all patients experienced a significant decrease and 28% of all patients experienced a significant increase in visual acuity of at least 3 lines. In 42% of all patients visual acuity remained stable [11]. The mean size of the CNV was 5 disc areas, which is comparable to the mean size of the CNV in this study (6.5 +/− 6.0 disc areas). Membranes included, however, were predominantly classic and 54% were associated with a subretinal hemorrhage. Prognosis of subretinal hemorrhage depends on the size of the hemorrhage, its location and the time of surgery and has been reported to lead to a decrease in visual acuity in only 5.6–20% [14].

Subgroup analysis revealed that after IPE translocation significant changes in visual acuity could be found in patients with either good or low visual acuity. No patient with a low initial visual acuity (<20/320) experienced a further significant decrease after one year. Although the mean level of initial visual acuity in this category was low (20/800, 1.6 logMAR units), those patients even showed a significant increase (20/250, 1.1 logMAR mean postperative visual acuity). Visual prognosis was not significantly correlated to CNV-type or size of the CNV. Part of the retinal function compromised by the CNV might have been restored after removal of the CNV together with subretinal exudations that may have formed a barrier to the transport of nutrients from the choriocapillaris. Visual restoration has been also reported after CNV removal and subretinal injection of tissue plasminogen activator in patients with large CNV (>2 disc areas) and low visual acuity (≤20/200) due to ARMD.

Five out of 7 patients (71.4%) with a good initial visual acuity (>20/100) experienced a significant decrease in visual acuity following IPE translocation. Other studies showed likewise that decreases in visual function are more likely in patients with exudative ARMD and good initial visual acuity. Obviously, removal of the CNV and IPE translocation was not able to preserve retinal function on an elevated functional level. On the other hand, some patients (4 cases, 7.1%) reached good final functional levels (>20/100) after IPE translocation. Consequently, other reasons than the surgical trauma might contribute to the low levels of postoperative visual acuity. Histopathologic studies of choroidal neovascular membranes have shown the photoreceptor cells and the choriocapillaris as part of the fibrovascular tissue [4]. Removal of such still functioning structures cannot be ruled out with any surgical membrane extraction and might result in a non-supportive environment for the translocated IPE cells.

Fixation was the second factor found to be significantly correlated to visual prognosis after IPE translocation. SLO perimetry revealed an area denuded of RPE at the posterior pole. In 25 patients (45%) postoperatively fixation could be localized within the RPE defect. It is well accepted that patients with geographic atrophy usually develop central scotomas from the RPE defect, accompanied by extrafoveal fixation at the margin of the atrophic area and only occasionally show fixation within the zone of atrophy [15]. Similar observations are reported after removal of submacular CNV [7].

Assuming that fixation within the RPE defect might reflect preserved photoreceptor function by translocated IPE cells, we would expect an advantage on visual acuity. Visual acuity, however, did not correlate with postoperative fixation, implicating that fixation within the surgically denuded area might be a more sensitive functional parameter than visual acuity in very low levels of visual acuity. Ophthalmoscopy and SLO perimetry revealed pigment clumps in some eyes within the field of RPE defect. As reported earlier, it is impossible to reveal its origin from RPE or from translocated IPE [9]. The injected IPE suspension consisted of cell clumps as well as of single cells. Single cells cannot be detected by ophthalmoscopy. Consequently, translocated IPE single cells cannot be documented. Resident retinal pigment epithelial cells repopulate RPE defects insufficiently after surgical CNV removal in ARMD [6]. In consequence, the RPE defect may not have been covered by resident RPE cells or by translocated IPE cells in some cases, resulting in a low postoperative visual acuity or extrafoveal fixation. In some eyes fixation was found on hyperpigmented spots within the area of RPE defect. This observation was confirmed by dynamic testing with the SLO fixation cross, when light perception was given in proximity to the pigmented material.

Fixation within the RPE defect was independent from the size of the defect. This observation rules out that fixation is affected by RPE from the margin of the defect. Patients with subfoveal RPE defects prefer to fixate extrafoveally, namely at the margin of the defect, as documented for 31 eyes (55%) in our series. Similary, patients with geographic atrophy fixate extrafoveally, at the margin of the atrophy zone independent from its size. Therefore, fixation in the area of RPE atrophy after IPE translocation in this study may signal a protective effect of IPE on retinal photoreceptors over one year. IPE cells have been shown to synthesize similar growth factors as RPE cells in vitro [Kociok, 1998 #11] and to be capable of phagocytosis of photoreceptor rod outer segments to some extent [Rezai, 1997 #12; Thumann, 1998 #13]. The supportive effect of translocated IPE cells within the RPE defect may be so weak that it does not result in a measurable improvement of visual acuity.

Interestingly, patients with preoperative extrafoveal fixation showed a significant increase in mean postoperative visual acuity despite persistent extrafoveal fixation. In those patients recovery of foveal fixation might have been hampered by irreversible preoperative damage of foveal photoreceptors. The surgical procedure of CNV removal and IPE translocation stabilized vision significantly at the low mean level of 20/200.

In our series the rate of CNV recurrence and persistence was 18% (10 cases) after one year. A similar rate of recurrence (24%) was reported after removal of predominantly classic CNV [11]. Other studies reported a recurrence rate of 46% after removal of classic subfoveal membranes [16]. In the Submacular Surgery Trial (SST) "late hyperfluorescence" was found in more than 50% of all surgically treated eyes at the 12-month examination. A possible explanation for this pronounced difference could be that only patients with recurrent CNVs after laser treatment of juxta- and extrafoveal choroidal membranes secondary to ARMD were included in the SST study. Laser treatment is not selective for the RPE and CNV but destroys retinal structures resulting in scar formation throughout the retina. Preoperative scar tissue may compromise the complete surgical removal of recurrent membranes. CNV recurrence was reported higher than in our series after laser photocoagulation of subfoveal and juxtafoveal CNV. Laser treatment for extrafoveal CNV in ARMD showed a recurrence in 59%. In our study 70% of patients with a recurrence or persistence showed a mixed CNV preoperatively. Histopathologic studies have demonstrated that the classic part of the CNV in fluorescence angiography correlates with choroidal neovascularization above the RPE cell layer wheras occult CNV grows beneath the RPE [5]. It might be possible that parts of the mixed CNV show different consistency and adherence to neighbouring RPE cells, leading to increased risk of persistence after CNV removal. Recurrences in this study did not result in a significant decrease in visual acuity after one year possibly due to their location outside the fovea and at the surgical margin of the RPE defect.

The rate of intra- and postoperative complications following IPE translocation was 14.2% (8 cases). Postoperative complications requiring additional re-pars plana vitrectomy included 3 cases (5.3%) which is considerably low, 1 of those patients (1.8%) was retreated by silicone oil for PVR. The SST study reported 9% of patients that received additional intraocular treatment due to retinal detachment and 9% due to submacular complications. The rate of intraoperative complications in this study was 9% (5 cases), resulting from subretinal bleeding after CNV-removal before injection of IPE cells.

Despite the obvious stabilization of visual acuity in many patients in this study after one year, the effect of IPE translocation to date is difficult to interpret. Since IPE cell as well as photoreceptor cell viability and survival cannot directly be tested, a prospective randomized trial could give more insight into significant results of this technique. The low rate of complications and the shortness of the surgical procedure encourage future efforts to investigate IPE translocation, e.g. to improve functional outcome by optimizing IPE cell attachment in the wounded area after CNV removal.

References

1. Algvere PV, Berglin L, Gouras P, Sheng Y, Kopp ED (1997) Transplantation of RPE in age-related macular degeneration: observations in disciform lesions and dry RPE atrophy. Graefes Arch Clin Exp Ophthalmol 235:149–58
2. Avery RL, Fekrat S, Hawkins BS, Bressler NM (1996) Natural history of subfoveal subretinal hemorrhage in age-related macular degeneration. Retina 16:183–9
3. Bressler NM, Bressler SB, Fine SL (1988) Age-related macular degeneration. Surv Ophthalmol 32:375–413
4. Green WR, Enger C (1993) Age-related macular degeneration histopathologic studies. The 1992 Lorenz E. Zimmerman Lecture. Ophthalmology 100:1519–35
5. Grossniklaus HE, Green WR (1998) Histopathologic and ultrastructural findings of surgically excised choroidal neovascularization. Submacular Surgery Trials Research Group. Arch Ophthalmol 116:745–9
6. Hsu JK, Thomas MA, Ibanez H, Green WR (1995) Clinicopathologic studies of an eye after submacular membranectomy for choroidal neovascularization. Retina 15:43–52
7. Hudson HL, Frambach DA, Lopez PF (1995) Relation of the functional and structural fundus changes after submacular surgery for neovascular age-related macular degeneration. Br J Ophthalmol 79:417–23
8. Lambert HM, Capone A Jr, Aaberg TM, Sternberg P Jr, Mandell BA, Lopez PF (1992) Surgical excision of subfoveal neovascular membranes in age-related macular degeneration. Am J Ophthalmol 113:257–62

9. Lappas A, Weinberger AW, Foerster AM, Kube T, Rezai KA, Kirchhof B (2000) Iris pigment epithelial cell translocation in exudative age-related macular degeneration. A pilot study in patients. Graefes Arch Clin Exp Ophthalmol 238:631–41

10. Machemer R (1998) Macular translocation. Am J Ophthalmol 125:698–700

11. Merrill PT, LoRusso FJ, Lomeo MD, Saxe SJ, Khan MM, Lambert HM (1999) Surgical removal of subfoveal choroidal neovascularization in age-related macular degeneration. Ophthalmology 106:782–9

12. Peyman GA, Blinder KJ, Paris CL, Alturki W, Nelson NC Jr, Desai U (1991) A technique for retinal pigment epithelium transplantation for age-related macular degeneration secondary to extensive subfoveal scarring. Ophthalmic Surg 22:102–8

13. Rezai KA, Lappas A, Farrokh-siar L, Kohen L, Wiedemann P, Heimann K (1997) Iris pigment epithelial cells of long evans rats demonstrate phagocytic activity. Exp Eye Res 65:23–9

14. Scheider A, Gundisch O, Kampik A (1999) Surgical extraction of subfoveal choroidal new vessels and submacular haemorrhage in age-related macular degeneration: results of a prospective study. Graefes Arch Clin Exp Ophthalmol 237:10–15

15. Sunness JS, Applegate CA, Gonzalez-Baron J (2000) Improvement of visual acuity over time in patients with bilateral geographic atrophy from age-related macular degeneration. Retina 20:162–9

16. Thomas MA, Dickinson JD, Melberg NS, Ibanez HE, Dhaliwal RS (1994) Visual results after surgical removal of subfoveal choroidal neovascular membranes. Ophthalmology 101:1384–96

17. Thomas MA, Kaplan HJ (1991) Surgical removal of subfoveal neovascularization in the presumed ocular histoplasmosis syndrome. Am J Ophthalmol 111:1–7

18. Thumann G (2002) Potential of pigment epithelium transplantation in the treatment of AMD. Graefes Arch Clin Exp Ophthalmol 240:695–7

19. Toonen F, Remky A, Janssen V, Wolf, S, Reim M (1995) Microperimetry in patients with central serous retinopathy. Ger J Ophthalmol 4:311–14

Correspondence: Bernd Kirchhof, Department of Ophthalmology, University of Cologne, Joseph Stelzmann Strasse 9, D-50935 Koeln, Germany, E-mail: BeKirchhof@aol.com

Transplantation of HLA-typed RPE in age-related macular degeneration – results after 6 months follow-up

G. Richard, K. Engelmann, M. Valtink, and J. Weichel

Klinik und Poliklinik für Augenheilkunde des Universitätsklinikums
Hamburg-Eppendorf, Germany

Abstract

Purpose: The retinal pigment epithelium (RPE) has been assumed to be causally involved in the pathogenesis of age-related macular degeneration (ARMD). The purpose of this prospective study was to determine the feasibility, safety and visual outcome of transplanting HLA-typed RPE cells in a series of patients suffering from ARMD with geographic atrophy of the RPE.

Patients and methods: RPE cells were isolated from donor eyes and cultured in a special medium. One part of the culture was subcultured for HLA-typing, the other part cryopreserved in a cell bank. In 9 eyes of 9 patients suffering from bilateral ARMD with geographic atrophy and visual deterioration, HLA-matched RPE cells were transplanted into the subretinal space. Patients underwent postoperative immunosuppressive therapy for six months.

Results: Throughout the follow-up of 6 months, no evidence of inflammation, infection or rejection of the graft was noted in any eye. There were no major retinal complications. In one treated eye, a retinal edema could be detected by fluorescein angiography and optical coherence tomography (OCT) that was due to the development of choroidal neovascularization (CNV). The vision slightly increased in four treated eyes, it remained stable in three treated eyes and declined in two treated eyes, whereas in none of the fellow eyes vision increased, remained unchanged in five eyes and decreased in four eyes.

Conclusion: The transplantation of adult human RPE cells in the subretinal space proved to be a safe surgical procedure. The use of HLA-matched RPE cells and postoperative immunosuppression seem to reduce the risk of graft rejection. The preliminary results of this study are encouraging with regard to the aim of RPE transplantation to arrest or delay the progression of the damage to the retina caused by geographic atrophy of the RPE.

Introduction

Age-related macular degeneration (ARMD) is characterized by a progressive deterioration of vision and constitutes a leading cause of legal blindness and severe central visual loss. It has been assumed that the retinal pigment epithelium (RPE) is causally involved in the pathogenesis of ARMD. The development of geographic atrophy of the RPE, the advanced form of atrophic ARMD, is associated with progressive pathological changes in the RPE

This study has been approved by the Ethics Committee of the Ärztekammer Hamburg, Germany (date of acceptance 2 September 1998).

and RPE loss which results in a secondary atrophy of the choriocapillaris and the photoreceptors [1, 2, 3].

Although several therapeutic strategies have been attempted in the past, there is currently no effective medical or surgical treatment for geographic atrophy. Regarding the pathogenesis of the disease, the transplantation of healthy RPE cells appears to be a causal therapy. However, first experimental studies on transplantation of fetal RPE in ARMD without immunosuppression revealed signs of graft rejection [4, 5]. Therefore, RPE immune rejection is considered a major concern for the success of allogenic grafting in patients with ARMD.

To obviate the risk of graft rejection, in the present study HLA-matched human adult RPE cells from the RPE cell bank of the University Eye Hospital of Hamburg were used for transplantation and patients additionally underwent a short-term postoperative immunosuppressive therapy. RPE cells stored in our cell bank have been demonstrated to maintain their specific morphologic and functional characteristics in vitro even after cryopreservation [6, 7]. The purpose of the present study was to evaluate the feasibility, safety and visual outcome of HLA-typed RPE transplantation in ARMD patients suffering from bilateral geographic atrophy of the RPE.

Material and methods

Isolation, cultivation, HLA-typing and cryopreservation of RPE cells

The cornea bank Hamburg, established in 1985, receives donor eyes from the Institutes of Pathology and Forensic Medicine at the University Hospital Hamburg-Eppendorf. The consent of organ donation is obtained according to the statutory principles of organ donation. Prior to transplantation, the donors were tested for infectious diseases including HIV and Hepatitis B and C. Since 1996, RPE cell cultures isolated from donor eyes have been stored cryopreserved in a cell bank.

After enucleation the corneoscleral disc is dissected according to standardized methods established for corneal organ culture. The choroidal sheets are carefully prepared off the sclera and treated with collagenase (Sigma, Germany) for 16 hours to loosen RPE cells. Isolated cells are seeded onto 24 well-plates with RPE growth medium F99$_{RPE}$ and cultured until confluency according to previously described methods [6]. The residual choroidal sheets are incubated in medium F99 + 1% FCS for four days to produce conditioned medium, an important supplement of the RPE growth medium [7]. At confluence, the cells are trypsinized and the cultures are partitioned: One part is cryopreserved in 1 ml FCS containing 7% DMSO (Sigma, Germany) and stored in liquid nitrogen until further use. The other part is subcultured for HLA-typing according to Ehrlich et al. [8] and for assessment of functional properties of the cells. Cells of every primary culture were loaded with autoclaved india ink at a concentration of 1 μl india ink/ml medium for three days to determine non-specific phagocytic activity.

Morphological appearance of the cultured cells was evaluated by phase contrast microscopy and documented by photography. Cell cultures contaminated with coisolated choroidal cells like melanocytes are not used for transplantation studies. Contaminating cells can easily be distinguished from RPE cells by their different morphological appearance. They are only sparsely seen and usually do not survive in medium F99$_{RPE}$.

Recultivation of cryopreserved cell cultures for transplantation

A cell culture that matches the HLA-type of a patient (correspondence on at least four MHC gene loci) was thawed and cultured as described above (choroid-conditioned medium as supplement is omitted). Cells were cultured until confluence. Sterility of the culture and morphology were monitored. Prior to transplantation the cells were trypsinized, centrifuged, and the pellet was resuspended in basal medium F99 (Table 2). Membrane integrity and cell number were determined by trypan blue dye exclusion test.

Patient recruitment / waiting list

Patients with bilateral ARMD with geographic atrophy and / or advanced drusen and visual deterioration were included.

Inclusion criteria were 1. bilateral geographic atrophy, 2. age 45 to 80 years, 3. no signs of occult or classic CNV, 4. absence of ocular diseases leading to further visual deterioration (glaucoma etc.), 5. absence of systemic disease possibly leading to visual deterioration (diabetes mellitus etc.), 6. informed consent.

Preoperatively, patients had a complete ophthalmological examination including visual acuity, intraocular pressure, slit-lamp biomicroscopy, fundus evaluation by binocular indirect ophthalmoscopy, and fundus photography. Additionally, fluorescein angiography, visual field testing, electroretinography (ERG), electrooculography (EOG), and optical coherence tomography (OCT) were performed. Vision testing was performed by independent investigators under constant circumstances.

The study was conducted in accordance with the World Medical Association's Declaration of Helsinki. The Ethics Committee of the Ärztekammer Hamburg, Germany, approved the protocol.

Surgical procedure

In all patients, except one, the worse eye was selected for transplantation of RPE cells. Standard three port vitrectomy was performed followed by a posterior vitreous detachment. Using a barbed microsurgical blade (Alcon Inc. Fortworth DX, USA) a small retinotomy was performed temporal or supratemporal of the macula. A 33 gauge subretinal spatula was introduced through the retinotomy. Then, the retina in the macular area was detached using balanced salt solution and the subretinal fluid was removed. Subsequently, the RPE cells were injected into the subretinal space slowly and under continuous visualization using an oil-hydraulic microinjection-pump [9]. Thereafter, a mild cryopexy was applied to the site of retinotomy and a fluid-gas exchange was performed. After suturing the sclera and the conjunctiva, a subconjunctival injection of gentamicin (5 mg) and dexamethasone (2 mg) was given. Postoperatively, the patients had to keep supine position for one hour to allow the injected cells to settle. Then, they had to stay in prone position for one week. All patients had routine postoperative care consisting of topical gentamicin q.i.d., topical prednisolone acetate q.i.d. and 1% topical cyclopentolate b.i.d. for two weeks. Additionally, as an oral steroid anti-inflammatory agent, methyl prednisolone was given with an initial dose of 1–2 mg/kg body weight on first day and gradually reduced over the following 6 days. Immunosuppressive therapy using cyclosporine A (3 mg/kg body weight) was started one day prior to transplantation surgery and was performed for six months. The serum level was adjusted to 80 to 120 ng per ml (monoclonal antibody test).

Postoperatively, the patients were examined daily during their hospital stay by indirect ophthalmoscopy. After discharge, follow-up examinations were performed at one, three, and six months. Examination included evaluation of visual acuity, applanation tonometry to measure intraocular pressure, slit-lamp microscopy, fundus evaluation using both indirect opthalmoscopy and three mirror funduscopy, fluorescein angiography and optical coherence tomography. Additionally, EOG, ERG and visual field testing were performed. All clinical testing was done by independent examiners.

Table 1. HLA-typing of donor and recipient: match on 1 (+) or 2 (+/+) alleles; mismatch on 1 (–) or 2 (–/–) alleles; 1 match / 1 mismatch on 2 alleles (+/–); empty field: recipient and/ or donor do not express the HLA gene locus

HLA-Locus	A	B	Cw	DRB1	DRB3	DRB4	DRB5	DQA1	DQB1	DPB1
Patient 1	+	+		+/+		+	+	+/+	+/+	+/–
Patient 2	+	+/–		+			+	+	+	+
Patient 3	+	+/–		+			+	+	–	+
Patient 4	–/–	–/–		+/+			+	+/+	+/+	+
Patient 5	+	+/–		+/+	+		+	+/+	+/–	+/–
Patient 6	–/–	–/–		+				+	+	+
Patient 7	+/+	+/+		+/–	+/–			+/+	+/–	+/–
Patient 8	+/–	+/–		+/–	–		+	+/+	+/–	+/–
Patient 9	+	–		+/–		+		–	+/+	–

Table 2. Characteristics of the transplanted RPE cells

Patient	Cell Number	Volume (µl)	Morphology of the cells prior to transplantation	Cell membrane integrity (%)
1	180.000	150	Elongated/epithelioid Few pigment granulae	99.5
2	123.000	150	Elongated/epithelioid Few pigment granulae	81.7
3	123.000	150	Elongated/epithelioid Few pigment granulae	81.7
4	123.250	100	Elongated/epithelioid Few pigment granulae	96.1
5	321.500	100	Elongated/epithelioid Few pigment granulae	93.0
6	39.500	100	Elongated/epithelioid Few pigment granulae	not determined
7	240.000	150	Elongated/epithelioid Few pigment granulae	88.0
8	149.250	90	Elongated/epithelioid Few pigment granulae	93.1
9	76.500	100	Epithelioid97.4 Few pigment granulae	

Results

RPE grafts

For RPE transplantation, HLA-matching donor cells were chosen from our RPE cell bank (Table 1). The average age of the donors used in this study was 56.6 ± 20.1 years, the average post mortem time before isolation of the cells was 40.9 ± 25.5 hours.

The determination of non-specific phagocytic activity in primary RPE cell cultures showed that only epithelioid cells take up carbon particles in high amounts whereas fibroblastoid cells display a drastically reduced uptake of carbon particles. Provided cell cultures partially retained their original pigmentation during expanding and displayed an epithelioid to fusiform morphology (Table 2).

Table 3. Patients' visual outcome

Patient	VA operated eye		Subjective assessment	VA fellow eye		Duration of visual deterioration	Progression
	Preop	6 months postop		Preop	6 months postop		
1	OS 20/200	20/200	+	20/100	20/125 ↓	18 months	fast
2	OD 20/40	20/40	=	20/32	20/50 ↓	6 months	slow
3	OS 20/400	20/125 ↑	+	20/20	20/20	3 months	fast
4	OS 20/400	20/400	=	20/200	20/200	6 months	slow
5	OS 20/400	20/200 ↑	++	20/80	10/400 ↓	6 years	slow
6	OS 20/200	20/100 ↑	=	20/400	20/400	4 years	slow
7	OD 20/125	20/400 ↓	–	20/32	20/32	5 years	slow
8	OS 20/32	20/125 ↓	– –	20/25	20/32 ↓	2 years	slow
9	OD 20/400	20/200 ↑	=	20/400	20/400	2 years	slow

Preoperative findings

The patients of this series consisted of one male and eight female individuals, aged 47 to 78 years at the time of operation. All patients had similar clinical conditions in both eyes. Therefore, the untreated contralateral eye served as control eye. Preoperatively, the visual acuity of the eyes assigned to transplantation was 20/400 to 20/125, one patient had a visual acuity of 20/32, another patient 20/40 (Table 3).

Postoperative findings

In all patients of this study the postoperative period was uneventful. During the follow-up, there were no signs of inflammation or infection in the vitreous or in the anterior chamber, and no leakage of fluorescein at the graft site indicating graft rejection. None of the patients developed retinal detachment, in none of the patients additional laser treatment was performed. In four patients cell clusters were visible on fundus examination which are supposed to be the grafted RPE cells. The pigmentation of these cell clusters did not change over time. We did not observe a disappearance of the grafted cells, but a fine granular pigmentation could be observed that may be a sign of continuous growth. Postoperative EOG, ERG and visual field testing revealed no significant change compared to preoperative findings. In one patient (patient 7) an edema was detected by fluorescein angiography and optical coherence tomography at three months which increased during the follow-up.

Six months postoperatively, vision had improved slightly in four of the treated eyes, remained stable in three eyes and decreased in two eyes (Table 3). In contrast, vision did not improve in five of the non-treated eyes and declined in four of these eyes.

Case reports

Patient 5

Preoperative characteristics of this 78-years-old man were geographic atrophy in both eyes, a visual acuity of 20/80 in the right eye and 20/400 in the left eye. Fluorescein angiography revealed geographic atrophy of the RPE with a partial loss of choriocapillaris.

RPE cells from a 44-years-old donor which had been cryopreserved for 790 days matched the HLA-type of the patient (Table 1). The assessment of the membrane integrity of the recultured cells by the trypan blue exclusion test revealed a vitality rate of 93%. Approximately 321.500 cells in 100 µl of cell suspension were injected into the submacular space of the left eye.

Three months after transplantation, a fine granulary hyperpigmentation was visible on fundus photography and on fluorescein photography which is supposed to represent the graft. At six months, the granular pigmentation in the macular area was increased. There was no leakage of dye from the graft area at any time and no sign of edema or new vessel formation in the host retina. The fundus picture remained unchanged on subsequent visits. ERG and visual evoked potential remained unchanged in both eyes during the follow-up period.

The visual acuity of the left eye improved from 20/400 to 20/200 whereas in the fellow eye the visual acuity deteriorated from 20/80 to 10/400 (Table 3).

Patient 7

A 68-years-old woman presented with geographic atrophy in both eyes. Her preoperative visual acuity in the right eye was 20/125, in the left eye 20/32. Fundus examination revealed focal areas of hypopigmentation, choriocapillaris loss and mineralisation. Drusen could be observed in the whole macular area.

RPE cells from a 63-years-old donor which had been cryopreserved for 291 days matched the HLA-type of the patient (Table 1). The assessment of the membrane integrity of the recultured cells by the trypan blue exclusion test revealed a vitality rate of 88%. Pars plana vitrectomy and subretinal transplantation of RPE cells was performed under local anaesthesia. 240.000 cells in 150 µl of cell suspension were injected into the subretinal space of the right eye.

After four weeks, slit-lamp microscopy showed hyperpigmented cell clusters within the atrophic area of the macula. On fluorescein angiography, there was no evidence of new vessel formation in the host retina and no leakage of the dye from the graft area. Visual acuity was unchanged.

Three months after transplantation, the visual acuity deteriorated slowly and a mild edema was visible in the macular area. At six months, fluorescein angiography revealed a hyperfluorescence in the macular area indicating an occult choroidal neovascularisation. The OCT confirmed an edema in the macular area. Visual acuity deteriorated to 20/400.

Discussion

This is the first study on transplantation of HLA-typed adult human RPE cells in ARMD patients suffering from geographic atrophy of the RPE. Throughout six months of follow-up, during which the patients were under immunosuppression, the procedure proved to be safe. None of the patients experienced graft rejection or any clinical signs of inflammation or infection. No severe side-effects or major intra- or postoperative complications, especially retinal tear formation, retinal detachment or proliferative vitreoretinopathy (PVR) which could be a result of the transplantation technique was noted. The fluorescein dye leakage in one of our patients seems to be due to a developing CNV. The origin of this remains unclear, but it can not be excluded that it was induced by a surgical injury of Bruch's membrane during the injection of RPE cells. However, CNV development is not uncommon in eyes with geographic atrophy [10, 11].

With regard to the visual outcome, RPE transplantation showed a limited success in 4 of 9 patients. In these patients visual acuity of the treated eyes slightly increased whereas the visual acuity of the fellow eyes remained stable or declined. Although we can not predict the long-term outcome, the preliminary results of this study are encouraging with regard to the aim of RPE transplantation to arrest or delay the progression of the retinal damage caused by RPE atrophy. We suppose that the precautions taken in this study to prevent graft rejection, the quality of cultured RPE cells and the surgical technique of their application in the subretinal space favour the outcome of RPE grafting.

Precautions taken to minimize the risk of immune rejection were the selection of ARMD patients with geographic atrophy, the use of HLA-matched RPE cells and a postoperative systemic immunosuppression. This is important because recent clinical trials and experimental studies in animal models have shown that the immune privilege of the subretinal space is not absolute and static [4, 5, 12, 13]. Algvere et al. [4] reported after transplanting a monolayer patch of human fetal RPE in five patients who underwent removal of subretinal fibrovascular membranes, the development of macular edema and fluorescein leakage concomitant with gradual reduction of visual acuity over 1 to 6 months. This may imply host-graft rejection which was supposed to be due to a breakdown of the blood-retina barrier after excision of a subfoveal neovascularization. In contrast, in patients with geographic atrophy, only one of four patch transplants was slowly rejected after 12 months. Human fetal RPE cell suspension transplants in four patients with non-exudative ARMD showed no evidence of rejection after a follow-up of 12 months [5]. The authors concluded that the intact blood-retina barrier in patients with non-exudative ARMD favours the successful outcome of transplantation. Our study in 9 patients with geographic atrophy supports this observation, but, nevertheless, we consider tissue typing and postoperative immunosuppression as necessary for transplantation of human adult RPE cells, because recent experiments in different animal models have shown that systemic immunity appears to exert a slow but significant influence in the subretinal space. Zhang and Bok [13] observed that subretinal RPE allografts in RCS rats underwent chronic rejection as evidenced by an increased loss of photoreceptors in immunologically challenged RCS rats. Grafts with disparity at major histocompatibility (MHC) class I and class II loci exhibited greater photoreceptor cell atrophy after donor spleen cell challenge than did grafts with disparity at MHC class II alone, although this effect was not as evident at longer transplant survival times. In contrast to the mouse studies of Jiang and coworkers [12], Zhang and Bok [13] did not observe a lymphocytic infiltration of the allogenic RPE grafts and suggested that this difference may be due to the fact that grafted mouse RPE was mis-matched at both, major and minor histocompatibility loci. They also showed that donor RPE cells which normally do not express MHC class II molecules, do so after transplantation into the subretinal space of RCS rats. After transplantation of human RPE cells into non-immunosuppressed monkeys, rejection was observed in 29% of the animals after 6 months [14]. These data suggest that inflammation or trauma induced by surgery could result in inflammatory cell infiltration near the graft and release of cytokines which could initiate graft rejection. Due to this risk it seems to be advisable, and the preliminary results of our study confirm this, to transplant only HLA-matched adult human RPE cells in patients suffering from geographic atrophy of the RPE and to give a postoperative immunosuppressive therapy. It remains unclear whether one of these factors or their combination contribute to the successful avoidance of immune rejection.

In this study, dispersed RPE cells were used for transplantation. The transplantation of RPE sheets requires a relatively large retinotomy and is therefore associated with an increased risk of RPE cell escape from the subretinal space into the vitreous and induction of proliferative vitreoretinopathy (PVR). In contrast to RPE sheets, cell suspensions can easily be injected into the subretinal space using an oil-hydraulic microinjection pump [9]. To support the settlement of the injected cells, we recommended the patients to stay in supine position for one hour after RPE transplantation. Subsequently, they had to stay in prone position for six days to ensure an effective tamponade of the retinotomy.

The quality and physiological features of cultured human RPE cells are regarded essential for the success of transplantation. In a previous study we have shown that under optimised cell culture conditions human RPE cell specific characteristics were maintained. Even after cryopreservation in a RPE bank, no loss of HLA expression was detectable in 12 of 14 cell strains studied. Moreover, patch-clamp experiments demonstrated that high-threshold L-type Ca^{2+} channels, which are typical for freshly isolated cells, could be detected in first passage and cryopreserved RPE cells [7]. Our results show that the optimisation and quality control of cell culture are important preconditions for successful cell transplantation.

The time of RPE transplantation surgery in patients with geographic atrophy of the RPE is an unsolved problem up to now. Our results do not justify to graft patients with good visual acuity. However, if visual acuity is to be restored, surgery must be contemplated at a stage of the disease when photoreceptor degeneration is not advanced and the damage may be still reversible. In the Royal College of Surgeons (RCS) rat, a model of inherited retinal dystrophy with functional defects of the RPE layer, it has been demonstrated that photoreceptor cells can be rescued when healthy RPE cells are transplanted into the subretinal space before an irreversible photoreceptor damage occurs [15–17]. In patients with geographic atrophy, it should be also considered a success when the further visual loss caused by RPE atrophy is prevented or delayed by RPE grafting before a substantial progression of irreversible photoreceptor damage occurs.

In summary, the preliminary results of this study are encouraging with regard to the aim of RPE transplantation to arrest or delay the progression of the damage to the retina caused by geographic atrophy of the RPE. Further research is required to determine the optimal cell number for transplantation and to develop methods for the identification of grafted RPE cells in the host retina. The evaluation of the long-term clinical outcome will offer the possibility to discuss the optimal time for RPE transplantation in the course of the disease.

References

1. Korte GE, Repucci V, Henkind P (1984) RPE destruction causes choriocapillary atrophy. Invest Ophthalmol Vis Sci 25:1135–45
2. Sarks SH (1976) Ageing and degeneration in the macular region: a clinico-pathological study. Br J Ophthalmol 60:324–41
3. Sarks SH (1980) Drusen and their relationship to senile macular degeneration. Aust J Ophthalmol 8:171–8
4. Algvere PV, Berglin L, Gouras P, Sheng Y (1994) Transplantation of fetal retinal pigment epithelium in age-related macular degeneration with subfoveal neovascularization. Graefe's Arch Clin Exp Ophthalmol 232:707–16
5. Algvere PV, Berglin L, Gouras P, Sheng Y, Kopp ED (1997) Transplantation of RPE in age-related macular degeneration: observations in disciform lesions and dry RPE atrophy. Graefe's Arch Clin Exp Ophthalmol 235:149–58

6. Valtink M, Engelmann K, Krüger R, Schellhorn ML, Löliger C, Püschel K, Richard G (1999) Aufbau einer Zellbank für die Transplantation von HLA-typisierten, kryokonservierten humanen adulten retinalen Pigmentepithelzellen. Ophthalmologe 96:648–52

7. Valtink M, Engelmann K, Strauß O, Krüger R, Löliger C, Sobottka-Ventura AC, Richard G (1999) Physiological features of primary cultures and subcultures of human retinal epithelial cells prior to and following cryopreservation for cell transplantation. Graefe's Arch Clin Exp Ophthalmol 237:1001–6

8. Ehrlich H, Bugawan T, Begovich AB, Scharf S, Griffith R (1991) HLA-DR, DQ and DP typing using PCR amplification and immobilized probes. Eur J Immunogen 18:33–55

9. Weichel J, Valtink M, Richard G, Engelmann K (1999) Optimization of a surgical approach for transplanting adult human retinal pigment epithelial cells into the subretinal space of RCS rats. Invest Ophthalmol Vis Sci 40[Suppl]:727

10. Macular Photocoagulation Study Group (1993) Five-years follow-up of fellow eyes of patients with age-related macular degneration and unilateral extrafoveal choroidal neovascularization. Arch Ophthalmol 111:1189–99

11. Algvere PV, Gouras P, Dafgard-Kopp E (1999) Long-term outcome of RPE allografts in non-immunosuppressed patients with AMD. Eur J Ophthalmol 9:217–30

12. Jiang L, Jorquera M, Streilein J (1994) Immunologic consequences of intraocular implantation of RPE allografts. Exp Eye Res 58:719–28

13. Zhang X, Bok D (1998) Transplantation of retinal pigment epithelial cells and immune response in the subretinal space. Invest Ophthalmol Vis Sci 39:1021–102

14. Gouras P, Algvere P (1996) Retinal cell transplantation in the macula: new techniques. Vision Res 36:4121–5

15. Li L, Turner JE (1988) Inherited retinal dystrophy in the RCS rat: prevention of photoreceptor degeneration by pigment epithelial cell transplantation. Exp Eye Res 47:911–17

16. Li L, Turner JE (1991) Optimal conditions for long term photoreceptor rescue in RCS rats: the necessity for healthy RPE transplants. Exp Eye Res 52:669–79

17. Lopez R, Gouras P, Kjeldbye H, Sullivan B, Reppucci V, Brittis M, Wapner F, Goluboff E (1989) Transplanted retinal pigment epithelium modifies the retinal degeneration in the RCS rat. Invest Ophthalmol Vis Sci 30:586–8

Correspondence: Prof. Dr. med. Gisbert Richard, Universitäts-Augenklinik Hamburg, Martinistrasse 52, D-20246 Hamburg, E-mail: richard@uke.uni-hamburg.de

Transplantation of autologous retinal pigment epithelium in eyes with neovascular age-related macular degeneration

S. Binder[1], I. Krebs[1], U. Stolba[1], A. Abri[1], H. Feichtinger[2],
R.-D. Hilgers[3], L. Kellner[1], C. Jahn[1], A. Assadoullina[1], and B. Stanzel[1]

[1] The Ludwig Boltzmann Institute for Retinology and Biomicroscopic Lasersurgery,
[2] Institute of Pathology and Bacteriology (Chairman: Prim. Hans Feichtinger M.D.)
Rudolf Foundation Clinic, Vienna, Austria
[3] Institute for Biometrie (Chairman: Prof. Ralf-Dieter Hilgers MS) Rheinisch-Westfälische
Technische Hochschule, Aachen, Germany

Introduction

Because of the higher life expectancy in the industrial world and increasing demands on life quality age related macular degeneration (AMD) has become one of the most important diseases in ophthalmologic research. While about 85% of patients are diagnosed with the "dry" atrophic form of AMD, 15% suffer from the "wet" form, which is responsible for the highest percentage of visual loss in these patients and mainly characterised by the development of choroidal neovascularisation [1]. Treatment modalities usually used f.e. laser photocoagulation, photodynamic therapy (PDT), or transpupillary therapy (TTT) are vasodestructive methods and have therefore a very limited potential to improve the retinal situation [2, 3, 4]. These methods also do not allow any visionary aspect for the treatment of the large group of patients with dry AMD.

The best proof of principle that foveal function can be regained on an extrafoveal pigment epithelium has been given by Machemer and de Juan with the retinal retinal rotation [5, 6]. In contrast to this currently with rather high intra- and postoperative complications loaded method [7] represents the procedure of retinal transplantation a relatively simple procedure, less likely for severe complications.

Transplantation in human eyes

The transplantation of RPE seemed to be a logical approach in restoring vision in patients with AMD. A full thickness rotation flap was transplanted by Peyman et al. in 1991 [8] for retinal pigment epithelial transplantation in two cases with terminal AMD. One flap was autologous in the second case also homologous material was used. In one eye improvement of vision was reported over several months, but also encapsulation of the transplants.

Along with the improvement of subretinal surgical techniques and instrumentation [9], a less traumatic approach for subretinal transplantation of cell suspensions or sheets could be used thereafter.

The disappointing visual results after membrane excision alone reported were explained by the mechanical removal of the RPE together with the membrane as well as the primary dysfunction of the RPE in these cases [10].

To compensate for the deficit 5 patients received a patch of previously cultured human fetal RPE placed in the foveal area after membrane excision. After 3 months four of the five lost fixation, a macular edema developed and fluorescein leakage was present sug-

gesting rejection. After 1 year most of the patients had experienced mild visual loss compared to their preoperative vision [11]. Then 4 eyes with atrophic "dry" macular degeneration received circular patches 0.6 mm in diameter again by Algvere's group. This time
the transplants were placed in non foveal areas. After 1 year, it was shown that the transplants had not disturbed visual function, there was some evidence of growth but no visual
improvement. A milder rejection was observed in these eyes and this was related to the
more intact blood-retinal barrier in "dry" AMD eyes [12]. Finally, to cover a larger area
including the fovea, a cell suspension of concentrated dissociated fetal human RPE has
been used in 7 subsequent cases of advanced but "dry" AMD. When 50 000 cells were
used, rejection was observed after 8–12 months, with 500 000 cells this event occurred
after 3 months. Eyes which received 20 000 and 200 cells respectively did nor show rejection at one year, but also no visual improvement [13].

Immunological aspects

Although the eye as a part of the central nervous system possesses the characteristics of
an immunologically privileged site, it was demonstrated, that RPE-transplants sensitised
their recipients to both alloantigens and RPE-specific autoantigens. Both can be considered potential barriers to successful transplantation and would make immune suppres-
sion regimens necessary. It was also demonstrated that the immunologic response is most
likely related to the amount of cells and increases with time [14].

Autologous transplantation

To overcome the immune reaction the search for autologous material became important.
Iris pigment epithelium cells, either fresh or cultured, have been used by groups in
Germany and Japan [15, 16]. Prevention of further loss of vision but also some improvement has been reported by Thumann et al. in eyes with different neovascular diseases
[17].

Full thickness RPE-transplants taken from adjacent areas of the CNV showed seques-
tration after a longer observation period [18], although some remaining functions were
demonstrated on micro perimetry [19]. Questions of basal lamina reconstruction, possible restoration of Bruch's membrane, proliferation of cells, and cell-interaction as well as
cell amounts necessary were nor answered so far.

Our approach

We felt, that the use of autologous RPE would offer a greater chance for restoring more
normal subretinal conditions and for gaining some visual function in patients with AMD
[20].

A cell suspension of freshly harvested RPE from an area not involved in the disease,
as the nasal retina is, and which allows also easy access and full control of the surgical
area was chosen.

In a *pilot study* [21] 14 eyes underwent subretinal surgery because of foveal CNV
with simultaneous transplantation of RPE harvested from the nasal subretinal area of
the same eye at the same time. Cell vitality was between 80–90% with Trypan blue
staining.

The harvesting efficacy, applied in a series of cadaver eyes [22] and systematically
evaluated showed that a reproducible cell amount between 11 000 to 29 000 (19 976 +−
6016) could be harvested from an area between 2–4 disc diameters with our technique.

Cell viability was high (82.0 +− 6.9%).

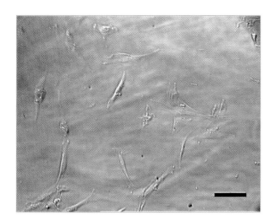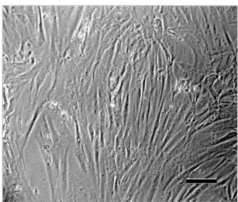

Fig. 1. Confluent monolayer of human RPE on plastic with a low CA++ DMEM medium, evaluation of the minimum cell number left: 24 h after plateling, right; confluence, spindle cell morphology due to proliferation directed culture medium

The minimal plateling density required for confluency was also evaluated. For adult human RPE using a CA++ adjusted DMEM/f12 amounts between 1400 and 2000 cells are needed to establish a confluent monolayer [23] (Fig. 1).

To answer the question about RPE conditions in the area of the membrane and its surrounding area, *RPE-cultures on excised subretinal membranes* were performed. In culture medium (DMEM+ 20% autologous Serum) the exised membranes showed growth of RPE in mono- and multi layers in 80% of the cases, they remained their epithelial characteristics for at least 4 months [24].

In an ongoing *prospective clinical trial* 48 eyes with NV AMD underwent surgery so far [25]. PDT was offered as an alternative treatment option for predominately classic fCNV. Briefly, patients with mainly very large predominately occult fCNV were candidates for surgery. Eyes were transplantation of RPE was not possible serves as controls. Cell viability was controlled with the Live-Death cell Viability Kit and showed between 70–80% viability (Fig. 2).

Visual outcome after 12 months follow – up showed in the transplantation group (n = 41) improvement two or more lines in 53% [22], remained the same +– one line in 34% [14] and showed visual loss of two or more lines in 12% [5] (Fig. 3).

In the control group (n = 7) were only membrane excision was performed 43% [3] had the same visual acuity before and after surgery 2 (28.5%) improved, 2 lost vision (Fig. 4).

While statistical significant improvement was demonstrable in the transplanted cases, no significance was observed in the controls. Complications observed were not higher than after vitrectomy with subretinal surgery alone, a retinal detachment occurred in 4 eyes (8.3%), and was treatable with a second vitrectomy in all eyes. Complications influencing the final visual outcome were observed in two eyes (4%), one developed a choroidal haemorrhage 48 hours after surgery and underwent a second vitrectomy with silicone tamponade and one developed a macular hole 3 months after surgery which was documented with OCT.

With fluorescein – and indocyanine green angiography we could show that the number of recurrent CNV with 3,2% (2/62) was extremely low in our two case series 14 + 48.

While most of the patients had no reading vision preoperatively (Jaeger 17) and most of them gained some improvement postoperatively (Jaeger 12–15) only 5 cases (8,6%)

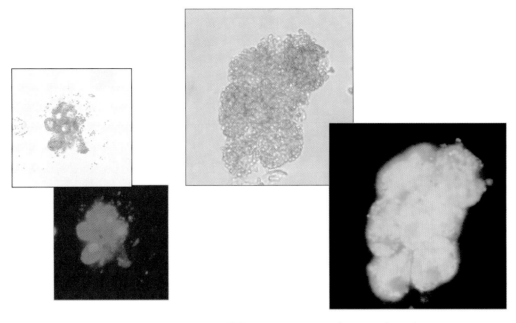

Fig. 2. RPE from Biopsie a 70–80% RPE viability was present in the transplanted suspension (Live-Dead Cell Viability Kit, red = dead cells, green = viable cells)

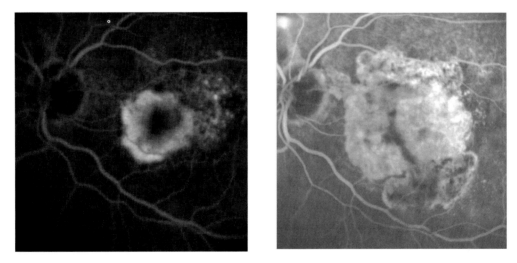

Fig. 3. Pre- and postoperative (12 months) fluorescein angiogramm of a patient with membrane removal alone (Control). VA 1/60 pre and postoperatively, the area of PE-atrophy has increased considerably

of the whole transplantation group gained useful reading vision between Jaeger I and IV.

Discussion and conclusions

In 85% of all AMD patients they suffer of the "dry" form of this disease [1]. Active therapies against this disease concentrated so far on the "wet" neovascular form [2, 3, 4].

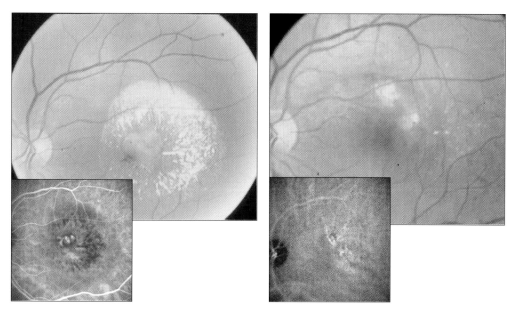

Fig. 4. Pre- and postoperative (12 months) photograph and late phase angiogramm (Insert) of a patient after membrane excision and RPE-transplantation. VA preop: 0.22 Jg 14, postop 1.22 Jg 1

The disadvantage of vasodestructive therapies however is that incidences of recurrences between 30–50% are reported [26]. In addition the moderate loss of vision after treatment is compared to severe visual loss in the natural course of the disease [3, 4]. Its seems better, that visual improvement is taken as the mayor criteria for successful treatment.

Treatments which try to achieve a more physiologic restitution of the retinal – subretinal foveal are retinal rotation and retinal transplantation. Along with reduction of complications and successfully used in "wet" exudative AMD both treatments can be potential treatment options also for "dry" AMD in the near future.

Our preliminary results indicate, that moderate visual improvement is possible with the help of autologous transplantation in more than half of the cases. These results are better when compared with the literature and our own control group with subretinal membraqne excision alone [27]. However, useful reading acuity – defined as reading acuity of a newspaper with normal reading glasses – was only observed in a small group of patients. The membrane size of this group was in general smaller (3000–4000 µm) than the overall medium size (6000 µm).

Although the comparison with the control group looks favourable so far, this number is too small to draw a final conclusion from this.

The low recurrence rate is also an interesting observation, because usually the first success after all other treatment modalities are lost again if a recurrent membrane grows. The effect of RPE on the inhibition of neovascularisation has been shown experimentally [28, 29].

The advantage of autologous RPE-transplantation, which are superior in the degradation of photoreceptor outer segment to IPE [30] freshly harvested cells is also faced with some disadvantages. First, the number of cells which can be transplanted is limited and aged cells are transplanted on a – at least partially – defect Bruch's membrane. Cell adhesion and survival are questions, we have to answer experimentally because of the lack of harmless markers in human eyes. However, in an experimental study Phillips and co-workers [31] could clearly demonstrate that RPE transplanted on debrided Bruch's membrane do in fact maintain photoreceptor and choriocapillaris structures when compared to abrasive areas alone and Tsukasha and co-workers have shown that uncultered RPE can attach to aged Bruch's membrane explants to a certain degree.

Summary

Although some favourable results have been observed in our experimental and clinical work and some questions answered, other questions and problems have to be addressed.

Better selection of cases with smaller defects can be one solution. The most challenging projects are probably the further improvement of transplantation techniques and the condition of the RPE cells to stimulate their growth and proliferation without changing their phenotype and the creation of an uniform layer of autologous RPE to improve the restoration of the Bruch's membrane defect.

References

1. Leibowitz HM, et al (1980) The Framingham Eye Study Monograph. Surv Ophthalmol 24[Suppl]:335–610
2. Macular Photocoagulation Study Group (1991) Argon laser photocoagulation for neovascular maculopathy: five year results from randomised clinical trial. Arch Ophthalmol 109:1109–14
3. Bressler NM (1998) Treatment of age related macular degeneration with Photodynamic Therapy (TAP) using verteporfin (BPD MA): Baseline characteristics and safety. Invest Opthalmol Vis Sci 39(4):242
4. Reichel E, Benocal AM, Ip M, et al (1999) Transpupillary thermotherapy of occult subfoveal choroidal neovascularization in patients with age-related macular degeneration. Ophthalmology 106:1908–14
5. Machemer R, Steinhorst R (1993) Retinal separation, retinotomy and macular relocation, a surgical approach for age related macular degeneration. Graefes Arch Clin Exp Opthalmol 231:635–41
6. de Juan E, Löwenstein A, Bressler N, et al (1998) Translocation of the retina for management of subretinal neovascularisation. Am J Ophthalmol 125:635–46
7. Eckardt C, Eckart U, Conrad HC (1999) Macular rotation with and without counter rotation of the globe in patients with age related macular degeneration. Graefes Arch Clin Exp Ophthalmol 237:313–25
8. Peyman GA, Blinder KJ, Paris KJ, et al (1991) A technique for retinal pigment epithelial transplantation for age related macular degeneration secondary to extensive subfoveal scarring. Ophthalmol Surg, pp 102–8
9. Thomas MA, Kaplan HJ (1991) Surgical removal of subfoveal neovascularisation in the presumed ocular histoplasmosis syndrome. Am J Ophthalmol 111:1–7
10. Thomas M, Dickinson J, Melberg N, et al (1996) Visual results after surgical removal of subfoveal choroidal neovascular membranes. Ophthalmology 101:1384–96
11. Algvere PV, Berglin L, Gouras P, et al (1994) Transplantation of fetal retinal pigment epithelium in age-related macular degeneration with subfoveal neovascularisation. Graefes Arch Clin Exp Ophthalmol 232:707–16
12. Algvere PV, Berglin L, Gouras P, et al (1997) Transplantation of RPE in age related macular degeneration; observations in disciform lesions and dry atrophy. Graefes Arch Clin Exp Opthalmol, pp 149–58
13. Algvere PV, Dafgard Kopp EME, Gouras P (1999) Long-term outcome of RPE allografts in non-immuno suppressed patients with AMD. Eur J Ophthalmol 9:217–30
14. Grisanti S, Misaki I, Kosiewitcz M, et al (1997) Immunity and immune privilege elicited by cultured retinal pigment epithelial cell transplants. Invest Opthalmol Vis Sci 38:1619–26
15. Thumann G, Heimann K, Schraemeyer U (1997) Quantitative Phagocytosis of rod outer segments by human nd poecine epithelial cells in vitro. Invest Ophthalmol Vis Sci 38(4):330
16. Tamai M, Abe T, Tomita, et al (1999) Autologous iris pigment transplantation in ager related macular degeneration. In: Das T (ed) Retina. Current practice and future trends. Hyderabad, India: Paras publishing, pp 151–61

17. Thumann G, Aisenbrey S, Schraemeyer U, et al (2000) Transplantation of autologous iris pigment epithelium after removal of choroidal neovascular membranes. Arch Ophthalmol 118(10):1350–5

18. Awylard GW, Kychenthal A, Stanga PE, et al (1999) RPE-transplantation a new surgical technique for treatment of choroidal NV in AMD. 12th Annual meeting of the Retina Society, Regensburg, Germany

19. Stanga PE, Kychenthal A, Fitzke F, et al (2002) Retinal pigment epithelium translocation after choroidal neovascular membrane removal in age-related macular degeneration. Ophthalmology 109:1492–8

20. Binder S, Stolba U, Krebs I, et al (2000) Zur Transplantation autologer Pigmentepithelzellen. Spektrum Augenheilkd 14/5:249–53

21. Binder S, Stolba U, Krebs I, et al (2002) Transplantation of autologous retinal pigment epithelium in eyes with foveal neovascularisation resulting from age-related macular degeneration: a pilot study. Am J Ophthalmol 133(2):215–25

22. Assadoulina A, Binder S, Stanzel B, et al (2003) Harvesting efficiancy and viability of rretinal pigment epithelial cells in aspirates from posterior retinal areas – a study on human eyes. Experimental Eye Research (submitted)

23. Stanzel BV, Huemer KH, Ahnelt PK, Feichtinger H, Binder S (2002) Minimal plateling density required for confluency of adult human RPE cells using a CA++ adjusted DMEM/F12 culture medium. Invest Ophthalmol Vis Sci 43(4):3437 (P 321)

24. Jahn Ch, Krugluger W, Binder S, Feichtinger H (2003) RPE-culture on exised subretinal membranes. Graefes Arch Clin Exp (submitted)

25. Binder S, Krebs I, Abri A, et al (2003) Outcome after transplantation of autologous retinal pigmentepithelium cells in age-related macular degeneration: a prospective study. Invest Ophthalmol Vis Sci (submitted)

26. Macular Photocoagulation Study Group (1994) Persistent and recurrent neovascularisation after laser photocoagulation of age-related macular degeneration. Arch Ophthalmol 112:489–99

27. Omerod ID, Puklin JE, Frank RE (1994) Long-term outcomes after surgical removal of advanced subfoveal neovascular membranes in age-related macular degeneration. Ophthalmology 101:1201–10

28. Seaton AD, Turner JE (1992) RPE transplants stabilize retinal vasculature and prevent neovascularisation in the RCS rat. Invest Opthalmol Vis Sci 33:83–9

29. Seaton AD, Sheedlo HJ, Turner JE (1994) A primary role for RPE transplants in the inhibition and regression of neovascularisation in the RCS rat. Invest Ophthalmol Vis Sci 35:162–9

30. Dintelmann T, Heimann K, Kayatz P, et al (1999) Comparative study of ROS degradation by IPE and RPE cells in vitro. Graefes Arch Clin Exp Ophthalmol 237:830–9

31. Philips SSS, Liu H, Tso M, Binder S (2003) Autologous transplantation of retinal pigment epithelium after mechanical debridement of Bruch's membrane. Exp Eye Research (in press)

32. Tsukasha I, Ninomiya S, Castellarin A, Yagi F, Sugino I, Zarbin M (2002) Early attachment of uncultured retinal pigment epithelium from aged donors onto Bruch's membrane explants. Exp Eye Research 74(2):255–66

Correspondence: Susanne Binder M.D., Professor and Chairman, Department of Ophthalmology, The Ludwig Boltzmann Institute for Retinology and Biomicroscopic Lasersurgery, Rudolf Foundation Clinic, Juchgasse 25, A-1030 Vienna, Austria, E-mail: susanne.binder@kar.magwien.gv.at

Retrospective analysis of subretinal surgery

C.I. Falkner[1], S. Binder[2], and H. Leitich[3]

[1,2] The Ludwig Boltzmann Institute of Retinology and Biomicroscopic Lasersurgery,
Department of Ophthalmology, Rudolf Foundation Clinic, Vienna, Austria
[3] Department of Obstetrics and Gynecology, University of Vienna, Vienna, Austria

Abstract

Background: Age-related macular degeneration (AMD) is the leading cause of legal blindness in people 50 years of age or older in the developed world. The treatment of AMD is still controversial and the search for a standard therapy for all forms of choroidal neovascularization (CNV) is on-going. Few randomized clinical trials are available regarding the surgical treatment of AMD. We performed a systematic review to determine the effectiveness of subretinal surgery for AMD and to summarize the reported results.

Methods: A MEDLINE search for the years 1992–2001 was conducted. Only original English- or German-language studies evaluating surgical interventions in AMD were assigned to one of four groups of surgical treatments. The main outcomes were improvement or deterioration of visual acuity (VA) after surgery.

Results: Sixty one studies met the inclusion criteria. The surgical procedures performed were removal of subfoveal choroidal neovascularization (CNV) (43%), macular translocation (25%), transplantation of pigment epithelium (10%) and removal of subretinal hemorrhage (23%). Thirty eight percent (range 0–87%) of all cases showed an improvement of VA and 26% (range 0–90%) a deterioration.

Conclusion: Compared to the natural course of AMD, subretinal surgery appears to be a promising method for the treatment of AMD. More randomized clinical studies are needed to draw unbiased conclusions and to allow for standard recommendations.

Introduction

Age-related macular degeneration (AMD) is the leading cause of legal blindness in people 50 years of age or older in the developed world [1]. The neovascular form of AMD occurs in approximately 20% of AMD patients, but is responsible for 90% of cases of severe irreversible central vision loss in patients with AMD [2, 3].

The treatment of AMD is still controversial and the search for a standard therapy for all forms of choroidal neovascularization (CNV) is on-going. Laser photocoagulation and photodynamic therapy (PDT) represent two therapeutic options for the management of neovascular AMD that have been proven effective in large-scale randomized clinical trials. Few randomized studies are available regarding the surgical treatment of AMD, including removal of subfoveal CNV, macular translocation, transplantation of pigment epithelium and removal of subretinal hemorrhage. The results of the randomized Submacular Surgery Trials (SST) have not yet been published [4].

We performed a systematic review to determine the effectiveness of subretinal surgery for AMD. The purpose of this assessment was to answer whether subretinal surgery is able to stabilize or reverse visual loss from AMD and which surgical intervention is most effective. Additionally, the results of the systematic review were compared to the natural course of AMD.

Material and methods

A literature search that was conducted in December 2001 consisted of a text word search in MEDLINE for the years 1992–2001. The year 1992 was chosen because Thomas et al. introduced the removal of subretinal membranes in patients with AMD in that year [5]. The terms AMD, (sub)macular, -retinal, -foveal, surgery, choroidal neovascularization, membrane removal, translocation, retinal or iris pigment epithelium, transplantation, hemorrhage and key word combinations were used. Eligibility criteria confined the analysis to original English- or German-language studies including surgical treatment and the diagnoses of AMD, a detailed visual outcome, including at least five cases and with a minimum follow-up of at least one week. Case reports, book articles, abstracts, nonclinical studies as well as "repeated" publications of the same case series were excluded. The references lists of those articles were consulted for additional citations.

A computer database was created as a fill-in-form to record all values. Two of the studies included were randomized clinical trials [4, 6], 9 prospective cohort studies [7–15] and 15 retrospective cohort studies [16–30]. Fifteen reports reviewed the results of large case series (n ≥ 31), 21 studies reported medium case series (11 ≤ n ≤ 30) and 25 studies small case series (n ≤ 10).

The variables year of publication, preoperative and final number of cases, total numbers and percentages with preoperative and final visual acuity (VA) of 20/200 or better, improvement and deterioration of VA, recurrence and complication rates as well as the minimum and maximum follow-up time (months) were extracted from each study. In addition, the studies included were assigned to one of four groups of surgical treatment. For each therapy group a descriptive statistical analysis was performed. To evaluate the functional outcome more precisely, an odds ratio (OR) was calculated for each included study. The OR compared the number of cases with a preoperative VA of 20/200 or better to the number of cases with a final VA of 20/200 or better. An OR ≤ 1 means that more cases achieved a VA of 20/200 or better after the operation and an OR ≥ 1 means that more cases had a VA of 20/200 or better before the surgical intervention. In 47 studies an improvement or deterioration of VA was defined as a change of 2 or more Snellen lines and in 2 studies as a change of 1 or more lines. The other studies did not contain any data referring to this.

Results

Sixty-one studies met the inclusion criteria and a total of 1273 cases was analyzed. The surgical procedures performed were removal of subfoveal CNV in 43% (26 studies), macular translocation in 25% (15 studies), pigment epithelium transplantation in 10% (6 studies) and removal of subretinal hemorrhage in 23% (14 studies). The median number of cases was 13 (range 5–102 cases), the median of the minimum follow-up time was 3 months (range 0,25–24 months) and the median of the maximum follow-up time was 18 months (range 2–73 months). Complications occurred in 55% of the cases (range 0–100%, missing in 7 studies). Thirty eight percent (range 0–87%) of all cases showed an improvement of VA after surgery and 26% (range 0–90%) a deterioration. A preoperative VA of

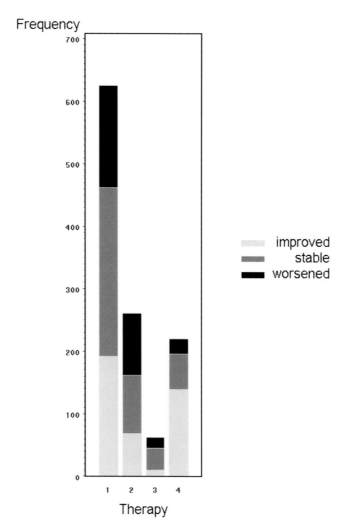

Frequency

Therapy

Fig. 1. Frequency of improved, stabilized and worsened cases for the 4 treatment groups (1 = removal of subretinal CNV, 2 = macular translocation, 3 = transplantation, 4 = removal of subretinal hemorrhage)

20/200 or better was seen in 37% (range 0–90%, missing in 3 studies), whereas a final VA of 20/200 or better was found in 42% (range 0–88%, missing in 3 studies).

The frequencies of improvement and deterioration of VA for the different treatment groups are shown in Fig. 1. A total of 647 cases after removal of subfoveal CNV [4–8, 16–23, 31–43] was analyzed. A preoperative VA of 20/200 or better was found with an overall crude rate of 29% (range of the individual study rates: 0–71%) and a final VA of 20/200 or better in 33% (range 0–80%) of these cases. Complications occurred in 48% (range 12–100%) and a recurrence of CNV was described in 25% (range 0–55%). At the last follow-up visit VA increased in 31% (range 0–80%) and decreased in 26% (range 0–60%) of a total of 625 cases (Table 1).

Three hundred thirty two cases after macular translocation [9–13, 24–27, 44–49] were included. A VA of 20/200 or better was described in 72% (range 30–90%) before the operation and in 60% (range 5–88%) after the operation. Complications were seen in 80% (range 50–100%) and a recurrence of CNV in 15% (0–43%). At the final

Table 1

Center	n	Follow up	VA ↑	VA ↓	Recurrence	OR
Abe T 2001	47	2–73	47%	19%		0,2 s
Berger AS 1992	19	0,25–10	21%	26%	16%	3,4
Bottoni F 1996	34	5–19	21%	26%	18%	0,1
Brindeau C 2001	8	4–48	0%	50%	13%	4,2
Corey RP 2001	10	6–26	20%	30%	30%	1,0
Eckardt C 1996	56	5–20	29%	18%	9%	0,9
Ehrt O 1999	23	1,5–2	57%	9%		0,5
Gandorfer A 1998	8	2–13,75	63%	13%	19%	0,3
Hudson HL 1995	6	6–14	67%	0%		1,0
Lewis H 1997	80	12	9%	38%	19%	4,7 s
Löwenstein A 1998	7	6	0%	43%		6,3
Merrill PT 1999	64	3–45	30%	28%	22%	1,3
Mietz H 1997	6	14–24	50%	50%	33%	0,5
Müller S 2000	5	3–24	60%	0%	40%	0,1
Nasir MA 1997	12	3–21	25%	33%		1,0
Ormerod LD 1994	10	14–28	80%	10%	40%	0,2
Park KH 1999	15	2–47	47%	33%		
Roth DB 1997	38	3–68	21%	29%	18%	1,7
Scheider A 1999	35	1,2–6	32%	16%	23%	0,4
SST-Pilot 2000	34	1–24	14%	50%	55%	2,9 s
Strmen P 1996	5	24–36	0%	60%	20%	1,0
Thach AB 1996	12	2–14	33%	42%		1,5
Thomas MA 1992	7	3–8	14%	14%	43%	0,5
Thomas MA 1994	41	2–39	12%	15%	27%	1,2
Tsujikawa M 1999	13	12–30	54%	23%	15%	0,5
Yuzawa M 2001	52	12	65%	19%	8%	0,4 s

Removal of subretinal CNV (n = number of cases; follow up = minimum and maximum follow up, months; VA ↑ = improvement of visual acuity; VA ↓ = deterioration of visual acuity; OR = odds ratio)

examination 26% (range 0–73%) of 261 cases showed an improved VA and 38% (range 0–90%) a worsened VA (Table 2).

In 63 cases transplantation of pigment epithelium [14, 50–54] was performed. A VA of 20/200 or better was seen in 45% (range 0–80%) before and 45% (range 20–67%) after the surgical procedure. The complication rate was 59% (range 29–100%) and the recurrence rate was 4% (range 0–8%). An improvement of VA was seen in 16% (range 0–86%) and a deterioration in 29% (range 0–75%) out of 63 cases (Table 3).

The results of removal of subretinal hemorrhage [8, 15, 28–30, 55–63] were evaluated in 231 cases. Fourteen percent (range 0–38%) had a preoperative VA of 20/200 or better, whereas 41% (range 11–79%) achieved this VA at the last follow-up examination. Complications were described in 42% (range 0–100%) and a recurrence of CNV occurred in 10% (range 0–25%). At the last follow-up visit VA increased in 63% (range 21–87%) and decreased in 11% (range 0–38%) of 220 cases (Table 4).

Additionally, the meta-analysis was compared to the natural course of AMD [64] and the results are shown in Table 5.

Discussion

This systematic review evaluated 61 studies comprising a total of 1273 cases, and the results allow to draw the following conclusions: In therapy group 4, the removal of

Table 2

Center	n	Follow up	VA ↑	VA ↓	Recurrence	OR
Akduman L 1999	20	2–12	5%	90%		35,3 s
Benner JD 2001	5	13–16	20%	20%		2,7
Buffenn AN 2001	11	0,33–21	73%	18%		1,0
Deramo VA 2001	9	2,75–17,5	22%	56%	33%	0,6
Eckardt C 1999	30	3–18	13%	7%	10%	1,3
Freedman SF 2000	15	1,5	0%	53%		
Glacet-Bernard A 2001	23	6–14	30%	52%	43%	1,0
Kim T 2001	8	1–17	13%	0%		1,0
Lewis H 1999	10	6	40%	60%	0%	2,3
Lewis H 2001	25	6	44%	40%	0%	1,2
Ohji M 1998	7	4–48	14%	57%		8,0
Ohji M 2001	51	6	18%	35%	21%	2,2
Pieramici DJ 2000	102	6	48%	19%		1,3
Wolf S 1999	7	6–16	29%	43%	0%	1,0
Wong D 2000	9	2,5–6	22%	44%	11%	6,4

Macular Translocation (n = number of cases; follow up = minimum and maximum follow up, months; VA ↑ = improvement of visual acuity; VA ↓ = deterioration of visual acuity; OR = odds ratio)

Table 3

Center	n	Follow up	VA ↑	VA ↓	Recurrence	OR
Abe T 2000	7	6–13	86%	0%		0,1
Algvere PV 1994	5	3	0%	60%		16,0
Algvere PV 1999	16	24–38	0%	75%		
Lappas A 2000	12	6	0%	8%	8%	1,0
Stanga PE 2001	6	1–10,5	0%	17%	0%	1,0
Thumann G 2000	17	6–11	24%	6%		0,5

Transplantation of pigment epithelium (n = number of cases; follow up = minimum and maximum follow up, months; VA ↑ = improvement of visual acuity; VA ↓ = deterioration of visual acuity; OR = odds ratio)

Table 4

Center	n	Follow up	VA ↑	VA ↓	Recurrence	OR
Chaudry NA 1999	5	3–24	80%	0%	20%	0,6
Claaes C 1996	15	5–31	87%	7%	0%	0,1
Haupert CL 2001	11	1–15	73%	18%	27%	0,5
Heiden-kummer HP 1995	8	2–48	75%	0%		0,9
Hesse L 1997	8	2–21	50%	13%		0,4
Ibanez HE 1995	39	0,25–19,75	21%	23%	5%	1,0
Kamei M 1995	22	7–31	82%	5%	18%	0,1 s
Krasnov MM 1992	32	6–32	81%		9%	0,0 s
Lambert HM 1992	10	6–10	70%	10%	0%	1,0
Lewis H 1994	24	6–30	83%	4%		0,0 s
Lim JI 1995	16	2–24	25%	38%	6%	1,4
Mandelcorn MS 1993	7	5–19	71%	0%	14%	0,1
Moriarty AP 1995	14	3–18	86%	7%	36%	0,0 s
Scheider A 1999	20	1,2–6	44%	11%	25%	2

Removal of subretinal hemorrhage (n = number of cases; follow up = minimum and maximum follow up, months; VA ↑ = improvement of visual acuity; VA ↓ = deterioration of visual acuity; OR = odds ratio)

Table 5

Therapy		VA ↑	VA ↓	Recurrence rate
Natural	≥1	7,2%	81,9%	65%
course	≥3	3,6%	68,6%	
Systematic review	≥2	37,7	26,5	15%

Comparison of the results of subretinal surgery to the natural course of AMD [64], with respect to the increase or decrease of visual activity (VA ↑, VA ↓)

subretinal hemorrhage [8, 15, 28–30, 55–63], the best visual outcome was achieved. The calculated estimates were 63% for improved vision and 10% for vision loss. This is not surprising as the preoperative VA was reduced to hand motions and counting fingers in most cases [15, 55–57, 60, 62, 63].

The rates of visual improvement after removal of subfoveal CNV [4–8, 16–23, 31–43] and macular translocation [9–13, 24–27, 44–49] were similar, whereas the rate of deterioration of VA was slightly lower in treatment group 1. The removal of subretinal CNV, however, included the largest number of studies (63% of all included studies), analyzed the largest case series (almost 43% of all cases) and showed a minimal mean variation. Consequently the functional outcome after this surgical procedure seems to be the most plausible.

Only six studies for the years 1994 to 2001 reporting the results of transplantation have been published so far [14, 50–54]. The development and research of this technique is still at the beginning, so the analyzed functional results are not quite convincing.

Large variations regarding the increase and decrease of visual outcome were observed between studies in all therapy groups. None of the tested variables, such as year of study publication, minimum and maximum follow-up time or the number of cases showed any significant influence. So the visual outcome seems to be dependent on the operating center, the selected patient population and other undetermined factors.

The included literature reported a significant rate of complications ranging from intra-operative complications, progression of cataract to retinal detachment with PVR and phthisis. Fifty-four of the 61 included studies reported of any complications [4–9, 11–24, 26–34, 36, 39, 41–44, 46–63] and only 33 studies contained information on the recurrence of CNV [4–9, 11–14, 16–19, 21, 23, 26, 32–34, 36, 39, 41–43, 46, 48, 49, 53, 56, 60–62]. The highest rate of complications (80%) was achieved after macular translocation [9–13, 24–27, 44–49], whereas the highest recurrence rate of CNV (25%) was described after removal of subfoveal membranes [4–8, 16–23, 31–43]. The available data reporting complications differed in each study and the overall complication rates ranged between 0% and 100%. Due to this limited data the occurrence of complications, particularly the recurrence of CNV could not be evaluated more precisely.

However, this systematic review has some bias. Most included studies contained information from small uncontrolled case series with limited follow-up time. Comparing results is difficult due to the variation in follow-up time, cases and preoperative VA. Additionally, the results are influenced by the evolving surgical techniques and the change in outcome measures.

Only 2 of the included studies were randomized clinical trials [4, 6]. These two relatively large studies (n = 34, n = 80) comparing removal of subretinal CNV to a control group showed considerably lower rates of improvement of VA after surgery (14% and 8.8%) and also considerably higher percentages of deterioration (50% and 37.5%).

Information about the effect of an intervention should be acquired by comparing a treated group to an untreated group similar in all important respects. Therefore a standardized study design is necessary comprising details about the patient population, the minimum number of cases and of follow-up intervals and the use of standardized VA measurements. The length of follow-up time is important to asses the recurrence of CNV in particular.

Compared to the natural course of AMD [64], subretinal surgery shows quite impressing functional results and proves to have a beneficial effect on the visual outcome of AMD. In conclusion, subretinal surgery evaluated in a total of 1273 cases showed a mean improvement of VA in 38% and a mean deterioration of VA in 26%, whereas a mean complication rate was observed in 55%. Current management options for patients with AMD include laser photocoagulation, photodynamic therapy and surgical treatment. Subretinal surgery seems to represent an innovative and promising method for the treatment of exsudative AMD. More randomized clinical trials are needed to draw unbiased conclusions, to estimate the relative risks and benefits of subretinal surgery compared to other treatment options and to allow for standard recommendations.

References

1. Klein R, Klein BEK, Jensen SC, Meuer SM (1997) The five-year incidence and progression of age-related maculopathy. The Beaver Dam Eye Study. Ophthalmology 104:7–21
2. Bressler NM, Bressler SB, Fine SL (1988) Age-related macular degeneration. Surv Ophthalmol 32:375–413
3. Votruba M, Gregor Z (2001) Neovascular age-related macular degeneration: present and future options. Eye 15:424–9
4. Submacular Surgery Trials Pilot Study Investigators (2000) Submacular Surgery Trials randomized pilot trial of laser photocoagulation versus surgery for recurrent choroidal neovascularization secondary to age-related macular degeneration: I. ophthalmic outcomes. Submacular Surgery Trials Pilot Study report number 1. Am J Ophthalmol 130:387–407
5. Thomas MA, Grand MG, Williams DF, et al (1992) Surgical management of subfoveal choroidal neovascularization. Ophthalmology 99:952–68
6. Lewis H, VanderBrug Medendorp S (1997) Tissue plasminogen activator-assisted surgical excision of subfoveal choroidal neovascularization in age-related macular degeneration. a randomized, double-masked trial. Ophthalmology 104:1847–51
7. Ormerod LD, Puklin JE, Frank RN (1994) Long-term outcomes after the surgical removal of advanced subfoveal neovascular membranes in age-related macular degeneration. Ophthalmology 101:1201–10
8. Scheider A, Gündisch O, Kampik A (1999) Surgical extraction of subfoveal choroidal new vessels and submacular haemorrhage in age-related macular degeneration: results of a prospective study. Graefes Arch Clin Exp Ophthalmol 237:10–15
9. Deramo VA, Meyer CH, Toth CA (2001) Successful macular translocation with temporary scleral infolding using absorbable suture. Retina 21:304–11
10. Freedman SF, Seaber JH, Buckley EG, et al (2000) Combined superior oblique muscle recession and inferior oblique muscle advancement and transposition for cyclotorsion associated with macular translocation surgery. J AAPOS 4:75–83
11. Glacet-Bernard A, Simon P, Hamelin N, et al (2001) Translocation of the macula for management of subfoveal choroidal neovascularization: comparison of results in age-related macular degeneration and degenerative myopia. Am J Ophthalmol 131:78–89
12. Lewis H, Kaiser PK, Lewis S, Estafanous M (1999) Macular translocation for subfoveal choroidal neovascularization in age-related macular degeneration: a prospective study. Am J Ophthalmol 128:135–46
13. Lewis H (2001) Macular translocation with chorioscleral outfolding: a pilot clinical study. Am J Ophthalmol 132:156–63
14. Lappas A, Weinberger AWA, Foerster AMH, et al (2000) Iris pigment epithelial cell transplantation in exudative age-related macular degeneration. A pilot study in patients. Graefes Arch Clin Exp Ophthalmol 238:631–41

15. Lewis H (1994) Intraoperative fibrinolysis of submacular hemorrhage with tissue plasminogen activator and surgical drainage. Am J Ophthalmol 118:559–68
16. Bottoni F, Airaghi P, Perego E, et al (1996) Surgical removal of idiopathic, myopic and age-related subfoveal neovascularization. Graefes Arch Clin Exp Ophthalmol 234:S42–S50
17. Corey RP, Scott IU, Flynn HW, et al (2001) Surgical removal of submacular choroidal neovascularization: a clinicopathologic study and factors influencing visual outcomes. Ophthalmic Surg Lasers 32:406–18
18. Merrill PT, LoRusso FJ, Lomeo MD, et al (1999) Surgical removal of subfoveal choroidal neovascularization in age-related macular degeneration. Ophthalmology 106:782–9
19. Mietz H, Merrill PT, Lambert HM, Font RL (1997) Combined subretinal and sub-retinal pigment epithelium neovascular membranes in age-related macular degeneration: a clinicopathologic study of six cases. Ophthalmic Surg Lasers 28:645–52
20. Nasir MA, Sugino I, Zarbin MA (1997) Decreased choriocapillaris perfusion following surgical excision of choroidal neovascular membranes in age-related macular degeneration. Br J Ophthalmol 81:481–9
21. Roth DB, Downie AA, Charles ST (1997) Visual results after submacular surgery for neovascularization in age-related macular degeneration. Ophthalmic Surg Lasers 28:920–5
22. Thach AB, Marx JL, Frambach DA, et al (1996) Choroidal hypoperfusion after surgical excision of subfoveal neovascular membranes in age-related macular degeneration. Int Ophthalmol 20:205–13
23. Thomas MA, Dickinson JD, Melberg NS, et al (1994) Visual results after surgical removal of subfoveal choroidal neovascular membranes. Ophthalmology 101:1384–96
24. Benner JD, Meyer CH, Shirkey BL, Toth CA (2001) Macular translocation with radial scleral outfolding: experimental studies and initial human results. Graefes Arch Clin Exp Ophthalmol 239:815–23
25. Kim T, Krishnasamy S, Meyer CH, Toth CA (2001) Induced corneal astigmatism after macular translocation surgery with scleral infolding. Ophthalmology 108:1203–8
26. Ohji M, Fujikado T, Kusaka S, et al (2001) Comparison of three techniques of foveal translocation in patients with subfoveal choroidal neovascularization resulting from age-related macular degeneration. Am J Ophthalmol 132:888–96
27. Pieramici DJ, de Juan E, Fujii GY, et al (2000) Limited inferior macular translocation for the treatment of subfoveal choroidal neovascularization secondary to age-related macular degeneration. Am J Ophthalmol 130:419–28
28. Haupert CL, McCuen BW, Jaffe GJ, et al (2001) Pars plana vitrectomy, subretinal injection of tissue plasminogen activator, and fluid-gas exchange for displacement of thick submacular hemorrhage in age related macular degeneration. Am J Ophthalmol 131:208–15
29. Hesse L, Meitinger D, Schmidt J (1997) Little effect of tissue plasminogen activator in subretinal surgery for acute hemorrhage in age-related macular degeneration. Ger J Ophthalmol 5:479–83
30. Lim JI, Drews-Botsch C, Sternberg P, et al (1995) Submacular hemorrhage removal. Ophthalmology 102:1393–9
31. Abe T, Yoshida M, Kano T, Tamai M (2001) Visual function after removal of subretinal neovascular membranes in patients with age-related macular degeneration. Graefes Arch Clin Exp Ophthalmol 293:927–36
32. Berger AS, Kaplan HJ (1992) Clinical experience with the surgical removal of subfoveal neovascular membranes. Short-term postoperative results. Ophthalmology 99:969–76
33. Brindeau C, Glacet-Bernard A, Coscas F, et al (2001) Surgical removal of subfoveal choroidal neovascularization: visual outcome and prognostic value of fluorescein angiography and optical coherence tomography. Eur J Ophthalmol 11:287–95
34. Eckardt C (1996) Chirurgische Entfernung von submakulären Neovaskularisationsmembranen. Ophthalmologe 93:688–93
35. Ehrt O, Scheider A, Gündisch O, et al (1999) Chirurgische Entfernung subfovealer choroidaler Neovaskularisationen bei AMD. Prä- und postoperative fundusperimetrische Befunde mit dem SLO. Ophthalmologe 96:421–7
36. Gandorfer A, Scheider A, Gündisch O, Kampik A (1998) Rezidivierende choroidale Neovaskularisationen bei altersbezogener Makuladegeneration. Fluoreszenzangiographische Morphologie nach chirurgischer Membranektomie. Ophthalmologe 95:408–12

37. Hudson HL, Frambach DA, Lopez PF (1995) Relation of the functional and structural fundus changes after submacular surgery for neovascular age-related macular degeneration. Br J Ophthalmol 79:417–23

38. Loewenstein A, Sunness JS, Bressler NM, et al (1998) Scanning laser ophthalmoscope fundus perimetry after surgery for choroidal neovascularization. Am J Ophthalmol 125: 657–65

39. Müller S, Ehrt O, Gündisch O, et al (2000) Funktionelle Ergebnisse nach CNV-Extraktion oder Photokoagulation bei alterskorrelierter Makuladegeneration. Ophthalmologe 97:142–6

40. Park KH, Yu HG, Yu YS, et al (1999) Surgical treatment of subretinal neovascular membrane. Korean J Ophthalmol 13:30–5

41. Strmeň P, Hasa J (1996) Surgical removal of large subretinal neovascular membranes: results and complications. Int Ophthalmol 20:165–9

42. Tsujikawa M, Tsujikawa K, Lewis JM, Tano Y (1999) Change in retinal sensitivity due to excision of choroidal neovascularization and its influence on visual acuity outcome. Retina 19:135–40

43. Yuzawa M, Isomae T, Mori R, et al (2001) Surgical excision versus laser photocoagulation for subfoveal choroidal neovascular membrane with age-related macular degeneration: comparison of visual outcomes. Jpn J Ophthalmol 45:192–8

44. Akduman L, Karavellas MP, Macdonald JC, et al (1999) Macular translocation with retinotomy and retinal rotation for exudative age-related macular degeneration. Retina 19:418–23

45. Buffenn AN, de Juan E, Fujii G, Hunter DG (2001) Diplopia after limited macular translocation surgery. J AAPOS 5:388–94

46. Eckardt C, Eckardt U, Conrad HG (1999) Macular rotation with and without counter-rotation of globe in patients with age-related macular degeneration. Graefes Arch Clin Exp Ophthalmol 237:313–25

47. Ohji M, Fujikado T, Saito Y, et al (1998) Foveal translocation: a comparison of two techniques. Sem Ophthalmol 13:52–61

48. Wolf S, Lappas A, Weinberger AWA, Kirchhof B (1999) Macular translocation for surgical management of subfoveal choroidal neovascularizations in patients with AMD: first results. 237:51–7

49. Wong D, Lois N (2000) Foveal relocation by redistribution of the neurosensory retina. Br J Ophthalmol 84:352–7

50. Abe T, Yoshida M, Tomita H, et al (2000) Auto iris pigment epithelial cell transplantation in patients with age-related macular degeneration: short-term results. Tohoku J Exp Med 191:7–20

51. Algvere PV, Berglin L, Gouras P, Sheng Y (1994) Transplantation of fetal retinal pigment epithelium in age-related macular degeneration with subfoveal neovascularization. Graefes Arch Clin Exp Ophthalmol 232:707–16

52. Algvere PV, Gouras P, Dafgård-Kopp E (1999) Long-term outcome of RPE allografts in non-immunosuppressed patients with AMD. Eur J Ophthalmol 9:217–30

53. Stanga PE, Kychenthal A, Fitzke FW, et al (2001) Retinal pigment epithelium translocation and central visual function in age related macular degeneration: preliminary results. Int Ophthalmol 23:297–307

54. Thumann G, Aisenbrey S, Schraermeyer U, et al (2000) Transplantation of autologous iris pigment epithelium after removal of choroidal neovascular membranes. Arch Ophthalmol 118:1350–5

55. Chaudhry NA, Mieler WF, Han DP, et al (1999) Preoperative use of tissue plasminogen activator for large submacular hemorrhage. Ophthalmic Surg Lasers 30:176–80

56. Claes C, Zivojnovic R (1996) Efficacy of tissue plasminogen activator (t-PA) in subretinal hemorrhage removal. Bull Soc Belge Opthalmol 261:115–18

57. Heidenkummer HP, Kampik A (1995) Chirurgische Extraktion subretinaler Pseudotumoren bei altersbezogener Makuladegeneration (AMD). Klinische, morphologische und immunhistochemische Ergebnisse. Ophthalmologe 92:631–9

58. Ibanez HE, Williams DF, Thomas MA, et al (1995) Surgical management of submacular hemorrhage. A series of 47 consecutive cases. Arch Ophthalmol 113:62–9

59. Kamei M, Tano Y, Maeno T, et al (1996) Surgical removal of submacular hemorrhage using tissue plasminogen activator and perfluorocarbon liquid. Am J Ophthalmol 121:267–75

60. Krasnov MM, Stolyarenko GE (1992) Surgical management of exsudative maculopathies: preliminary report. Eur J Ophthalmol 2:122–8

61. Lambert HM, Capone A, Aaberg TM, et al (1992) Surgical excision of subfoveal neovascular membranes in age-related macular degeneration. Am J Ophthalmol 113:257–62
62. Mandelcorn MS, Menezes AV (1993) Surgical removal of subretinal hemorrhage and choroidal neovascular membranes in acute hemorrhagic age-related macular degeneration. Can J Ophthalmol 28:19–23
63. Moriarty AP, McAllister IL, Constable IJ (1995) Initial clinical experience with tissue plasminogen activator (tPA) assisted removal of submacular haemorrhage. Eye 9:582–8
64. Treatment of age-related macular degeneration with Photodynamic Therapy (TAP) Study Group (2001) Photodynamic therapy of subfoveal choroidal neovascularization in age-related macular degeneration with verteprofin. Two-year results of 2 randomized clinical trials-TAP Report 2. Arch Ophthalmol 119:198–207

Correspondence: C.I. Falkner, M.D., The Ludwig Boltzmann Institute of Retinology und Biomicroscopic Lasersurgery, Department of Ophthalmology, Rudolf Foundation Clinic, Juchgasse 25, A-1030 Vienna, Austria.

Subfoveal neovascular membranes – membrane morphology and outcome after combined subretinal surgery and autologous RPE transplantation

A. Assadoullina[1], H. Feichtinger[2], S. Binder[1], and A. Abri[1]

[1] The Ludwig Boltzmann Institute of Retinology and Biomicroscopic Laser Surgery, Department of Ophthalmology, and [2] Institute of Pathology and Bacteriology, Rudolf Foundation Clinic, Vienna, Austria

Abstract

Purpose: We have recently described combined subretinal surgery and simultaneous autologous transplantation of RPE as a therapeutic option for the treatment of CNV in patients with advanced AMD. The purpose of the present study was to determine whether the size and morphology of the membranes were correlated with patient outcome.

Methods: We examined 19 AMD patients, which underwent combined subretinal surgery and autologous transplantation of RPE. All patients had improved or stabilized visual acuity in follow-up after surgery. The membranes were prepared for conventional histology and evaluated for their morphological composition on serial sections applying a semiquantitative score of 0, 1+, 2+ and 3+ to the following parameters: amount of acellular matrix, neovascularization/microvascular density (MVD), cellularity with special reference to inflammatory cells, and presence of RPE. These data including membrane size as determined preoperatively by fluorescein angiography (FLA) were correlated with postoperative visual acuity.

Results: By preoperative FLA all lesions were classified as clinically predominantly occult. Regarding postoperative outcome we divided all patients in two groups. Group I with visual improvement of 2 and more lines comprised 7 patients, and group II with unchanged/stabilized visual acuity of +/−1 line the remaining 12 patients. Mean membrane size was 6,19 +/− 1,33 mm in the group of patients with, and 6,41 +/− 1,87 in the group without visual improvement, respectively. Recurrences did not occur.

Histology: All 19 membranes contained a significant amount of acellular matrix (scores 2+/3+); a prominent neovascularization/high MVD was present in 13/19 specimens and was usually associated with a high degree of cellularity, i.e. a moderate or marked inflammatory component predominated by lymphocytes (14/19). 6/19 membranes presented as minimally vascularized and acellular scars. In 15/19 cases a significant amount of RPE cells was present in the excised membranes; this prevalence was especially high in the group II.

Outcome: When compared to the development of visual acuity after therapy, neither FLA findings, nor histopathologic features of the membranes were predictive.

Conclusion: In a pilot study of 19 patients with advanced AMD/CNV treated with combined subretinal surgery and autologous RPE transplantation features other than membrane morphology and membrane size seem to determine patient outcome. The tendency for a higher amount of RPE cells in the group with no improvement should be further investigated.

Introduction

In industrialized countries, age related macular degeneration is one of the major causes of blindness in elderly patients [1]. Current therapies are laser treatment including coagulation and photodynamic therapy, but also surgical removal of the neovascular choroidal membrane has been an option [2–4]. We have recently developed a new treatment modality combining membrane surgery with autologous RPE-transplantation [5]. The advantages of this approach are minor traumatic effect compared with rotation technique and the simultany of surgery and transplantation. 57% of treated patients improved their visual acuity for 2 and more lines [5]. The question of this study was, whether size and morphological composition of membranes could influence functional results of therapy.

Material and methods

19 patients with advanced AMD who underwent combined CNV membrane excision and autologous transplantation of RPE and had improved or stabilized visual acuity in follow-up were included in the study. Membrane size was determined preoperatively by fluorescein angiography (FLA). The surgical membrane specimens were routinely processed for light microscopy and stained with hematoxylin-eosin (HE) and periodic-acid schiff (PAS). The membranes were evaluated for their morphological composition on serial sections applying a semiquantitative score of 0, 1+, 2+, and 3+ to the following parameters: amount of acellular matrix, neovascularization/microvascular density (MVD), cellularity with special reference to inflammatory cells, and the presence of RPE. In addition, the amount of acellular matrix was determined by means of an image analysis system (LUCIA). The morphologic parameters and membrane size were then correlated with the postoperative changes of visual acuity for distance. Visual acuity was measured before treatment, 1 month and 3 months postoperatively, and every 3 months thereafter using ETDRS charts and transfer of the respective values to logarithms of minimal angle of resolution (logMAR).

Details of the surgical method were described earlier [5]. Briefly, the patients underwent pars plana vitrectomy with removal of the posterior hyaloid. The first retinotomy was performed temporally or nasally superior to the membrane. After mobilisation and gentle hydrodissection with Ringer's solution, the subfoveal membrane was slowly removed with a subretinal forceps. A second retinotomy was then created nasal to the optic disk with a subretinal pick and a shallow retinal detachment was achieved by subretinal injection with Ringer's solution. Consecutively, RPE's were gently mobilized over an area of 2 to 4 disc diameters, aspirated, and slowly transplanted by means of the first retinotomy into the subretinal space. Surgery was completed with an air or gas tamponade.

Results

Clinical findings: 11 patients were female, 8 male. Mean age of patients was 76 years (range, 64 to 87 years). The follow-up of patients was 18–36 months. By preoperative FLA all lesions were classified as predominantly occult. Regarding postoperative outcome all patients were divided in two groups; 7 patients showed a visual improvement of 2 and more lines (group I), the remaining 12 patients (group II) presented unchanged visual acuity of +/–1 line. Mean membrane size was 6,19 +/– 1,33 mm in the group of patients

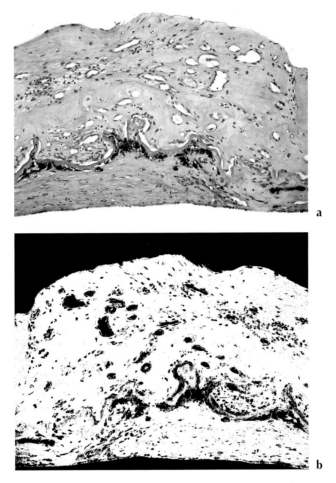

Fig. 1. Patient 10: choroidal neovascular membrane, classified as neovascularization 2+, matrix 3+, cellularity 2+, RPE 3+ (**a** PAS; **b** binary image captured by image analysis – white area corresponds to the amount of matrix and conducted 80,39%)

with improved, and 6,41 +/– 1,87 in the group with stabilized visual acuity, respectively. A significant progression of visual impairment and recurrences did not occur.

Histology: All 19 membranes were rich in matrix (scores 2+/3+); 13/19 membranes exhibited a prominent vascularity usually associated with a high degree of cellularity, i.e. a moderate or marked inflammatory infiltrate predominated by lymphocytes (14/19). 6/19 membranes corresponded to minimally vascularized and acellular scars. In 15/19 cases the excised membranes contained numerous RPE cells and this feature was more often seen in group II patients.

Outcome: When compared to the development of visual acuity after therapy, neither membrane size nor histopathologic features of the membranes showed a significant correlation.

Results are summarized in Tables 1 and 2.

Discussion

Age-related macular degeneration is a serious health problem in the old population. Laser coagulation and photodynamic therapy (PDT) are methods of choice in cases of classic

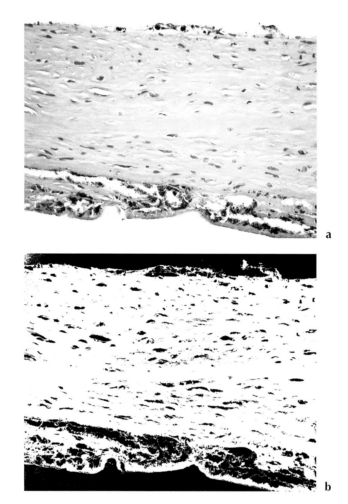

Fig. 2. Patient 7: choroidal neovascular membrane, classified as neovascularization 0, matrix 3+, cellularity 0, RPE 1+ (**a** PAS; **b** binary image captured by image analysis – white area corresponds to the amount of matrix)

Table 1. Patients with improved visual acuity

Patient nr.	Age	Visual acuity change*	Morphology					Preoperative membrane size (mm)**
			Matrix		MVD	Cellularity	RPE	
			Score	%	Score	Score	Score	
1	64	7,00	3+	86,90	1+	1+	2+	5,28
2	74	7,00	3+	n.s.	0	1+	1+	7,41
3	74	8,00	3+	92,23	2+	2+	2+	8,60
4	76	3,00	3+	88,79	3+	3+	0	5,24
5	78	10,00	3+	94,90	2+	2+	2+	5,85
6	81	2,00	2+	82,65	3+	3+	2+	6,01
7	73	3,00	3+	n.s.	0	0	1+	4,97
Mean								6,19+/−1,33

* LogMAR
** as determined by preoperative FLA

Table 2. Patients with unchanged/stabilized visual acuity

Patient nr.	Age	Visual acuity change*	Morphology					Preoperative membrane size (mm)**
			Matrix		MVD	Cellularity	RPE	
			Score	%	Score	Score	Score	
8	70	−1,00	3+	90,21	2+	2+	3+	4,44
9	77	−1,00	2+	74,12	2+	2+	1+	6,53
10	82	−1,00	3+	80,39	2+	2+	3+	6,15
11	81	0,00	3+	82,10	2+	3+	3+	8,41
12	68	0,00	3+	83,98	1+	2+	2+	4,91
13	73	0,00	2+	n.s.	3+	3+	2+	5,57
14	85	0,00	3+	n.s.	1+	2+	2+	9,10
15	77	0,00	3+	79,50	3+	3+	3+	5,24
16	79	0,00	2+	73,10	2+	1+	2+	5,34
17	87	1,00	2+	n.s.	1+	1+	3+	10,20
18	79	1,00	3+	74,94	2+	2+	3+	6,44
19	78	1,00	2+	60,93	3+	3+	3+	4,59
Mean								6,41+/−1,87

* LogMAR
** as determined by preoperative FLA

membranes [2, 3]. All patients in our study had advanced disease with subfoveal, predominantly occult membranes with only small classic parts not suitable for these established therapies and were therefore treated by combined membrane surgery and autologous RPE transplantation. In contrast to laser treatment [6], PDT [7] or membrane excision along [8] with recurrence rates of up to 55%, no such recurrences of CNV were seen in our group of patients within a follow-up period of 18 to 36 months. Nevertheless, based on the postoperative development of visual acuity the 19 patients could be divided into two subgroups: group I with visual improvement of 2 and more lines, and group II with stabilized visual acuity of +/−1 line, respectively. In view of these clinical findings we investigated, whether a simply determinable preoperative parameter like membrane size did correlate with the postoperative visual function; furthermore we looked whether the morphologic composition of the membranes possibly reflecting disease activity was influential.

Postoperative visual acuity was independent of membrane size as determined by FLA. The morphologic parameters of membranes like amount of matrix, microvascular density, cellularity reflected in the degree of inflammatory infiltration and the amount of RPE cells were scored semiquantitatively. When compared with the postoperative development of visual function no significant correlation with any of the morphologic characteristics evaluated became evident. The higher scores concerning the amount of RPE cells found in membranes of patients with unchanged visual acuity was only a tendency. It should also be mentioned that the evaluation of RPE content must be seen with caution, since the mostly superficial localization of these cells makes them especially sensible to artifacts due to mechanical manipulations during and after surgery and the consecutive steps necessary for the histological preparation of the specimens.

The results presented refer to a group of highly selected patients, who generally profited from the actual therapy with either improvement or stabilization of visual acuity in contrast to the natural course of the disease [9]. In a larger series of 68 patients, 8 (11,9%) showed postoperative visual deterioration. For these cases only date on membrane size were available, which, similar to the study cases revealed no significant difference [10].

In conclusion, the results of this study suggest that factors other than membrane morphology and the size seem to be responsible for differences in the postoperative development of visual function observed in AMD patients treated with subretinal surgery and autologous RPE transplantation.

References

1. Evans J, Wormald R (1996) Is the incidence of registrable age-related macular degeneration increasing? Br J Ophthalmol 80(1):9–14
2. Macular Photocoagulation Study Group (1993) Five-year follow-up of fellow eyes of patients with age-related macular degeneration and unilateral extrafoveal choroidal neovascularization. Arch Ophthalmol 111(9):1189–99
3. Treatment of age-related macular degeneration with Photodynamic Therapy (TAP) Study group (1999) Photodynamic therapy of subfoveal choroidal neovascularization in age-related macular degeneration with verteporfin: one-year results of 2 randomized clinical trials–TAP report. Arch Ophthalmol 117(10):1329–45
4. Berger AS, Kaplan HJ (1992) Clinical experience with the surgical removal of subfoveal neovascular membranes. Ophthalmology 99:969–75
5. Binder S, Stolba U, Krebs I, Kellner L, Jahn C, Feichtinger H, Pavelka M, Frohner U, Kruger A, Hilgers RD, Krugluger W (2002) Transplantation of autologous retinal pigment epithelium in eyes with foveal neovascularization resulting from age-related macular degeneration: a pilot study. Am J Ophthalmol 133(2):215–25
6. Macular Photocoagulation Study Group (1994) Persistent and recurrent neovascularisation after laser photocoagulation for subfoveal choroidal neovascularisation of age-related macular degeneration. Arch Ophthalmol 112:489–99
7. Schmidt-Erfurth U, Michels S, Barbazetto I, Laqua H (2002) Photodynamic effects on choroidal neovascularization and physiological choroid. Invest Ophthalmol Vis Sci 43(3):830–41
8. Thomas M, Dickinson J, Melberg N, et al (1996) Visual results after surgical removal of subfoveal choroidal neovascular membranes. Ophthalmology 101:1384–96
9. Stevens TS, Bressler NM, Maguire MG, Bressler SB, Fine SL, Alexander J, Phillips DA, Margherio RR, Murphy PL, Schachat AP (1997) Occult choroidal neovascularization in age-related macular degeneration. A natural history study. Arch Ophthalmol 115(3):345–50
10. Binder S, Krebs I, Stolba U, Jahn Ch, Kellner L, Feichtinger H, Abri A, Assadoullina A, Stanzel B (2003) Incidence of recurrent membrane growth after surgical excision of foveal choriodal neovascularization combined with transplantation of autologous retinal pigment epithelium. Invest Ophthalmol Vis Sci 44(4):20

Correspondence: Adele Assadoullina, MD, The Ludwig Boltzmann Institute of Retinology and Biomicroscopic Laser Surgery, Department of Ophthalmology, Rudolf Foundation Clinic, Juchgasse 25, A-1030 Vienna, Austria, E-mail: adele.assadoullina@kar.magwien.gv.at

Current status of macular translocation surgery

E. de Juan, Jr, G. Y. Fujii, K.-G. Au Eong, M. S. Humayun,
and R. R. Lakhanpal

The Retina Institute, Doheny Eye Institute, The Keck School of Medicine,
University of Southern California, Los Angeles, CA, USA

Abstract

Macular translocation surgery remains the only treatment with potential for significant visual improvement. Indications are expanding and the surgical technique is continuously improving. The knowledge of the fixation and microperimetry pattern enables better understanding of the macular dysfunction in eyes with subfoveal choroidal neovascularization and should be useful for evaluation of baseline retinal cell viability in order to optimise patient selection. Improved surgical technique and appropriate patient selection result in higher effectiveness and decreased complications.

Introduction

Choroidal neovascularization (CNV) secondary to age-related macular degeneration (AMD), pathologic myopia, ocular histoplasmosis syndrome (OHS), and related disorders are accountable for a large proportion of impaired vision and blindness in the adult general population. In fact, AMD alone is the leading cause of blindness in elderly individuals 60 years and older in many developed countries [1]. Approximately 90% of the blindness due to AMD is attributable to CNV.

Extensive research on the treatment of neovascular maculopathy has resulted in several major developments recently. The development of photodynamic therapy with verteporfin for subfoveal CNV is particularly significant. Photodynamic therapy has been shown to effectively reduce the risks of visual loss in eyes with subfoveal predominantly classic CNV [2] as well as pure occult CNV [3] secondary to AMD. In addition, it has also been demonstrated to safely increase the chance of stabilizing or improving vision in patients with subfoveal CNV secondary to pathologic myopia [4]. Unfortunately, multiple retreatments are usually necessary and improvement in vision following treatment is uncommon. Although the complications associated with photodynamic therapy are relatively few and minor, the potential for significant visual improvement is also low.

Prior to this recent development, the only treatment modality that has been proven to be effective for the treatment of subfoveal CNV due to AMD, OHS and idiopathic causes was laser photocoagulation [5, 6]. The Macular Photocoagulation Study (MPS) proved that laser photocoagulation of the entire area of age-related subfoveal CNV is beneficial with regards to long-term visual acuity when compared to observation [7]. However, the treatment was associated with an immediate average reduction of three Bailey-Lovie lines in visual acuity and the benefits of treatment over the natural history of the condition only became apparent six months later. Retention or recovery of good vision rarely occurred in treated patients. For these reasons, even before the advent of photodynamic therapy, laser photocoagulation was not well accepted as a modality of treatment for subfoveal

CNV in some countries [8]. It has now been superceded by photodynamic therapy in most centers.

Another major recent advance is the development of a novel surgical approach to neovascular maculopathy. Known as macular translocation, it may be defined as any surgery that has a primary goal of relocating the central neurosensory retina or fovea intraoperatively or postoperatively specifically for the management of macular disease [9]. Unlike photodynamic therapy, the single greatest benefit of macular translocation is its potential to significantly improve vision in some patients. This article reviews the current status of macular translocation and highlights some aspects of patient selection that may predict good postoperative outcome.

Past, present and future

Lindsey and associates first experimented with retinal relocation to study the anatomic dependency of the foveal retina on foveal retinal pigment epithelium and choroid in 1983 [10]. In 1985, Tiedeman and associates proposed using retinal relocation as a treatment for subfoveal CNV [11]. This proposal was not pursued for some time until Machemer and Steinhorst finally demonstrated its feasibility in humans in 1993 [12].

Machemer and Steinhorst's original technique involves lensectomy, complete vitrectomy, planned retinal detachment by transscleral infusion of fluid under the retina, 360° peripheral retinotomy, rotation of the retina around the optic disc and retinal reattachment with silicone oil tamponade [12]. Some investigators have since modified this technique [13, 14], including performing a large but less than 360° retinotomy [15, 16].

In an effort to reduce the incidence and severity of proliferative vitreoretinopathy that has been reported to occur with macular translocation with large or 360° retinotomy, Imai and de Juan described a new technique without any retinotomy in 1996 [17]. They detached the retina by transscleral subretinal hydrodissection and performed anteroposterior scleral shortening near the equator to create a relative redundancy of the retina to allow macular translocation. Since its initial description in 1996, de Juan and associates and others have made several modifications to their technique [18–26]. These include chorioscleral outfolding, radially orientated chorioscleral shortening, and use of scleral titanium clips and absorbable sutures for chorioscleral shortening.

A recent experimental study by Hayashi and associates evaluated the retinal changes after macular translocation in dog eyes [27]. Histologic studies disclosed the retina was normal where it had reattached to the retinal pigment epithelium, but retina involved in retinal folds showed loss of photoreceptor cells.

As more surgeons performed macular translocation and introduced refinements and modifications, a proliferation of nonstandardized terms followed. This makes direct comparison between studies difficult and creates potential for confusion. In an effort to facilitate communication within the scientific community, Au Eong and associates proposed a standardized terminology and classification for macular translocation, thus unifying the various techniques that are currently in use [9]. In addition, key concepts such as minimum desired translocation (MDT), postoperative foveal displacement, and the pattern of retinal displacement with various techniques were also introduced to aid understanding of the new surgery. Hopefully, the use of a common standardized terminology will enhance further research in this area although the definitions, terms, classification, and concepts concerning macular translocation are likely to continue to evolve as it undergoes further modifications and refinements.

Rationale

The objective of macular translocation is to move the fovea in an eye with a recent-onset subfoveal lesion such as CNV to a new location with presumably healthier bed of retinal pigment epithelium-Bruch's membrane-choriocapillaris complex devoid of the lesion. The rationale is that this displacement reestablishes a more normal subretinal environment beneath the fovea and allows the fovea to recover or maintain its visual function. In addition, relocating the fovea overlying a lesion such as CNV to an area outside the border of the CNV allows its ablation with conventional laser photocoagulation without destroying the fovea, thereby preserving central vision and arresting the progression of the CNV. When combined with submacular surgery, macular translocation also allows the fovea to be relocated to an area outside the retinal pigment epithelial defect often associated with CNV removal.

Terminology and classification

An international panel of experts has proposed definitions for several terms relating to macular translocation [9]. These are shown below.

The several different techniques currently in use for macular translocation may be classified according to the size of the retinotomy/retinotomies used as follows:

(i) *macular translocation with punctate or no retinotomy/retinotomies* (also known as *limited macular translocation*).
   This group may be further subdivided into those performed
      (a) *with* chorioscleral shortening, or
      (b) *without* chorioscleral shortening.
         Chorioscleral shortening may be effected by *chorioscleral infolding* (imbrication or inpouching) or *chorioscleral outfolding* (outpouching). These may be either *circumferentially* or *radially* orientated.
(ii) *macular translocation with large curvilinear "incisions" of retina.*
   This group may be further subdivided into
      (a) *macular translocation with 360° retinotomy*
      (b) *macular translocation with large (but less than 360°) retinotomy.*

Indications

Currently, the most common indication for macular translocation is subfoveal CNV. Given that CNV is most frequently age-related, AMD is the most common condition treated with this procedure [22, 28–39]. Other causes of CNV that have been treated with macular translocation include pathologic myopia [29, 40–44]. Ocular Hystoplasmosis Syndrome [28, 40], angioid streaks [40, 45], multifocal choroiditis [40], and idiopathic cases [40].

Recently, macular translocation has been used to treat polypoidal choroidal vasculopathy [46]. We have also demonstrated the feasibility of using macular translocation to manage subfoveal retinal pigment epithelial loss following submacular surgery [47]. It is possible that the spectrum of conditions in which macular translocation is clinically useful may expand in the future.

Surgical techniques

A) Macular translocation with punctate or no retinotomy/retinotomies
(limited macular translocation)

Our current technique for macular translocation with punctate retinotomies has been described elsewhere in detail [18, 21, 22, 48]. Very briefly, for inferior macular translocation, we pre-place five nonabsorbable mattress sutures in the superotemporal quadrant for chorioscleral infolding prior to a standard 3-port pars plana vitrectomy. Following vitrectomy, we detach the retina temporal to the optic disc by subretinal infusion of balanced salt solution (BSS) through several punctate retinotomies with a 41-gauge retinal hydrodissection cannula (MADLAB retinal hydrodissection cannula, Bausch & Lomb Surgical, St Louis, MO). The use of a calcium- and magnesium-free solution for subretinal hydrodissection has been shown to facilitate the retinal detachment [49, 50]. Intravitreal irrigation with calcium- and magnesium-free BSS Plus solution (Alcon Laboratory, Fort Worth, TX) may also alter the adhesion between the retinal pigment epithelium microvilli and retinal outer segments, making planned retinal detachment less traumatic [51]. Once the retina is detached, we tighten and tie the mattress sutures to effect chorioscleral infolding, causing redundancy of the retina relative to the eyewall. We then carry out a 75–90% fluid-air exchange before closing the sclerostomies. Postoperatively, the patient keeps his head upright for several days. In this position, the gravitational force of the subretinal fluid and the floatation force of the intravitreal air bubble will be aligned (in different directions) to effect inferior macular translocation.

Since de Juan and associates' report on macular translocation with punctate retinotomies [18], many surgeons have proposed modifications to their original technique. Recently, several investigators have used either sutures or titanium clips for chorioscleral outfolding to increase the redundancy of the retina relative to the eyewall. In an experiment on human cadaver eyes, chorioscleral outfolding shortened the inner eyewall more effectively than chorioscleral infolding [52], thus increasing the likelihood of effective macular translocation.

Benner and associates reported successful retinal translocation in 8 rabbit eyes using modified stainless titanium ligating clips (Ligaclip extra LT200, medium; Ethicon, Endo-Surgery, Norderstedt, Germany) for radial chorioscleral outfolding [25]. They noted, however, greater anterior segment inflammation in rabbit eyes treated with clips than in macular translocation surgeries performed using sutures for chorioscleral infolding. This observation deterred them from using clips for their initial macular translocation with chorioscleral outfolding in humans.

Lewis used titanium clips (DuraClose™, Surgical Dynamics, Inc., Norwalk, Connecticut) for chorioscleral outfolding and compared the postoperative foveal displacement effected by those placed circumferentially to those arranged in a radial fashion in 25 patients [24]. He found the median postoperative foveal displacement among patients who had circumferential chorioscleral outfolding was 614 μm (range, 0–1326 μm) compared to 1629 μm (range, 0–3200 μm) achieved by those who had radial outfolding.

Deramo and associates reported using absorbable suture for chorioscleral infolding [28]. They found that the postoperative foveal displacement achieved in the early postoperative period did not regress after resolution of the chorioscleral infolding although induced postoperative oblique corneal astigmatism resolved. The resolution of the corneal astigmatism coincided with the disappearance of peripheral retinal elevation due to the infolding.

For limited macular translocation, the technique for superior displacement of the fovea is still not perfected and therefore inferior displacement is preferred in most cases.

We consider superior limited macular translocation only in cases when the MDT for a superior displacement is very small but that for inferior displacement is large. With a large subretinal lesion in which inferior limited macular translocation is not possible and the MDT for a superior displacement is large, macular translocation with 360° may be considered.

Nasal macular translocation is feasible and may be considered in patients with subfoveal CNV centered temporally relative to the fovea [20]. The technique is similar to inferior limited macular translocation except for the placement of the mattress sutures and the postoperative head positioning. The mattress sutures are placed temporally and the head is held such that the temporal retina is uppermost (i.e. the patient lies on his unoperated side). This modification adds a new direction in which the fovea may be displaced during macular translocation, and may be a viable option for selected patients who may otherwise be poor candidates for superior or inferior macular translocation [20].

It is possible to achieve effective macular translocation without chorioscleral shortening or large retinotomy [19, 39]. Stretching of the retina is thought to produce the redundancy required for effective macular translocation [9].

B) Macular translocation with large or 360° retinotomy

Machemer and Steinhorst's original macular translocation technique utilizes a 360° retinotomy to mobilize the retina [12]. The operation consists of essentially five steps: (1) vitrectomy with lensectomy, (2) planned total retinal detachment, (3) 360° peripheral retinotomy, (4) removal of subretinal blood and membranes, and (5) retinal reattachment with rotation of the retina around the optic nerve. The initial surgeries look some 5 to 6 hours to complete, and were performed under general anesthesia. Because the postoperative foveal displacement achievable with this technique is huge, postoperative cyclotropia is a significant problem. To reduce this complication, Eckardt and associates developed simultaneous macular translocation with 360° retinotomy and extraocular muscle surgery to counter-rotate the eye in the opposite direction [13]. Their results and that of others showed that when combined with simultaneous extraocular muscle surgery, the postoperative subjective tilt and cyclotorsional diplopia were less severe [13, 53].

Instead of 360° peripheral retinotomy, Ninomiya and associates proposed a large retinotomy outside the temporal vascular arcades to translocate the macula [16]. Unfortunately, the results from this technique has not been as satisfactory as that performed with 360° retinotomy [15].

Ohji and associates compared thee techniques of macular translocation (limited macular translocation, macular translocation with large retinotomy, and macular translocation with 360° retinotomy) in 51 consecutive patients [54]. They found the mean postoperative foveal displacement was greater in the macular translocation with 360° retinotomy (3340 μm) than in the limited macular translocation (1120 μm, P < .001) and the macular translocation with large retinotomy (1060 μm, P < .001).

Patient selection

Minimum desired translocation (MDT)

One of the most important factors to achieving a good postoperative outcome in macular translocation is patient selection. Since current techniques of limited macular translocation have a median postoperative foveal displacement of about 1200 microns, the magnitude of the MDT is a very important factor in determining whether a proposed macular translocation procedure is likely to be effective i.e. whether the proposed procedure is likely to displace the foveal center to a new location outside the border of the subretinal lesion. Surgeons planning to perform limited macular translocation on a particular patient should be aware of the median postoperative foveal displacement they have achieved in their previous cases. Knowledge of one's median postoperative foveal displacement, when considered together with the MDT for a particular eye, can give some idea of the likelihood of achieving effective macular translocation. For example, if the MDT in an eye is *equal* to the median postoperative foveal displacement normally achieved by the surgeon, barring any complication, the eye has an approximately 50:50 chance of achieving effective macular translocation after the surgery. If the MDT is less than the median postoperative foveal displacement, the eye has a greater than 50% chance of achieving effective macular translocation and vice versa [9, 35].

Scanning laser ophthalmoscopic (SLO) microperimetry

One major concern in eyes with neovascular maculopathy is whether there are viable photoreceptors that can be rescued from the diseased subretinal environment to a new location with a healthier retinal pigment epithelium-Bruch's membrane-choriocapillaris complex so that they can regain or maintain their function. In a recent study, we found that good visual acuity ($\geq$ 20/100) is a good predictor for a favorable visual outcome following effective macular translocation [55]. However, poor visual acuity (< 20/100) was not predictive of an unfavorable postoperative visual outcome. This is because impaired vision does not necessarily mean an absence of viable foveal photoreceptors, but may be due to such factors as subretinal hemorrhage and fluid. In eyes with poor visual acuity, a detailed evaluation of the visual function is recommended to determine the presence of viable foveal retinal cells before one can exclude them from a rescue procedure. We have found that SLO microperimetry with fixation pattern evaluation provides optimum positive and negative predictive values, with good sensitivity and specificity [55].

For the purpose of evaluating fixation patterns, we have created a classification to assist in differentiating between eyes with good, moderate, and poor fixation [55]. We have looked specifically at two parameters, fixation location and fixation stability, and have proposed the following grading:

A) Fixation location: (Fig. 1)

(1) *Predominantly central fixation*: eyes with most ($\geq$ 50%) of the preferred fixation points located within a limit area of variation of 2°-diameter circle centered on the fovea.

(2) *Poor central fixation*: eyes with less than 50% but more than 25% of the preferred fixation points located within the 2° circle.

(3) *Predominantly eccentric fixation*: eyes with less than 25% of the preferred fixation points located within the 2° circle.

B) Fixation stability: (Fig. 2)

(1) *Stable fixation*: eyes with 75% or more of the fixation points located within a predetermined limit area of variation of a 2°-diameter circle centered in the gravitational center of all fixation points, regardless of the position of the foveal center.

(2) *Relatively unstable fixation*: eyes with less than 75% of the fixation points located within a 2° circle, but with 75% or more of the fixation points located within a 4° circle the fixation, being both centered in the gravitational center of all fixation points.

(3) *Unstable fixation*: eyes with less than 75% of the fixation points located within a 4° circle centered in the gravitational center of all fixation points.

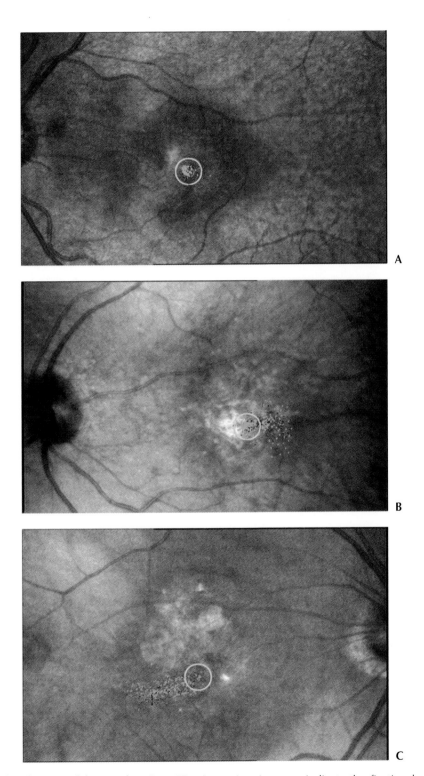

Fig. 1. Classification of fixation location: (Fixation points in green indicate the fixation location during each perceived stimulus presentation. Fixation points in red indicate the fixation location during non-perceived stimulus presentation.) **A** The location of fixation was defined as *predominantly central fixation* when more than 50% of the preferred fixation points were located within a pre-determined limit area of variation of 2°-diameter circle centered in the fovea. **B** The location of fixation was classified as *poor central fixation* when less than 50% but more than 25% of the preferred fixation points were located within the 2°-diameter circle. **C** The location of fixation was classified as *predominantly eccentric fixation* when less than 25% of the preferred fixation points located within the 2°-diameter circle

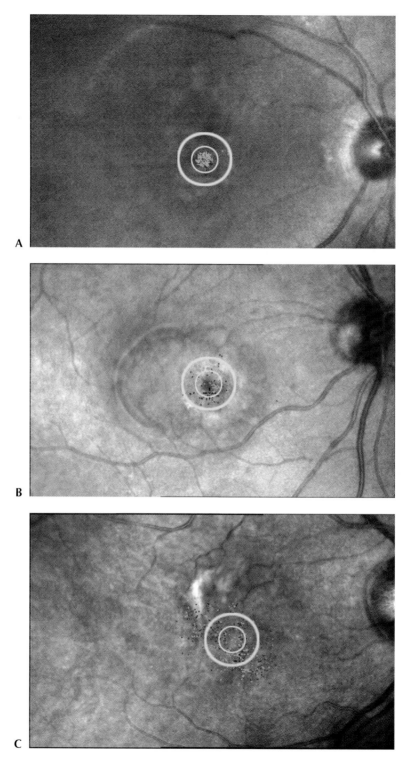

Fig. 2. Classification of fixation stability: **A** The location of fixation was defined as *stable fixation* when more than 75% of the fixation points were located within a pre-determined limit area of variation of a 2°-diameter circle centered in the gravitational center of all fixation points, regardless of the position of the foveal center. **B** The location of fixation was classified as *relatively unstable fixation* when less than 75% of the fixation points were located within a 2°-diameter circle, but more than 75% of the fixation points were located within a 4°-diameter circle. **C** The location of fixation was classified as *unstable fixation* when less than 75% of the fixation points were located within a 4° circle

Based on this fixation grading, we evaluated the correlation between fixation pattern and postoperative visual acuity of eyes that achieved effective macular translocation.

We found that eyes with predominantly central and stable fixation (i.e. without dense central scotoma) had the highest chance of achieving good vision ($\geq 20/100$) after effective macular translocation (84% and 91%, respectively). Conversely, eyes with predominantly eccentric and unstable fixation had the lowest chance of achieving good visual acuity following effective translocation (22% and 33%, respectively). Eyes with poor central and relatively unstable fixation had a moderate chance of achieving good visual acuity after effective translocation (33% and 58%) [55]. Thus, this concept of foveal viability evaluation enhances the patient selection process and predicts more accurately whether a particular eye is likely to do well after surgery.

Visual outcomes

The greatest advantage of macular translocation over other current treatment modalities is the potential for significant visual acuity improvement following successful treatment. By moving viable retinal cells in the fovea to a healthier bed of retinal pigment epithelium-Bruch's membrane-choriocapillaris complex, the cells may recover their visual function.

Subfoveal choroidal neovascularization due to AMD

The largest series of eyes treated with macular translocation to date was by Pieramici, de Juan, Fujii and associates [35, 56]. This study reported the outcomes of 102 consecutive eyes with neovascular AMD in 101 patients aged 41–89 years (median, 76 years) that underwent inferior limited macular translocation by a single surgeon for new or recurrent subfoveal CNV. After surgery, 62% of the cases achieved effective macular translocation with a median postoperative foveal displacement of 1200 µm (range, 200–2800 µm). At 3 and 6 months postoperatively, 31% and 49% of the eyes respectively achieved a visual acuity better than 20/100 while 37% and 48% of the eyes respectively experienced 2 or more Snellen lines of visual improvement [35]. Sixteen percent of the eyes experienced 6 or more Snellen lines of visual improvement [35]. The most recent data we have collected on these 102 eyes show that by 12 months postoperatively, 40.7% of eyes achieved a visual acuity of 20/100 or better [56]. Thirty-nine and a half percent of the eyes experienced two or more Snellen lines of visual improvement, 29.0% remained unchanged visual acuity; and 31.4% lost two or more lines of visual acuity [56]. These data demonstrate that the beneficial effects of macular translocation are sustained over a period of at least one year.

In this era of photodynamic therapy, there is concern if the potential benefits of macular translocation outweigh the surgical risks involved. There is currently no available data from randomized clinical trials comparing the efficacy of macular translocation and photodynamic therapy directly. Current data suggest the potential risks and benefits of photodynamic therapy and macular translocation to be quite different. Photodynamic therapy is a relatively low-risk procedure aimed at maintaining the presenting visual acuity while improving the visual acuity is a realistic goal for the higher-risk macular translocation. A pilot multicenter clinical trial is currently underway to evaluate the feasibility of conducting a larger randomized clinical trial comparing the two modalities of treatment. However, since most patients are likely to make up their minds on which treatment modality is more acceptable to them, it may be difficult to enroll suitable patients who are willing to be randomized to receive one of these two treatments.

Subfoveal choroidal neovascularization due to causes other than AMD

We reported the results of inferior limited macular translocation in 23 eyes of 22 patients with subfoveal CNV secondary to pathologic myopia (11 eyes), ocular histoplasmosis syndrome (OHS) (4 eyes), angioid streaks (4 eyes), idiopathic causes (3 eyes), and multifocal choroiditis (1 eye) [40]. In this heterogenous group, the preoperative visual acuity was 20/100 or better in 11 of the 23 eyes (47.8%). After a mean follow-up of 9.8 months (range, 6–18 months), the postoperative visual acuity was 20/100 or better in 7 of the 11 eyes (63.6%) with pathologic myopia. In eyes with OHS, 3 out of 4 eyes (75%) achieved a postoperative visual acuity of 20/100 or better after a mean follow-up of 12.8 months (range, 9–18 months). After a mean follow-up of 14.3 months (range, 9–18 months), the postoperative vision was 20/100 or better in 2 out of 4 eyes (50%) with angioid streaks. Two of the 3 eyes (66.6%) with idiopathic CNV and one eye with multifocal choroiditis achieved a postoperative visual acuity of 20/100 or better after a mean follow-up of 8.3 months (range, 6–12 months). This series suggests that macular translocation can restore vision in a significant number of patients with subfoveal CNV secondary to causes other than AMD. Although the precise indications for surgical intervention are still to be determined, these initial results are encouraging [40].

Complications

A number of surgical complications are associated with limited macular translocation. However, by avoiding the creation of large retinotomies, as is performed in macular translocation with large or 360° retinotomy, the incidence of retinal detachment and proliferative vitreoretinopathy is significantly decreased. We retrospectively reviewed 153 consecutive cases of limited macular translocation to study their complications and factors relating their development [57]. This series included the early cases of limited macular translocation, allowing us to examine the existence of a learning curve for the procedure.

Of 153 eyes, the intraoperative complications identified included macular hole (12), retinal break (8), subretinal hemorrhage (7), vitreous hemorrhage (3), scleral perforation (3), and choroidal hemorrhage (1). The postoperative complications included retinal detachment (25), retinal breaks (13), macular fold (7), vitreous hemorrhage (4), new CNV at retinotomy site (2), choroidal hemorrhage (1), and suspected endophthalmitis (1). Eyes that developed retinal detachment, subretinal hemorrhage, or macular fold had significantly greater loss of vision than eyes without these complications ($P < .05$) [57].

The most common serious postoperative complication is retinal detachment. The incidence of retinal detachment, hemorrhage or any complication decreased significantly during the study period ($P = .03$), suggesting the existence of a learning curve [57]. Proliferative vitreoretinopathy and retinal breaks were found in a significant number of eyes. When a retinal break is identified during the surgery, laser retinopexy or cryoretinopexy intraoperatively or in the early postoperative period is indicated. This will reduce the risk of persistent retinal detachment in the postoperative period. Retinal break detected postoperatively may or may not be associated with retinal detachment. In the absence of retinal detachment, laser retinopexy is advised to reduce the risk of its subsequent occurrence. Postoperative retinal detachment requires surgical intervention. Pneumoretinopexy is suitable in cases where the retinal break(s) is in the superior two-thirds of the retinal periphery but in most cases, a repeat operation is indicated. Currently, our incidence of retinal detachment following limited macular translocation is approximately 5–10%.

Other findings in this study were that the presence of predominantly classic CNV, the occurrence of an intraoperative retinal break, any intraocular hemorrhage, or macular fold formation were significantly associated with retinal detachment ($P < .03$). As expected, eyes that developed retinal detachment, subretinal hemorrhage, or macular fold had significantly more visual loss than eyes without these complications [57].

Interestingly, transient formed visual hallucinations have been reported to occur in two patients following macular translocation [58]. These hallucinations of people, faces, and animals occurring in the presence of normal cognition, orientation, and insight are suggestive of Charles Bonnet syndrome. They began within 24 hours following macular translocation and resolved after the retina became reattached. This temporal association of the state of retinal attachment and/or acute change of vision with the onset and cessation of hallucinations provides the strongest support to date for the "sensory deprivation" theory of hallucination. It has been suggested that a reduction of sensory input to specific areas of the brain allows previous perceptions into consciousness as hallucinations.

Recurrence and persistence

In our study, the incidence of persistent and recurrent CNV in eyes that achieved effective macular translocation and received laser photocoagulation was 34.6% at 12 months, demonstrating that eyes continue to be at risk of recurrent CNV after surgery and laser ablation [56]. In the group with effective macular translocation, recurrence occurred more frequently in the subfoveal location (64.7%) than in the juxta- or extra-foveal location (35.3%). Therefore, it is important that patients continue to monitor their central vision with an Amsler grid to detect early recurrences as a proportion of them may still be amenable to laser ablation because of their juxta- or extra-foveal location.

Overall, at 12 months postoperatively, the group of patients with persistent or recurrent CNV showed a trend towards worse median change in visual acuity than the group with no recurrence [56].

When the recurrent CNV is either extrafoveal or juxtafoveal, additional laser photocoagulation to ablate the lesion is indicated. When the recurrent CNV is subfoveal, we recommend photodynamic therapy if the angiographic characteristics qualifies it for treatment although the effects of prior macular translocation on the response of the CNV to photodynamic therapy is currently unknown. Observation and submacular surgery are other management options. We do not recommend repeat macular translocation because of a high risk of retinal detachment and proliferative vitreoretinopathy.

Conclusion

Macular translocation is a procedure that has the potential for visual acuity improvement. Appropriate patient selection optimizes the visual outcomes with this procedure. By establishing effective forms of retinal function evaluation in eyes with subfoveal CNV, it is possible to better select patients with higher chances of visual improvement and avoid surgery in eyes without viable foveal cells. Complications can be minimized by surgeon experience and improved surgical techniques. Several contributions in the literature over the past few years indicate that, with appropriate surgical technique and careful patient selection, eyes with subfoveal CNV may benefit from macular translocation.

References

1. Hawkins BS, Bird A, Klein R, West SK (1999) Epidemiology of age-related macular degeneration. Mol Vis 5:26

2. Bressler NM (2001) Photodynamic therapy of subfoveal choroidal neovascularization in age-related macular degeneration with verteporfin: two-year results of 2 randomized clinical trials-tap report 2. Arch Ophthalmol 119:198–207

3. Verteporfin therapy of subfoveal choroidal neovascularization in age-related macular degeneration: two-year results of a randomized clinical trial including lesions with occult with no classic choroidal neovascularization–verteporfin in photodynamic therapy report 2 (2001). Am J Ophthalmol 131:541–60

4. Photodynamic therapy of subfoveal choroidal neovascularization in pathologic myopia with verteporfin (2001) 1-year results of a randomized clinical trial–VIP report no. 1. Ophthalmology 108:841–52

5. Macular Photocoagulation Study Group (1991) Laser photocoagulation of subfoveal neovascular lesions in age-related macular degeneration. Results of a randomized clinical trial. Arch Ophthalmol 109:1220–31

6. Macular Photocoagulation Study Group (1994) Visual outcome after laser photocoagulation for subfoveal choroidal neovascularization secondary to age-related macular degeneration. The influence of initial lesion size and initial visual acuity. Arch Ophthalmol 112:480–8

7. Macular Photocoagulation Study Group (1993) Laser photocoagulation of subfoveal neovascular lesions of age-related macular degeneration. Updated findings from two clinical trials. Arch Ophthalmol 111:1200–9

8. Beatty S, Au Eong KG, McLeod D, Bishop PN (1999) Photocoagulation of subfoveal choroidal neovascular membranes in age related macular degeneration: the impact of the macular photocoagulation study in the United Kingdom and Republic of Ireland. Br J Ophthalmol 83:1103–4

9. Au Eong KG, Pieramici DJ, Fujii GY, Ng EW, Humayun MS, Maia M, Harlan JB, Jr, Schachat AP, Beatty S, Toth CA, Thomas MA, Lewis H, Eckardt C, Tano Y, De Juan E (2001) Macular translocation: unifying concepts, terminology, and classification. Am J Ophthalmol 131:244–53

** A panel of ophthalmologists with expertise in macular translocation reviewed available data and developed some unifying concepts, terminology, and classification of macular translocation to facilitate communication within the scientific community

10. Lindsey P, Finkelstein D, D'Anna S (1983) Experimental retinal rotation. ARVO abstracts Invest Ophthalmol Vis Sci 24:242

11. Tiedeman J, de Juan E, Machemer R, Hatchell DL, Hatchell MC (1985) Surgical relocation of the macula. ARVO abstracts. Invest Ophthalmol Vis Sci 26:59

12. Machemer R, Steinhorst UH (1993) Retinal separation, retinotomy, and macular relocation: II. A surgical approach for age-related macular degeneration? Graefes Arch Clin Exp Ophthalmol 231:635–41

13. Eckardt C, Eckardt U, Conrad HG (1999) Macular rotation with and without counter-rotation of the globe in patients with age-related macular degeneration. Graefes Arch Clin Exp Ophthalmol 237:313–25

14. Wirostko WJ, Mittra RA, Rao PK, Borrillo JL, Dev S, Mieler WF (2000) A combination light-pipe, soft-tipped suction, and infusion cannula instrument for macular translocation. Am J Ophthalmol 129:549–51

15. Akduman L, Karavellas MP, MacDonald JC, Olk RJ, Freeman WR (1999) Macular translocation with retinotomy and retinal rotation for exudative age-related macular degeneration. Retina 19:418–23

16. Ninomiya Y, Lewis JM, Hasegawa T, Tano Y (1996) Retinotomy and foveal translocation for surgical management of subfoveal choroidal neovascular membranes. Am J Ophthalmol 122:613–21

17. Imai K, de Juan E, Jr (1996) Experimental surgical macular relocation by scleral shortening. ARVO abstracts. Invest Ophthalmol Vis Sci 37[Suppl]:S116

18. de Juan E, Jr, Loewenstein A, Bressler NM, Alexander J (1998) Translocation of the retina for management of subfoveal choroidal neovascularization II: a preliminary report in humans. Am J Ophthalmol 125:635–46

19. de Juan E, Jr, Vander JF (1999) Effective macular translocation without scleral imbrication. Am J Ophthalmol 128:380–2

20. Fujii GY, De Juan E, Au EK, Harlan JB (2001) Effective nasal limited macular translocation. Am J Ophthalmol 132:124–6

21. Fujii GY, de Juan E, Jr, Hartranft CD, Jensen PS (2000) Limited macular translocation. In: Ryan S (ed) Retina. St Louis: CV Mosby, 2580–96

22. de Juan E, Jr, Fujii GY (2001) Limited macular translocation. Eye 15:413–23

23. Kamei M, Roth DB, Lewis H (2000) Macular translocation using scleral clips to create an out-pouching radial fold of the sclera, choroid and retinal pigment epithelium [abstract]. ARVO abstracts. Invest Ophthalmol Vis Sci 41:S540

24. Lewis H (2001) Macular translocation with chorioscleral outfolding: a pilot clinical study. Am J Ophthalmol 132:156–63

25. Benner JD, Meyer CH, Shirkey BL, Toth CA (2001) Macular translocation with radial scleral ouffolding: experimental studies and initial human results. Graefes Arch Clin Exp Ophthalmol 239:815–23

26. Fujikado T, Ohji M, Hosohata J, Hayashi A, Oda K, Tano Y (2000) Comparison of visual function after foveal translocation with 360 degrees retinotomy and with scleral shortening in a patient with bilateral myopic neovascular maculopathy. Am J Ophthalmol 130:525–7

27. Hayashi A, Usui S, Kawaguchi K, Fujioka S, Kusaka S, Fujikado T, Ohji M, Tano Y (2000) Retinal changes after retinal translocation surgery with scleral imbrication in dog eyes. Invest Ophthalmol Vis Sci 41:4288–92

28. Deramo VA, Meyer CH, Toth CA (2001) Successful macular translocation with temporary scleral infolding using absorbable sture. Retina 21:304–11

29. Glacet-Bernard A, Simon P, Hamelin N, Coscas G, Soubrane G (2001) Translocation of the macula for management of subfoveal choroidal neovascularization: comparison of results in age-related macular degeneration and degenerative myopia. Am J Ophthalmol 131:78–89

30. Kim T, Krishnasamy S, Meyer CH, Toth CA (2001) Induced corneal astigmatism after macular translocation surgery with scleral infolding. Ophthalmology 108:1203–8

31. Lewis H, Kaiser PK, Lewis S, Estafanous M (1999) Macular translocation for subfoveal choroidal neovascularization in age- related macular degeneration: a prospective study. Am J Ophthalmol 128:135–46

32. Lin SB, Glaser BM, Gould D, Baudo TA, Lakhanpal RR, Murphy RP (2000) Scleral outfolding for macular translocation. Am J Ophthalmol 130:76–81

33. Ohji M, Fujikado T, Saito Y, Hosohata J, Hayashi A, Tano Y (1998) Foveal translocation: a comparison of two techniques. Semin Ophthalmol 13:52–62

34. Ohtsuki H, Shiraga F, Hasebe S, Kono R, Yamane T, Fujiwara H (2001) Correction of cyclover-tical strabismus induced by limited macular translocation in a case of age-related macular degeneration. Am J Ophthalmol 131:270–2

35. Pieramici DJ, De Juan E, Fujii GY, Reynolds SM, Melia M, Humayun MS, Schachat AP, Hartranft CD (2000) Limited inferior macular translocation for the treatment of subfoveal choroidal neovascularization secondary to age-related macular degeneration. Am J Ophthalmol 130:419–28

36. Potter MJ, Chang TS, Lee AS, Rai S (2000) Improvement in macular function after retinal translocation surgery in a patient with age-related macular degeneration. Am J Ophthalmol 129:547–9

37. Toth CA, Freedman SF (2001) Macular translocation with 360-degree peripheral retinectomy impact of technique and surgical experience on visual outcomes. Retina 21:293–303

38. Wong D, Harding S, Grierson I (2000) Foveal translocation with secondary confluent laser for subfoveal CNV in AMD: 12 month follow up. Br J Ophthalmol 84:670–1

39. Wong D, Lois N (2000) Foveal relocation by redistribution of the neurosensory retina. Br J Ophthalmol 84:352–7

40. Fujii GY, Humayun MS, Pieramici DJ, Schachat AP, Au Eong KG, de Juan E Jr (2001) Initial experience of inferior limited macular translocation for subfoveal choroidal neovascularization resulting from causes other than age-related macular degeneration. Am J Ophthalmol 131:90–100

41. Fujikado T, Ohji M, Hayashi A, Kusaka S, Tano Y (1998) Anatomic and functional recovery of the fovea after foveal translocation surgery without large retinotomy and simultaneous excision of a neovascular membrane. Am J Ophthalmol 126:839–42

42. Fujikado T, Ohji M, Saito Y, Hayashi A, Tano Y (1998) Visual function after foveal translocation with scleral shortening in patients with myopic neovascular maculopathy. Am J Ophthalmol 125:647–56

43. Ichibe M, Imai K, Ohta M, Hasebe H, Yoshizawa T, Abe H (2001) Foveal translocation with scleral imbrication in patients with myopic neovascular maculopathy. Am J Ophthalmol 132:164–71
44. Kadonosono K, Takeuchi S, Iwata S, Uchio E, Itoh N, Akura J (2001) Macular fold after limited macular translocation treated with scleral shortening release and intravitreal gas. Am J Ophthalmol 132:790–2
45. Roth DB, Estafanous M, Lewis H (2001) Macular translocation for subfoveal choroidal neovascularization in angioid streaks. Am J Ophthalmol 131:390–2
46. Terasaki H, Miyake Y, Suzuki T, Nakamura M, Nagasaka T (2002) Polypoidal choroidal vasculopathy treated with macular translocation: clinical pathological correlation. Br J Ophthalmol 86:321–7
47. Fujii GY, De Juan E, Thomas MA, Pieramici DJ, Humayun MS, Au Eong KG (2001) Limited macular translocation for the management of subfoveal retinal pigment epithelial loss after submacular surgery. Am J Ophthalmol 131:272–5
48. Haller JA, Hartranft CD, Fujii GY, Pieramici D, Humayun MS, de Juan E Jr (2000) Limited macular translocation for neovascular maculopathy. Semin Ophthalmol 15:81–7
49. Faude F, Wendt S, Biedermann B, Gartner U, Kacza J, Seeger J, Reichenbach A, Wiedemann P (2001) Facilitation of artificial retinal detachment for macular translocation surgery tested in rabbit. Invest Ophthalmol Vis Sci 42:1328–37
50. Faude F, Wiedemann P, Reichenbach A (1999) A "detachment infusion" for macular translocation surgery. Retina 19:173–4
51. Fang XY, Hayashi A, Cekic O, Morimoto T, Ohji M, Kusaka S, Kamei M, Fujikado T, Tano Y (2001) Effect of Ca(2+)-free and Mg(2+)-free BSS Plus solution on the retinal pigment epithelium and retina in rabbits. Am J Ophthalmol 131:481–8
52. Kamei M, Roth DB, Lewis H (2001) Macular translocation with chorioscleral outfolding: an experimental study. Am J Ophthalmol 132:149–55
53. Freedman SF, Seaber JH, Buckley EG, Enyedi LB, Toth CA (2000) Combined superior oblique muscle recession and inferior oblique muscle advancement and transposition for cyclotorsion associated with macular translocation surgery. J AAPOS 4:75–83
54. Ohji M, Fujikado T, Kusaka S, Hayashi A, Hosohata J, Ikuno Y, Sawa M, Kubota A, Hashida N, Tano Y (2001) Comparison of three techniques of foveal translocation in patients with subfoveal choroidal neovascularization resulting from age-related macular degeneration. Am J Ophthalmol 132:888–96
55. Fujii GY, De Juan E, Sunness JS, Humayun MS, Pieramici DJ, Chang TS (2002) Patient selection for macular translocation surgery using scanning laser ophthalmoscope. Ophthalmology 109:1737–44
56. Fujii GY, de Juan EJr, Pieramici DJ, Humayun MS, Phillips S, Reynolds SM, Melia M, Schachat AP (2002) Inferior limited macular translocation for subfoveal choroidal neovascularization secondary to age-related macular degeneration: one-year visual outcome and recurrence report. Am J Ophthalmol 134:69–74
57. Fujii GY, Pieramici DJ, Humayun MS, Schachat AP, Reynolds SM, Melia M, De Juan E (2000) Complications associated with limited macular translocation. Am J Ophthalmol 130:751–62
58. Au Eong KG, Fujii GY, Ng EW, Humayun MS, Pieramici DJ, de Juan E Jr (2001) Transient formed visual hallucinations following macular translocation for subfoveal choroidal neovascularization secondary to age-related macular degeneration. Am J Ophthalmol 131:664–6

Correspondence: Eugene de Juan, Jr, MD, The Retina Institute, Doheny Eye Institute, The Keck School of Medicine, University of Southern California, 1450 San Pablo St, DEI-3600, Los Angeles, CA 90033, USA, E-mail: dejuan@usc.edu

Two-year results after macular translocation with 360° retinotomy

S. Aisenbrey[1], G. Thumann[2], and K. U. Bartz-Schmidt[1]

[1] Center of Ophthalmology, Eberhard-Karls University, Tübingen, Germany
[2] Department of Ophthalmology, University of Cologne, Germany

Abstract

Background: Macular rotation surgery comprises surgical extraction of choroidal neo-vascular membranes in age-related macular degeneration (AMD) and translocation of the foveal neural retina over adjacent retinal pigment epithelium.

Objective: To determine whether macular translocation with 360° retinotomy can stabilize and/or improve visual acuity in patients with subfoveal choroidal neovascularization (CNV) secondary to AMD.

Design: This study consisted of a standardized surgical procedure on a series of 90 consecutive patients and follow-up examinations at fixed intervals for 24 months.

Participants: All patients in this study had experienced recent visual loss resulting from subfoveal CNV caused by AMD. Twenty-six patients had major macular subretinal hemorrhage, 39 patients had occult subfoveal CNV, and 25 patients had classic subfoveal CNV.

Methods: Macular translocation surgery was performed between 1997 and 1999. The patients were examined preoperatively and at 3, 6, 12 and 24 months postoperatively; examination included visual acuity, microperimetry, angiography, and orthoptic assessment.

Results: Visual acuity increased by 15 or more letters in 24 patients, remained stable in 37 patients, and deteriorated by 15 or more letters in 29 patients at 12 months; at 24 months, visual acuity improved in 16 patients, remained stable in 24 patients, and worsened in 38 patients. A secondary procedure was necessary in 17 patients because of severe complications; proliferative vitreoretinopathy was observed in 17 eyes, macular pucker in 5 eyes, and macular hole in one patient.

Conclusions: Macular translocation is a technically demanding surgical procedure. Although the procedure has a high rate of surgical and postoperative complications, the functional and anatomical results appear to be promising for selected patients with subfoveal CNV secondary to AMD.

Introduction

Age-related macular degeneration (AMD) is the leading cause of severe visual loss among the elderly in Western societies. Approximately 10 to 20% of patients with AMD develop the exudative type of this disease, which is characterized by choroidal neovascularization (CNV). Growth of new vessels from the choroid through Bruch's membrane and into the subretinal space causes exudation and hemorrhagic lesions accompanied by progressive visual loss, resulting in the formation of disciform scars with loss of photoreceptors.

Treatment options for subfoveal CNV are limited. Until the approval of photodynamic therapy (PDT), the only proven therapy for subfoveal CNV was laser photocoagulation. PDT is now suggested for patients with relatively small, predominatly classic or 100% occult lesions; however, the majority of patients with exudative AMD are not candidates for PDT [23]. Conventional surgical extraction of subfoveal neovascular membranes is not particularly helpful because the underlying RPE is invariably removed resulting in poor visual outcome. Furthermore, several studies have shown progression of atrophy after membrane extraction and recurrence of CNV in 30 to 40% of patients [4, 5, 6, 9, 13, 18, 21]. Several modifications of the simple extraction have been suggested to improve its success rate. Transplantation of iris (IPE) or retinal pigment epithelial (RPE) cells after removal of the CNV may be beneficial, but only a limited number of pilot studies are available [1, 14, 22].

Macular translocation is a new surgical technique for the treatment of exudative macular degeneration. The idea of translocating the neurosensory retina away from the subfoveal abnormalities to a healthier appearing RPE and choriocapillaris was first proposed in 1983 by Lindsey et al. [16]. Machemer and Steinhorst reported the results of this surgical procedure in humans in 1993 [17]. The technique used in our series is a modification of the original macular translocation proposed by Machemer. In this surgical approach the retina is detached from the RPE and rotated such that the fovea is relocated in contact with an area of healthy RPE. Theoretically, if the fovea is relocated in contact with healthy RPE there is the potential for improved visual function. Currently two different surgical approaches are used to achieve translocation of the macula, namely macular translocation with large retinotomies of up to 360° or limited rotation using scleral shortening or scleral imbrication [2, 3, 7, 8, 10, 11, 12, 15, 19, 20, 24]. Macular translocation with a large retinotomy allows the treatment of larger lesions than the technique of limited rotation, which was first described by de Juan. In order to compensate for induced cyclotropia, Eckardt and Eckardt suggested the combination of macular translocation with counterrotation of the globe in 1998.

The goal of our study was to evaluate visual and anatomical outcomes in a prospective case series of 90 patients suffering from exudative AMD. After publishing the 1-year results of this study in 2002, we now report the functional outcomes at 2 years after macular translocation with 360° retinotomy.

Methods

Patients

Between December 1997 and December 1999, 90 eyes of 90 patients were followed in a prospective consecutive case series. Criteria for inclusion consisted of (1) age of 50 years or older, (2) best-corrected visual acuity of 20/50 or less in the eligible eye, (3) evidence of drusen, (4) new or recurrent choroidal neovascularization that involved the geometric center of the foveal avascular zone or subfoveal hemorrhages secondary to adjacent choroidal neovascularization and (5) informed consent. Ocular criteria for exclusion consisted of disciform lesions, pigment epithelial tears, polypoidal vasculopathy, deep retinal anomalous complexes, and eyes with recurrent membranes after conventional membrane extraction or laser photocoagulation. The age of the patients (29 men and 61 women) ranged from 58 to 90 years with a mean of 75 years of age. The affected eye was the right eye in 53 patients and the left eye in 47 patients. In 23 patients, the eye that underwent surgery was the eye with the worst visual acuity, whereas in 67 patients the eye that underwent surgery had a visual acuity better than the contralateral eye.

Examination

Preoperatively, all patients underwent a comprehensive ophthalmologic examination, including anterior segment biomicroscopy, intraocular pressure measurement, and fundus examination with slit-lamp biomicroscopy. Best-corrected distance visual acuity was measured by a certified visual examiner with the use of the Early Treatment Diabetic Retinopathy Study (ETDRS) chart according to a fixed protocol. Color photographs of the macula and the disc of each eye as well as a fluorescein and an indocyanin green angiogram were taken and microperimetry of the macula of the study eye was performed by scanning laser ophthalmoscopy. Orthoptic examinations usually included measurements of subjective monocular cyclorotation by Maddox rod cylinder at a distance of 40 cm, the light bar of Harms screen at a distance of 1 m, and additionally the Hirschberg test, the cover test, the test with Bagolini striated glasses and the Titmus fly test. Based on a review of the angiograms, patients were assigned to one of three groups: hemorrhagic CNV of at least one disc area involving the fovea, predominantly occult CNV, and predominantly classic CNV.

Patients were scheduled to return for follow-up at 3,6,9,12 and 24 months after surgery; at each follow-up visit the examinations were the same as preoperatively. The primary efficacy outcome was the change in visual acuity (logMAR) of the study eye at 2 years after surgery compared with the visual acuity at the baseline examination.

Surgery

Macular translocation surgery was performed under general anesthesia. In phakic eyes, the lens was removed by means of phacoemulsification and a foldable acrylic posterior chamber lens was implanted. In all patients a three-port pars plana vitrectomy was performed, a posterior vitreous detachment was induced and the peripheral vitrectomy was completed as far as possible. To induce the retinal detachment, BSS was injected through a small retinotomy usually performed in 'the inferior midperiphery' using a specially designed "detachment" cannula. Once the retina was detached, liquid perfluorcarbon was injected into the vitreous cavity and a 360° peripheral retinotomy was performed just posterior to the ora serrata. The perfluorcarbon was subsequently removed. Using a silicone tipped extension needle, the temporal retina was lifted and pulled nasally. With care, the neovascular membrane was extracted and detached from the underlying Bruch's membrane with micro-forceps. Any hemorrhage from feeder vessels was coagulated by bipolar diathermy. Liquid semifluorane was injected into the vitreous cavity to stabilize the posterior retina. The retina was translocated to its new position with a silicone-tipped extrusion needle. Rotation of the fovea was usually performed superiorly, only in a few cases the fovea was rotated inferiorly. Once the fovea was rotated to the desired position, the retina was entirely unfolded by injection of perfluorocarbon liquid. Laser retinopexy was applied around the midperipheral retinotomies and adjacent to the border of the 360° peripheral retinotomy. The perfluorocarbon-semifluorane liquid mixture was exchanged for silicone oil of 5000 cSt.

In a first series of patients, the excyclorotation of the eye was performed in combination with the primary vitrectomy. If subjective cyclorotation persisted, surgical revision on the eye muscles was done together with silicone oil removal. In a second series of patients,

eye muscle surgery was not performed together with primary retinal surgery but with silicone oil removal. In these cases, subjective cyclorotation caused by retinal rotation could
be assessed before muscle surgery and thus ocular counterrotation could be better
adjusted.

Results

Ninety eyes in 90 patients with CNV due to AMD were treated with macular translocation. Preoperatively, best corrected visual acuity ranged from hand-movement to 20/63
(median 20/200), and patients with occult CNV had significantly better visual acuity
compared to patients with hemorrhages. Preoperative fluorescein angiography showed
classic subfoveal choroidal neovascularization in 25 eyes and occult or mixed subfoveal
choroidal neovascularization in 39 eyes. Subfoveal hemorrhage secondary to CNV was
observed in 26 eyes. The two-year follow-up was completed in 78 of the 90 patients.

Twelve months after macular translocation, best-corrected visual acuity ranged from
hand-movements to 20/40. Twenty-four patients showed improvement of visual acuity of
3 lines or more from baseline on the ETDRS chart, 42 patients retained stable visual acuity
with a change of less than 3 lines and 34 patients showed decreased visual acuity of 3
lines or more. At 24 months, best-corrected visual acuity ranged from light perception to
20/40. Sixteen patients showed improvement of visual acuity of 3 lines or more from
baseline on the ETDRS chart, 24 patients remained within 0.2 logMAR units of their preoperative score, and 38 patients showed decreased visual acuity of 3 lines or more.

After muscle surgery the angle of subjective cyclorotation was less than 7 degrees in
the operated eye in 26% of patients. In one third of these patients we obtained a positive test for binocular single vision using Bagolini striated glasses. One of these patients
even had a positive Titmus fly test. In 74% of the patients subjective cyclorotation measured more than 7 degrees; in 18 patients cyclorotation measurement was not performed
postoperatively. A total of 28% of patients complained of persistent diplopia.

In preoperative angiograms, the size of the choroidal neovascular complex varied from
0.5 to 4.5 disc diameters in patients with classic CNV, 0.75 to 7.5 disc diameters in
patients with occult CNV and 1 to 9 disc diameters in patients with subretinal hemorrhages. Postoperatively, the extent of the atrophic lesion was 1.5 to 6.5 disc diameters for
the first group, 1 to 4.5 disc diameters for the second group and 1.5 to 4 disc diameters
for the last group. At 12 months, seventy-eight patients showed conspicuous areas of
hyper- and hypopigmentation reflecting alterations of the RPE within the arcades. Chronic
macular edema with late phase hyperfluorescence without evidence of persistent or
recurrent neovascularization was observed in 36 eyes. A recurrent choroidal neovascularization with progressive leakage in the late phase was detected by angiography in three
patients. At 12 months, retinal rotation was sufficient to relocate the foveal center out of
the atrophic zone in 77 of 89 patients (Fig. 1), in 12 of 89 eyes the fovea was still located
within an area of retinal atrophy; most of these 12 eyes belonged to patients with massive
subretinal hemorrhage preoperatively. Comparison of preoperative and postoperative fluorescein and indocyanine green angiography allowed the calculation of the direction and
angle of macular translocation: the foveal center was displaced superiorly in 94 eyes and
inferiorly in 6 eyes. The extent of translocation varied from 10 to 60 degrees (median 31
degrees). All eyes showed corneal erosion immediately following surgery secondary to
the corneal abrasion that was done to improve intraoperative visibility. In two patients
acrylic intraocular lenses implanted during the original surgical procedure had to be
exchanged because of dislocation and iris capture. In one eye, silicone oil droplets
adhered to a previously implanted silicone intraocular lens; these silicone oil droplets on
the lens were removed using semifluorinated alcanes (F_6H_8). Two eyes showed persistent

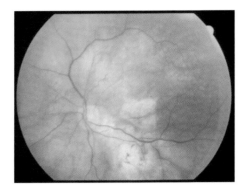

Fig. 1. Postoperative fundus photograph of the left eye of an 80 years old female patient 42 months after macular translocation, demonstrating the new center relocated outside the center of choroidal atrophy

ocular hypotony after macular translocation and silicone oil removal with intraocular pressure not rising over 8 mmHg. One patient developed persistent corneal decompensation and required a corneal transplant. Recurrent CNV occurred in 3 patients, with the vessels always growing towards the new foveal center; in two of these patients the recurrent membrane complex was removed surgically, in the other patient the CNV was treated by photocoagulation since the CNV was excentric to the new foveal center. Primary proliferative vitreoretinopathy developed in 9 eyes following vitrectomy; secondary proliferative vitreoretinopathy with retinal detachment following silicone oil removal was observed in 10 eyes; macular pucker was observed in 5 eyes; peripheral epiretinal membranes in 7 eyes and a persistent macular hole in one eye. All these patients were treated surgically to reattach the retina or remove neovascular membranes. All of these complications were observed in the first year after surgery and no further complications occurred during the second year after surgery.

Discussion

For the first time we present a large consecutive series of patients that underwent macular translocation with 360° retinotomy for the treatment of exudative age-related macular degeneration with a follow-up of two years.

At present, macular translocation seems to be a promising therapeutic option, which offers the possiblity of improving vision in patients suffering from AMD.

In our series, two years after surgery 16/78 patients showed significant improvement of vision and another 24 patients retained stable visual acuity. However, approximately half of the patients showed deteriorated VA at 24 months. A secondary procedure due to severe complications was necessary in 25 cases. In 19 of the 25 eyes the complications were due to PVR, a rate which theoretically could be reduced by improving the surgical technique and shortening the duration of surgery.

A significant number of patients experienced deterioration of visual function, although they did not have any complications and showed a healthy-appearing funduscopic picture. Possibly in these cases, a significant part of the pigment epithelium was translocated along with the retina, as previously described in the literature. Other explanations might be associated with the type of the original neovascular membrane, the preoperative condition of the pigment epithelium and the adhesion between pigment epithelium and retina.

The precise indications for macular translocation are not yet well defined. However, we found a significantly better functional outcome after macular translocation in patients with classic CNV or hemorrhages than in patients with occult CNV. Furthermore, the rate of retinal detachment representing the most significant retinal complication was lower in patients with classic CNV than in patients with occult CNV. In the two eyes with recurrent subfoveal choroidal neovascularization after laser photocoagulation we could not separate the sensory retina from the photocoagulation scar without mechanical manipulation and creation of a large RPE defect. Thus, macular translocation should not be recommended for patients previously treated with laser photocoagulation for choroidal neovascular membranes.

In a small series of our patients who underwent macular translocation we performed conventional and multifocal electroretinograms pre- and one month postoperatively. The electrophysiological data indicated a reduction of photopic and scotopic amplitudes for all patients after macular translocation with 360° retinotomy.

Macular translocation with 360° retinotomy offers the possibility to treat patients with classic CNV as well as occult CNV or massive hemorrhages and CNV of a larger size, compared to laser photocoagulation and photodynamic therapy.

Macular translocation with 360° retinotomy is a promising new surgical technique for the treatment of subfoveal CNV and it is not limited by the size, the nature, or the potential obscuration of the lesion. Our study indicates that macular translocation can stabilize, and sometimes improve visual acuity in the majority of patients. A clearer picture of the role of macular translocation with 360° retinotomy in the treatment of subfoveal neovascularization will emerge when the results from an international randomized, multicenter trial, the MARAN study, will become available.

References

1. Abe T, Yoshida M, Kano T, Tamai M (2001) Visual function after removal of subretinal neovascular membranes in patients with age-related macular degeneration. Graefe's Arch Clin Exp Ophthalmol 239:927–36
2. Aisenbrey S, Lafaut BA, Szurman P, Grisanti S, Fricke J, Neugebauer A, Thumann G, Walter P, Bartz-Schmidt KU (2002) Macular translocation with 360° retinotomy for exudative age-related macular degeneration. Arch Ophthalmol 120:451–9
3. Akduman L, Karavellas M, MacDonald C, Olk J, Freeman W (1999) Macular translocation with retinotomy and retinal rotation for exudative age-related macular degeneration. Retina 19: 418–23
4. Benson MT, Callear A, Tsaloumas M, China J, Beatty S (1998) Surgical excision of subfoveal neovascular membranes. Eye 12:768–74
5. Berger AS, Kaplan HJ (1992) Clinical experience with the surgical removal of subfoveal neovascular membranes. Ophthalmology 99:969–75
6. Berglin L, Algvere P, Olivestedt G, Crafoord S, Stenkula S, Hansson LJ, Tomic Z, Kvanta A, Seregard S (2001) The Swedish national survey of surgical excision for submacular choroidal neovascularization (CNV). Acta Ophthalmol Scand 79:580–4
7. De Juan E, Loewenstein A, Bressler NM, Alexander J (1998) Translocation of the retina for management of subfoveal choroidal neovascularization II: A preliminary report in humans. Am J Ophthalmol 125:635–46
8. De Juan E, Vander JF (1999) Effective macular translocation without scleral imbrication. Am J Ophthalmol 128:380–2
9. Eckardt C (1996) Surgical removal of submacular neovascularization membranes. Ophthalmologe 93:688–93
10. Eckardt C, Eckardt U, Conrad HJ (1999) Macular rotation with and without counter-rotation of the globe in patients with age-related macular degeneration. Graefe's Arch Clin Exp Ophthalmol 237:313–25

11. Fujikado T, Ohji M, Hayashi A, Kusaka S, Tano Y (1998) Anatomic and functional recovery of the fovea after foveal translocation surgery without large retinotomy and simultaneous excision of a neovascular membrane. Am J Ophthalmol 126:839–42

12. Lai JC, Lapolice DJ, Stinnett SS, Meyer CH, Arieu LM, Keller MA, Toth CA (2002) Visual outcomes following macular translocation with 360° peripheral retinotomy. Arch Ophthalmol 120:1317–24

13. Lambert HM, Capone AJ, Aaberg TM, Strenberg PJ, Mandell BA, Lopez PF (1992) Surgical excision of subfoveal neovascular membranes in age-related macular degeneration. Am J Ophthalmol 113:257–62

14. Lappas A, Weinberger AWA, Foerster AMH, Kube Th, Kirchhof B (2000) Iris pigment epithelium translocation in age-related macular degeneration. Graefe's Arch Exp Clin Ophthalmol 238:631–41

15. Lewis H, Kaiser P, Lewis S, Estafanous M (1999) Macular translocation for subfoveal choroidal neovascularization in age-related macular degeneration: A prospective study. Am J Ophthalmol 128:135–46

16. Lindsey P, Finkelstein D, D'Anna S (1983) Experimental retinal relocation. ARVO abstracts. Invest Ophthalmol Vis Sci 24[Suppl 3]:242

17. Machemer R, Steinhorst UH (1993) Retinal seperation, retinotomy, and macular relocation: II. A surgical approach for age-related macular degeneration. Graefes Arch Clin Exp Ophthalmol 231:635–41

18. Merrill PT, LoRusso FJ, Lomeo MD, Saxe SJ, Khan MM, Lambert HM (1999) Surgical removal of subfoveal choroidal neovascularization in age-related macular degeneration. Ophthalmology 106:782–9

19. Ninomiya Y, Lewis JM, Hasegawa T, Tanoi Y (1996) Retinotomy and foveal translocation for surgical management of subfoveal choroidal neovascular membranes. Am J Ophthalmol 122:613–21

20. Pertile G, Claes C (2002) Macular translocation with 360 degree retinotomy for management of age-related macular degeneration with subfoveal choroidal neovascularization. Am J Ophthalmol 134:560–5

21. Scheider A, Gündisch O, Kampik A (1999) Surgical extraction of subfoveal choroidal new vessels and submacular hemorrhage in age-related macular degeneration: results of a prospective study. Graefe's Arch Clin Exp Ophthalmol 237:10–15

22. Thumann G, Aisenbrey S, Schraermeyer U, Lafaut B, Esser P, Walter P, Bartz-Schmidt KU (2000) Transplantation of autologous iris pigment epithelium transplantation after removal of choroidal neovascular membranes. Arch Ophthalmol 118:1350–9

23. Verteporfin in Photodynamic Therapy Study Group (2001) Verteporfin therapy of subfoveal choroidal neovascularization in age-related macular degeneration: Two-year Results of a randomized clinical trial including lesions with occult with no classic choroidal neovascularization. Verteporfin in Phtodynamic Therapy Report No. 2. Am J Ophthalmol 131:541–60

24. Wolf S, Lappas A, Weinberger A, Kirchhof B (1999) Macular translocation for surgical management of subfoveal choroidal neovascularizations in patients with AMD: first results. Graefe's Arch Clin Exp Ophthalmol 237:51–7

Correspondence: Dr. Sabine Aisenbrey, Center of Ophthalmology, Eberhard-Karls University Tübingen, Schleichstrasse 12–15, D-72070 Tübingen, Germany, E-mail: s.aisenbrey@uni-koeln.de

Cataract extraction in age-related macular degeneration: the ECAM-Study – an ongoing trial*

S. Brunner, C. I. Falkner, I. Krebs, A. Abri, and S. Binder

The Rudolph Foundation Hospital in Vienna, Department of Ophthalmology (Head: Prof. S. Binder), The Ludwig-Boltzmann-Institute for Retinology and Biomicroscopic Laser Surgery, Vienna, Austria

Introduction

Survey on AMD and cataract

At the end of the Millennium 6.5% of the population were older than 75 years [26], that means 500.000 people for Austria and 5.3 million for Germany, respectively.

Senile cataract and age-related macular degeneration (AMD) both belong to the most common causes of decreased vision and blindness in persons over 60 years.

These two age-related eye diseases do have a growing frequence because of the higher life expectancy in the civilized countries; e.g. the prevalence rate of AMD in persons over 40 is about 9.4% [1], rising up to 30% [6], and over 52% [31, 34] in the group between 70 and 90 years; variations belong to the selection of age groups and to different definitions of AMD.

In persons from 65–85 years, the cataract prevalence rates are about 53–80% [2], but only 44% in cases of coexistent age-related macular degeneration [6] – see Fig. 1.

Despite the fact that senile cataract is more common in elderly persons than AMD and even more often the cause of bilateral visual impairment, AMD definitely is the leading cause for blindness in industrialized nations in recent times.

Cataract surgery has proved to be a very efficient and safe procedure in recent years as a consequence of dramatic improvements in microsurgical techniques. In the decade from 1985–1995 cataract extractions worldwide rose up to 300%, as international statistics show. In particular, extractions in patients over 80 had an especially high increase (e.g. there was a 4-fold increase counted at the Singapore National Eye Centre).

Surgical rates in 1997 (i.e. number of cataract operations per million inhabitants per year) were 5000 for the USA and 3000 for western European countries, respectively. Tendency is going up further.

A growig coincidence is seen in case of cataract and AMD. Therefore, scientists are most interested to search for a possible uniform etiology to understand and influence both of the diseases.

Discussion on etiology

The reports on the influence of cataract extraction on the progression of preoperatively diagnosed AMD, are inconsistent for now. Thus, the mechanisms for postoperative (p.o.) macular edema or – degeneration are poorly understood [36–39].

---

*In accordance to the results of the round table discussion of Study Representatives of the 4 partner clinics on Nov. 25th, 2000 at the Bristol Hotel, Vienna, as well as to the correction of the IMS.

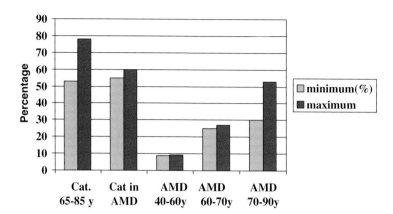

Fig. 1. Prevalence rates of Cataract and AMD in the second half of life. Compare [1, 2, 6, 24]

The course of (seldom) exsudative AMD seems to aggravate in the first six months after cataract surgery [9], however, but in cases of more common "dry" AMD, scientific opinions are highly conflicting.

Pollack [10] was looking for the clinical course of AMD during the first 3 years after cataract surgery. He noticed that AMD was increasing more often in operated eyes, as compared to the partner eyes, which was probably caused by phototoxicity.

Van der Schaft [11], on the other hand, did not call for the same theory. No significant changes in macular degenerations could be found in 82 post-mortal eyes, even if pseudophakic eyes with/without UV-filters were compared to each other.

The Beaver-Dam-Study [12] reported on a big longitudinal trial in 3684 adults from 43 to 86 years. The conclusion was that pseudophakic eyes may have a 2.8-fold risk for a progression in AMD after five years.

Other results were found out in Rotterdam study [13], where 6417 right eyes were investigated: on an average, no higher prevalence rates for atrophic or exsudative forms of AMD could be seen in eyes after cataract surgery when compared to phakic eyes.

In this context, it seems to be necessary to look not only for morphologic changes, since at least the same importance has to be contributed to patient's satisfaction and visual function.

Shuttleworth [14] was reporting on 99 patients having AMD, of whom 80% were discovering a significant improvement in vision after cataract extraction. Not less than 17% of them said that eye surgery had not been helpful to them.

More recently, Armbrecht and colleagues [26] were conducting a bi-centric, non-randomized trial on 187 cases of AMD. They found a clear improvement in vision after cataract surgery in "mild" to "moderate" forms of AMD.

However, investigative methods were not exactly the same in the two ophthalmologic centers.

Conclusions

There is still much to work and learn on our topic; especially large, prospective trials are needed. They might show us new pathogenetic factors or could contradict to older theories. All this would be very helpful for the ophthalmic professional to determine the optimal time for cataract surgery in his AMD-patient.

Nevertheless, this decision is influenced by many other factors, such as the patient's informed consent or his physical condition in general.

The co-operation to our patients indeed is of greatest importance to finally achieve a better quality of vision (and life) for them.

We were sure that the issues in ECAM-I may just be answered by pre-operative randomisation of our patients, since few literature has been published to this topic. Additionally, there are statistical deficits in most of the specific papers [9–14, 21, 26].

Therefore we started on a multi-centric trial (with further participation of three other ophthalmologic centers) in May 2002, in the way that has been described.

Study design

The trial *Extracapsular cataract extraction and course of age-related macular degeneration (ECAM-1)* shall describe the clinical course of pre-existent, non-exsudative forms of age-related macular degeneration (AMD) in the context of routine extracapsular cataract extraction by phacoemulsification.

The *main goal* of the ECAM-study is to test for a hypothetic association between cataract surgery and a faster progression of pre-existent AMD.

Furthermore, consequences for visual function and quality of life of our patients will be assessed.

Possible new risk factors for AMD as well as the influence of post-operative abnormalities on the promotion of AMD may be described.

It is our challenge now to contribute for an optimal point of time in cataract surgery of AMD-patients, in order to raise quality of vision and life for them.

Treatment options

Patients with advanced senile cataract and non-exsudative AMD will be randomized after looking for inclusion and exclusion criteria in ECAM-1.

Hence, 2 groups will be formed:

Group I: Control group with no surgery but observation for 6 months; 1 week after surgery, a final examination will be done. Just one eye per patient can be included.

Group II: Immediate cataract surgery (just one eye per patient); subsequently, there will be 6 months of observation.

Final variables

The main final variable is size of AMD (in percent of a well-defined region) after six months compared to the size at inclusion. The value of the main variable at the beginning of the trial will be taken into account as a co-variable.

Other final variables are changes in: visual acuity (distance and reading), gradings of cataract (LOCS-III), qualitative gradings of AMD, and a quality of life assessment by a modified VF 14-questionnaires.

Other variables are changes of: low contrast sensitivity (by acuity charts), visual acuity meter results, intraoculor pressure (AT), vitreous behaviour (ultrasound examinations) and inflammatory reactions (slit lamp).

Inclusion/exclusion criteria

Inclusion criteria

– Moderate forms of senile cataract in one or both eyes. Grading has to be done by the LOCS-III system [15, 33] and SL-pictures. *At minimum*, a grading of 2.1 has to be

reached in at least one sub-classification – nuclear, cortical or posterior subcapsular cataract.
– *Fundus insight* must be sufficient enough for fundus imaging, as FLA, SLO and digitized colour pictures.
– Non-exsudative, age-related macular degeneration with clinical importance (drusen with/without pigmentary anomalies, or circumscribed atrophy of pigment epithelium). The AMD shall match with the term "early AMD" in some international classifications [32]. *At minimum*, one point in our ECAM-scheme has to be reached.
– *Age* > 19 years.

Exclusion criteria

– Vascular retinopathy (diabetic and hypertensive retinopathies, former central retinal artery/vein occlusions)
– Late AMD-forms following the international classifications (exsudative AMD or final geographic macular atrophy)
– Atrophy of the optic nerve
– Glaucoma
– Mature cataract (no sufficient fundus insight)
– Former ophthalmic surgery or trauma in the same eye
– Myopia ≥ 10 diopters
– Patients with no compliance and/or suffering from multiple diseases

Methods

Statistical structure, randomization

In ECAM-I, 320 patients shall be randomized. That is, 160 patients in both of the groups (I or II) or 40 patients per group and clinical center.

ECAM-I will run for about 2 years, taking part in up to 4 ophthalmic centers.

At first, this is necessary to get the high sample size of 320 patients soon, which is needed for statistically significant results.

Secondly, we wish to avoid bias error from a specific surgical technique ("surgeon factor"). The participation of patients from different regions should also add to the scientific power of the trial.

Finally, an *observer-blinded analysis* and quantification of the main variable (Size of AMD) will be provided by participation of an independent, fifth Study Center.

Statistical analysis

The main variable (size of AMD after 6 months) will undergo Co-variance analysis (according to randomization) with the following fix factors:

Center (I-IV); Age ($\leq$65/>65); Cataract-Grading (<3/$\geq$3);
AMD-Grading (<3/$\geq$3); Treatment group (I/II).
The size of AMD at the beginning will be calculated as Co-variable.

Analysis of ordinal scaled or dichotomic variables will be done by the "Proportional-Odds-Model" or by logistic regression with respect to the same influence factors.

An explorative prognosis model will try to identify potential risk factors for a progression of AMD (we are thinking of a positive correlation to a progression in AMD in the following cases: postoperative bulbus hypotension, postoperative cyclitis and central vitreous traction).

The main criterion will be tested for therapeutic effects on the two-sided significance level of alpha = 0.05. Sample size will be calculated from the according numbers in the two-sided T-test for comparison of parallel groups.

With a sample size of 160 patients in each group, a systematic difference of therapies can be found in an amount of 1/3 of standard deviation with a probability of ≥0.8 (Power ≥ 80%).

Examinations (visual acuity, fundus imaging)

Distance acuity has to be tested by ETDRS-charts [16, 29] that have been proved in many trials.

For near acuity, RADNER-charts are needed [30]. *Contrast sensitivity* has to be tested by auto-refraction or other systems, such as the Pelli Robson Contrast Sensitivity charts. Every V.A. testing shall include an examination by V.A.-meter or retinometer.

Image angles should range from 30–40° (ideally, 35°) in mydriasis, after looking for sharpness and elimination of dispersion or reflexes.

We have developed a special scheme for AMD-classes (the ECAM-scheme) for a clinical differentiation of the three major types of dry AMD: drusen, confluent drusen and pigment epithelial atrophy.

Grading

All cataracts will be graded by the standardized LOCS-III-System [15, 33].

The patient's cataract has to be compared with the standardized retro-illuminated slides to get reproducible grading results. Grading must be done in 4 different categories, all of which the grading result has to be 2.1 or more in at least one category.

Digitized fundus images (SLO, FLA or infrared pictures) will be analyzed by semi-quantitative, computer-assisted processing. Pictures will be filtered by a special software with amplification of contrast in the green canal after removing shadows. AMD-related findings within a well-defined *region of interest* (=ROI) or *area of interest* (=AOI) of the retinal center will then be graded (aspect, number and size of pathologic findings).

The ROI/AOI is defined as a circle, centered in the fovea, with a diameter of 1,500 to 3,000 micrometers [19] or a 256 × 256-pixel area in the digitized fundus images.

Finally, all the lesions being typical for AMD, such as drusen, atrophic or exsudative changes, will be indicated in percent of ROI (see Fig. 2).

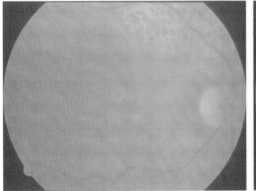 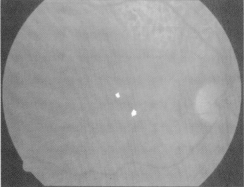

Fig. 2. Left Image: Colour photograph with early AMD showing two singular drusen. Right Image: After digitizing, total drusen area may be indicated as 1556/33250 pixels (i.e. 0.47%) of the ROI (region of interest)

Many advantages are calling for such a technique: First, the production of highly reproducible results with a specificity of 90%. Second, sensitivity does also correlate with conventional qualitative grading in 60–90%. Third, it is a time-and cost-saving system with an overall advantage for statistical analysis.

Surgical methods, p.o. medication

Surgical technique and postoperative medication in ECAM-I were brought into conformity with all participating Centers in November, 2000 in Vienna, as following:

- Local anaesthesia (subconjunctival or parabulbar)
- Small incision surgery (corneoscleral tunnel or *clear corneal incision*)
- Phacoemulsification, with implantation of a foldable lens in the capsular bag, no sutures if possible.
- Postoperative medication: Steroidal eye drops and/or ointment in the first week (eventually combined with NSAR = non-steroidal antirheumatics), followed by steroids and/or antiphlogistics for another three weeks.

Timetable for examinations

Timetable for Group I (late surgery):

	E-1 Admission	E-2 After 1 month	E-3 After 3 months	E-4 After 6 months	E-5 1 week postop.
Vis. Acuity (D/R), V.A. Meter,	X	X	X	X	X
Contrast Sensitivity, Slit Lamp	X	X	X	X	X
Grading AMD	X	X	X	X	X
Grading of Cataract, LOCS-III	X			X	
Images, semi-quantitat. Grad	X			X	X
FLA (SLO), Questionn, (Ultrasd.)	X			X	X

Timetable for Group II (early surgery):

	E-1 Admission	E-2 1 week postop.	E-3 1 month postop.	E-4 3 months postop.	E-5 6 months popstop.
Vis. Acuity (D/R), V.A. Meter,	X	X	X	X	X
Contrast Sensitivity, Slit Lamp	X	X	X	X	X
Grading AMD	X	X	X	X	X
Grading of Cataract, LOCS-III	X				
Images, Semi-quantit. Grad.	X	X			X
FLA (SLO), Question, (Ultrasd.)	X	X			X

Legend to timetables:
(postop. = postoperatively; E-1 to E-6 = Examination points; Vis. Acuity (D/R) = Visual acuity for distance and reading; FLA = Fluorescein Angiography Imaging, SLO = Scanning Laser Ophthalmoscopy, SL = Slit Lamp examinations (i.o. pressure, signs for inflammation, . . .).
Ultrasd. = A + B mode ultrasound of the vitreous body.

Actually included patients and discussion

Until September 2002, 11 patients (8 women and 3 men) had been included into the ECAM study. The average age was 80 years, and cataracts were predominantly nuclear in 6 cases and cortical in 5 cases. The average grading value was 3.5 in the LOCS-III-system.

In the first observation period, 40% of patients of the "early surgery" group had improvements in contrast sensitivity, whereas all of them had good improvements in visual acuity (distance and near acuity) of more than three lines as well as in the quality of life index.

The question on how to deal with cataracts in AMD patients is still an unsolved issue.

There were some studies suggesting no AMD-progression and a clear visual benefit after cataract extraction (Shuttleworth, Armbrecht, the Rotterdam study), however, some of the larger epidemiologic trials (Beaver Dam) found an increased risk for pseudophakic patients to develop late(r) AMD stages.

In general, there is pretty much scientific evidence that more advanced AMD stages have a higher tendency to progress after cataract surgery than earlier stages would do.

But where are the borders? And how could we define a highly reproducible and time-saving grading system to test for these borders?

Finally, what can we tell to our patients, seeking for medical support, and not a controversial discussion? We must take into account, that in cases of confirmed non-exsudative AMD, many patients will get a clear advantage in acuity, contrast sensitivity as well as their quality of life index, at least in the first 6 months. Moreover, most of these patients are far over 60 with a decreased life expectancy.

So we are curiously waiting to get more results published in the coming years.

Acknowledgements

Participating Eye Centers
- Univ.-Clinic for Opthalmology, Vienna (scheduled)
- The Rudolph Foundation Hospital, Vienna, Ophthalmic Department
- Univ.-Clinic for Ophthalmology, Innsbruck (scheduled)
- Univ. Eye Clinic of the Ludwig-Maximilians-University, Munich (scheduled)

Co-ordination
- The Rudolph Foundation Hospital, Vienna, Ophthalmic Department (Prof. Dr. S. Binder. Coordinator: Dr. S. Brunner)
- Univ.-Institute f. Medical Statistics, Vienna (IMS) (Prof. Dr. P. Bauer)

AMD-Grading Center (scheduled)
Dept. of Medical Physics, University of Aberdeen (Dr. A. Manivannan), Forresterhill, Aberdeen AB 25 2 ZD, Scotland, U.K.

Financial support
The study has been supported by the "Vienna's Headmaster Fund" as well as by ALCON-Int. company.

Ethical commission
The ECAM study passed the ethical commission board of the Rudolph Foundation hospital in Nov. 2000.

References (ECAM-I)

1. Klein R, Klein BEK, Jensen SC, Mares-Perlman JA, Cruickshanks KJ, Palta M (1999) Age-related maculopathy in a multiracial United States population. Ophthalmology 106:1056–65

2. Sperduto RD, Seigel D (1980) Senile lens and senile macular changes in a population-based sample. Am J Ophthalmol 90:86–91

3. Klein R, Wang Q, Klein BEK, Moss SE, Meuer SM (1995) The relationship of age-related maculopathy, cataract and glaucoma to visual acuity. Invest Ophthalmol Vis Sci 36:182–91

4. De la Paz MA (1998) Age-related macular degeneration: update and controversies. Advanced vitreous surgery course in: Duke University Eye Center

5. Young RW (1988) Solar radiation and age-related macular degeneration. Surv Ophthalmol 32:252–69

6. Gjessing HGA (1953) Gibt es einen Antagonismus zwischen Cataracta senilis und Haabscher seniler Makulaveränderungen? Acta Ophthalmol 31:401–21

7. Liu IY, White L, LaCroix AZ (1989) The association of age-related macular degeneration and lens opacities in the aged. Am J Public Health 79:765–9

8. Klein R, Klein BEK, Wang Q, Moss SE (1994) Is age-related maculopathy associated with cataracts? Arch Ophthalmol 112:191–6

9. Stolba U, Binder S, Velikay M (1989) Does cataract surgery with lens implantation influence the course of age-related macular degeneration? J Fr Ophthalmol 12:897–901

10. Pollack A, Markovich A, Bukelman A, Oliver M (1996) Age-related macular degeneration after extracapsular cataract extraction with intraocular lens implantation. Ophthalmology 103:1546–54

11. Van der Schaft TL, Mooy CM, de Bruijn WC, Mulder PGH, Pameyer JH, de Jong PTVM (1994) Increased prevalence of disciform macular degeneration after cataract extraction with implantation of an intraocular lens. Br J Ophthalmol 78:441–5

12. Klein R, Klein BEK, Jensen SC, Cruickshanks KJ (1998) The relationship of ocular factors to the incidence and progression of age-related maculopathy. Arch Ophthalmol 116:506–13

13. Vingerling JR, Klaver CCW, Hofman A, de Jong PTVM (1997) Cataract extraction and age-related macular degeneration: the Rotterdam study. Invest Ophthalmol Vis Sci 38(4):472

14. Shuttleworth GN, Luhishi EA, Harrad RA (1998) Do patients with age related maculopathy and cataract benefit from cataract surgery? Br J Ophthalmol 82:611–16

15. Chylack LT, Leske MC, Sperduto R, Khu P, McCarthy D (1988) Lens opacities classification system. Arch Ophthalmol 106:330–4

16. Vanden Bosch MA, Wall M (1997) Visual acuity scored by the letter-by-letter or probit methods has lower retest variability than the line assignment method. Eye 11:411–17

17. Halliday BL, Ross JE (1983) Comparison of 2 interferometers for predicting visual acuity in patients with cataract. Br J Ophthalmol 67:273–7

18. Klein RK, Davis MD, Magli YL, Segal P, Klein BEK, Hubbard L (1991) The Wisconsin age-related maculopathy grading system. Ophthalmology 98:1128–34

19. Shin DS, Javornik NB, Berger JW (1999) Computer-assisted, interactive fundus image processing for macular drusen quantitation. Ophthalmology 106:1119–25

20. Kirkpatrick JNP, Spencer T, Manivannan A, Sharp A (1995) Quantitative image analysis of macular drusen from fundus photographs and scanning laser ophthalmoscope images. Eye 9:48–55

21. Blair CJ, Ferguson J (1979) Exacerbation of senile macular degeneration following Cataract extraction. AJO 87:77–83

22. Barrett BT, Davison PA, Eustace P (1995) Clinical comparison of three techniques for evaluating visual function behind cataract. Eye 9:722–7

23. Munier A, Gunning T, Kenny D, O'Keefe M (1998) Causes of blindness in the adult population of the Republic of Ireland. Br J Ophthalmol 82(6):630–3

24. Ho T, Law MN, Goh LG, Yoong T (1997) Eye diseases in the elderly in Singapore. Singapore Med J 38(4):149–55

25. Reidy A, Minassian DC, Vafidis G, Joseph J, Farrow S, Wu J, Desai P (1998) Prevalence of serious eye disease and visual impairment in a north London population: population-based, cross-sectional study. BMJ 316(7145):1643–6

26. Armbrecht AM, Findlay C, Kaushal S, Aspinall P, Hill AR (2000) Is cataract surgery justified in patients with age related macular degeneration? A visual function and quality of life assessment. Br J Ophthalmol 84(12):1343–8

27. Steinberg EP, Tielsch JM, Schein OD, Javitt JC, Sharkey P, Cassard SD (1994) The VF-14 – An Index of functional impairment in patients with cataract. Arch Ophthalmol 112:630–8

28. Linder M, Chang TS, Scott IU, Hay D, Chambers K, Sibley LM, Weis E (1999) Validity of the Visual Function Index (VF-14) in patients with retinal disease. Arch Ophthalmol 117:1611–16

29. Early Treatment Diabetic Retinopathy Study (1985) Manual of Operations, Chapter 12

30. Radner W, Willinger U, Obermayer W, Mudrich C, Velikay-Parel M, Eisenwort B (1998) A new reading chart for simultaneous determination of reading vision and reading speed. Klin Monatsbl Augenheilkd 213(3):174–81

31. Vingerling JR, Dielemans I, Hofman A, Grobbee DE, Hijmering M (1995) The prevalence of age-related maculopathy in the Rotterdam study. Ophthalmology 102(2):205–10

32. Bird AC, Bressler NM, Bressler SB, Chisholm IH, Coscas G, Davis M, Jong PT, Klaver CC, Klein BE, Klein R, et al (1995) An international classification System for age-related maculopathy and age-related macular degeneration. The international ARM Epidemiological Study Group. Surv Ophthalmol 39(5):367–74

33. Chylack LT, Wolfe JK, Singer DM, Leske MC, Bullimore MA, Bailey IL (1993) The Lens Opacities Classification System III. Arch Ophthalmol 111:831–6

34. Dickinson AJ, Sparrow JM, Duke AM, Thompson JR, Gibson JM (1997) Prevalence of age-related maculopathy at two points in time in an elderly British population. Eye 11(Pt 3):301–14

35. Klaver CC, Vingerling JR (1997) Epidemiologie. In: Holz FG, Pauleikhoff D (Hrsg) Altersabhängige Makuladegeneration. Berlin, Heidelberg: Springer

36. Barraquer J, Troutman RC, Rutllan (1965) Die Chirurgie des vorderen Augenabschnittes, vol I. Stuttgart: Ferd. Enke Verlag

37. Wilkinson CP (1982) The natural course of CME occurring in pseudophakic eyes. 24th International Congress of Ophthalmology. San Francisco

38. Falcone PM (1996) Vitreomacular traction syndrome confused with pseudophakic cystoid macular edema. Ophthalmic Surg Lasers 27(5):392–4

39. Vinores SA, Amin A, Derevjanik NL (1994) Immunhistochemical localisation of blood-retinal barrier and breakdown sites associated with post-surgical macular edema. Histochem J 26(8):655–65

Correspondence: Dr. Simon Brunner, The Rudolph Foundation Hospital, Department of Ophthalmology, The Ludwig-Boltzmann-Institute for Retinology and Biomicroscopic Laser Surgery, Juchgasse 25, 1030 Vienna, Austria.

Combined phacoemulsification and lens implantation with vitreous surgery in macular disorders

C.E. Jahn, S. Binder, I. Krebs, U. Stolba, C. Mihalics, and A. Abri

Department of Ophthalmology, The Ludwig Boltzmann Institute for Retinology and
Biomicroscopic Laser Surgery, Rudolf Foundation Hospital, Vienna, Austria
(Chairman: Prof. Dr. Susanne Binder)

Introduction

Combined surgery became safer during the last years, because surgical techniques and new materials reached a high level of development in anterior and posterior segment surgery. Patients with cataract in combination with vitreoretinal diseases, especially with macular disorders, profit from these improvements.

Until 1992, when Malbran reported about his results in combined cases, surgery was usually restricted to indications like cataract with vitreous opacities and cataract with vitreous haemorrhage in eyes with less severe retinopathy, or simple vitreous haemorrhages after branch vein occlusion or spontaneous vascular rupture [1].

In this time there was the opinion, that an intraocular lens (IOL) should be not implanted, if the retinal situation showed active, proliferative disease and / or a retinal detachment. The decision whether an IOL should be implanted or not was made at the end of vitreous surgery, when the retinal situation could be jugded properly. The need of an intraocular tamponade was considered as a contraindication for a polymethyl-metacrylate (PMMA) – IOL, which necessitated an enlargement of the incision. This was due to the fear of lens dislocation, iris capture or wound dehiscense with irisprolaps and consequent delayed wound healing. Suturing a large wound always distores the corneal shape and makes view during vitreous surgery more difficult.

In 1994 and 1995 new foldable silicon lenses were implanted via a small incision, but soon it was realized, that they cannot be combined with a silicon oil tamponade. Biochemical alterations of these lenses can cause swelling and opacification of the implant, when the posterior capsule is open [2].

It has been noted that cataract extraction on eyes with previous vitrectomy is often more complicated because of various anatomic changes within the eye [3]. Other study groups have described deeper anterior chambers [4, 5], unstable lens capsules [4, 5, 6] and posterior capsular plaques [7].

The new generation of foldable acrylic lenses enlarged the indications for combined surgery because they allow an optimal view during surgery to the retina, can be implanted with a small incision and make the combination with intravitreal gas- or silicon oil tamponade possible.

The purpose of our report is to describe our experiences and complications related to combined phacoemulsification of the lens with posterior chamber lens-implantation and pars plana vitrectomy in a consecutive series of patients with macular disorders.

Material and methods

A total of 118 eyes, operated between august 1995 and january 2001 (74 right and 44 left eyes) of 116 patients were included in the study. 55 patients were male and 61 were female with an age ranging between 17 and 89 years (medium 70,3 years).

We recorded the indications for combined surgery, age of the patients at surgery, surgical procedure and postoperative complications.

A complete eye examination of the anterior and posterior segment was made preoperativly, postoperativly and after 1,3 and 6 months. Ultrasonography and / or fluorescein angiography were made when necessary.

Techniques

Every patient underwent phacoemulsification of the lens via a small incision and implantation of a foldable intraocular lens. A standard three port pars plana vitrectomy was made under monitored intubation anaesthesia. Then a fornix-based conjunctival flap was dissected medial and lateral the limbus.

Sclerotomy sites were marked 3.0–3.5 mm posterior the limbus inferotemporaly, superionasaly and superiotemporaly. A suture was preplaced for the inferotemporal sclerotomy site.

In most of the cases a clear corneal superior temporal incision was used. In the other eyes first a partial-depth corneal incision, 1 to 2 mm posterior to the superior limbus and then a stab incision of 3,0–3,2 mm within the corneoscleral groove was made. The anterior chamber was filled with hyaluronate sodium (Healon©).

Continous tear capsulorhexis was performed, followed by hydrodissection with balanced salted solution. The lens nucleus was removed with phacoemulsification. Residual cortical material was aspirated with the tip of the irrigation-aspiration instrument.

The anterior chamber and capsular bag were reformed with viscoelastics, and a foldable acrylic intraocular lens was inserted through a small incision – 3,2 mm. If an intravitreal tamponade was planned, the wound was temporarely sealed with a 10,0 nylon suture.

The infusion cannula was placed inferotemporal and connected to the irrigation solution (balanced salt solution, BSS). Via two superiorly located sclerotomies the endoilluminator and the vitrectomy instrument were introduced.

The vitreous surgery was performed either with a mechanical cutter in 107 eyes (90,7%) or with an Erbium-Yag-Laser Vitrectomy Machine in 11 eyes (9,3%).

Scatter laser photocoagulations and / or endodiathermy was added when necessary. After fluid silicon oil or gas exchange the sclerotomies were closed. Acetylcholin was injected into the anterior chamber to constrict the pupil and the viscoelastic was removed. All patients were treated with combined topical antibiotic-corticosteroid ointment and atropine ointment.

Results

Indications for a combined surgery were cataract and preretinal membranes in 18 eyes (15,2%), subretinal membranes in 38 cases (32,2%), macular holes in 19 patients (16,1%) and 43 cases of retinal detachment with macular envolvement (36,5%) (Fig. 1).

In 45 cases (38,1%) silicon oil and in 21 eyes (17,8%) an expanding gas (SF6, C2F6) was used as an intravitreal tamponade.

Surgery was uneventful in all eyes. Complications related to the combined procedure were listed and devided into immediate and late.

Immediate complications occurred in a duration period of 1 to 3 weeks in 7 cases (5,9%). These were keratopathy in 3 eyes (2,5%), shallow anterior chamber in 3 cases (2,5%) and 1 irritation of the pupillomotoric function (0,9%) (Fig. 2).

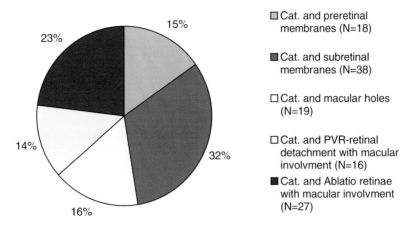

Fig. 1. Indications for combined surgery (N = 118)

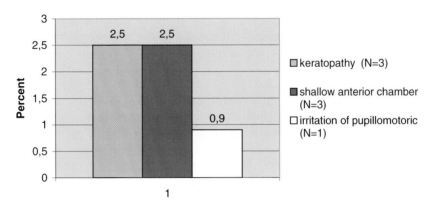

Fig. 2. Immediate complications 1–3 weeks (N = 7) 5,9%

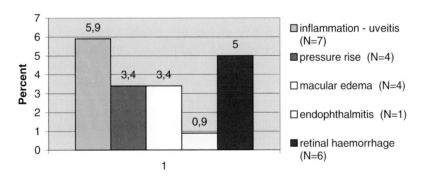

Fig. 3. Late complications 4 weeks–6 month (N = 22) 18,6%

Late complications, defined as complications in a period of 4 weeks to 6 months postoperatively, were observed in 22 cases (18,6%) – uveitis and inflammation in 7 eyes (5,9%), transient intraocular pressure rise and macular edema in 4 cases (3,4%) each. A retinal haemorrhage occurred in 6 eyes (5,0%). Only in 1 case (0,9%) an endophthalmitis occurred about one month postoperatively (Fig. 3). This inflammation vanished completely under topical and systemic antibiotic treatment.

Discussion and conclusion

Modern surgical techniques and new lens materials have made combined surgery much safer. Cataract formation and progression is a well-known consequence of pars-plana vitrectomy (PPV).

There was always a dilemma what to do first. On the one hand, if vitrectomy is done behind the cataract, the retinal situation will be judged very hard, due to a cataractous lens, and cataract surgery becomes more difficult. On the other hand, if cataract surgery is made in the first line, the retinal disorders will be changed for the worse.

When cataract extraction is delayed after vitrectomy, the absence of vitreous support for the posterior capsule may complicate the removal of the nucleus and cause excessive capsule movement during cortical aspiration, increasing the risk of an inadvertent posterior capsular tear [12].

To avoid some of these problems Blankenship et al. [13] described a method of combined lensectomy and vitrectomy similar to that of Girard [14], in which a posterior chamber lens is placed at the end of the surgery. With two 19-gauge needles through the pars plana the posterior lens capsule is excised, leaving the anterior capsule and zonules intact, and the cataractous lens is aspirated. After vitrectomy a posterior chamber lens is inserted through a limbal wound into the ciliary sulcus anterior to the anterior lens capsule. Finally a large central discission in the anterior lens capsule is created [13].

The disadvantages of this technique include sulcus fixation of the posterior chamber lens and large discission in the anterior and posterior capsule with the potential risk of developing keratopathy if silicon oil is used as tamponade.

Some study groups found that about 80% of eyes undergoing vitrectomy for macular pucker develop nuclear sclerosis over an average period of 6 to 29 months [8, 9]. These results were similar to other reports of increased nuclear sclerosis after PPV for repair of macular pucker and macular holes [8, 10, 11]. The average interval between phacoemulsification and PPV was about 20 months [6, 7].

Chang et al. described in their report, that 74% of the vitrectomiced eyes had predominatly nuclearsclerotic cataract compared with 42% of the control eyes [3].

Based on our experiences phacoemulsification of the lens first, via a small incision through the anterior chamber, inserting an foldable acryllic intraocular lens and vitrectomy with retinal surgery as a second step seems to be the safer method to treat patients with cataract and macular disorders. Visual results after vitreous surgery, like macular hole surgery and epi-/subretinal surgery, can be better compared, if the cataractous lens has been removed. Results of our study suggest that cataract surgery and IOL do not hinder complete vitreoretinal surgery in combination with tamponades, which were made in 66 cases (55,9%).

The purpose of our study was to confirm that in combined cataract and vitreous surgery early complications are transient and late complications occure with the same intensity and frequency than expected in vitrectomy and retinal surgery alone.

Not only moderate complications, like significant posterior capsular opacification and glaucoma, but also mild complications, like mild opacification at the capsule occurred in a similar period, rate and frequency than our data suggest.

Furthermore combined surgery offers a lot of advantages for the patient. The primary advantages are only one surgical procedure, one anaesthesia, better access to the vitreous base, a low rate of complications and prevention of contact of silicon-oil with the corneal endothelium, in order to reduce risk of keratopathy. Combined surgery with modern foldable IOLs offers faster visual rehabilitation without increasing the risk.

References

1. Malbran ES (1992) Pan-American Association of Ophthalmology 1991 presidental address. Ophthalmology 99(1):160–1
2. Stolba U, Binder S, Velikay M, Wedrich A (1996) Intraocular silicon lenses in silicon oil: an experimental study. Graefes Arch Exp Ophthalmol 234(1):55–7
3. Chang MA, Parides MK, Chang S, Braunstein RE (2002) Outcome of phacoemulsification after pars plana vitrectomy. Ophthalmology 109:948–54
4. Lacalle VD, Garate FJO, Alday NM, et al (1998) Phacoemulsification cataract surgery in vitrectomized eyes. J Cataract Refract Surg 24:806–9
5. McDermott ML, Puklin JE, Abrams GW, Eliott D (1997) Phacoemulsification for cataract following pars plana vitrectomy. Ophthalmic Surg Lasers 28:558–64
6. Pinter SM, Sugar A (1999) Phacoemulsification in eyes with past pars plana vitrectomy: case control study. J Cataract Refract Surg 25:556–61
7. Grusha YO, Masket S, Miller KM (1998) Phacoemulsification and lens implantation after pars plana vitrectomy. Ophthalmology 105:287–94
8. Cherfan GM, Michels RG, de Bustros S, et al (1991) Nuclear sclerotic cataract after vitrectomy for idiopathic epiretinal membranes causing macular pucker. Am J Ophthalmol 111:434–8
9. Freeman WR, Azen SP, Kim JW, et al (1997) Vitrectomy for the treatment of full-sickness stage 3 or 4 macular holes. Results of a multicentered randomized clinical trial. Arch Ophthalmol 115:11–21
10. de Bustros S, Thompson JT, Michels RG, et al (1988) Nuclear sclerosis after vitrectomy for idiopathic epiretinal membranes. Am J Ophthalmol 105:160–4
11. Schaumberg DA, Dana MR, Christen WG, Glynn RJ (1998) A systematic overview of the incidence of posterior capsule opacification. Ophthalmology 105:1213–21
12. Koenig SB, Mieler WF, Han DP, Abrams GW (1992) Combined phacoemulsification, pars plana vitrectomy, and posterior chamber intraocular lens insertion. Arch Ophthalmol 110:1101–4
13. Blankenship GW, Flynn HW, Kokame GT (1989) Posterior chamber intraocular lens insertion during pars plana lensectomy and vitrectomy for complications of proliferative diabetic retinopathy. Am J Ophthalmol 108:1–5
14. Girard LJ (1984) Posterior chamber implant after pars plana lensectomy. In: Emory JM, Jacobson AC (eds) Current concepts in cataract surgery: selected Proceedings of the Eighth Biannual Cataract Surgical Congress. East Norwalk, Conn: Appleton & Lange, 71

Correspondence: C.E. Jahn, Department of Ophthalmology, The Ludwig Boltzmann Institute for Retinology and Biomicroscopic Laser Surgery, Rudolf Foundation Hospital, Juchgasse 25, A-1030 Vienna, Austria.

Photodynamic therapy (PDT) in eyes with pathologic myopia

I. Krebs, S. Binder, U. Stolba, and A. Abri

Department of Ophthalmology, The Ludwig Boltzmann Institute of Retinology and
Biomicroscopic Laser Surgery, Rudolf Foundation Hospital, Vienna, Austria
(Chairman: Prof. Dr. Susanne Binder)

Introduction

Pathologic Myopia has been reported to be a major cause of blindness, especially in younger patients [1]. Pathologic myopia is characterized by excessive axial length and secondary degenerative changes in the periphery and in the posterior pole. Choroidal neovascularisation (CNV) occurs in 5–10% [2, 3] of these patients and extends under the centre of the foveal avascular zone in about 50% [4, 5]. Thermal photocoagulation of subfoveal CNV results in an immediate permanent decrease of vision with an absolute scotoma in the centre [6, 7]. Two multicenter, double-masked, placebo-controlled, randomised clinical trials-the Verteporfin in Photodynamic Therapy Study (VIP-study) [8] and the Treatment of Age-related Macular Degeneration With Photodynamic Therapy Study (TAP-study) [9] showed a better outcome for distance acuity in cases of pathologic myopia than in cases with age-related macular degeneration (AMD). The purpose of our study was to examine more precisely a series of eyes with pathologic myopia and sCNV treated with PDT and work out characteristics of the myopic membranes.

We included in our study eyes with pathologic myopia and subfoveal choroidal neovascularisation with a distance acuity of at least 0,1. Pathologic myopia was defined as an eye requiring a distance correction of at least −6,0 dioptres or with an axial length of more than 26,5 mm [10, 11]. We excluded patients with general contraindication against Verteporfin like porphyria or porphyrin sensitivy and severe liver disease. Eyes with any significant ocular disease other than sCNV or pathologic myopia, or surgery within 2 months could not be included. Eyes with signs of age-related macular degeneration such as large drusen or with signs of multifocal choroiditis were excluded.

Patients and methods

Besides medical history, biomicroscopy of the anterior and posterior segment was performed. The best corrected distance acuity was tested with ETDRS Charts in 4 m distance, the test was repeated in 2 m distance when the patient could read less than 1 line [12]. The reading acuity was tested with JÄGER Charts in a distance of 20 cm with an additional correction of +3,0 to +5,0 dioptres (this additional correction must not be changed at the follow up examinations). For the 10 degree static threshold perimetry the Macular2 (M2) program of the Octopus 101 perimeter was used [13, 14]. The fluorescein angiography and the measurement of the lesion size was performed with the Heidelberg Retina Angiograph. The Optical Coherence Tomography (OCT) was performed with enlarged pupils with the Optical Coherence Tomography-Scanner (Zeiss). The multifocal Electroretinography (mERG) with the Retiscan (Roland Consulting) completed our examinations. All these examinations were repeated after 6 weeks, three months and afterwards every three months.

Table 1. Decimal distance acuity with ETDRS Charts

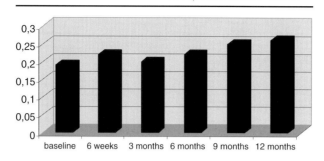

Table 2. Reading acuity Jäger Charts

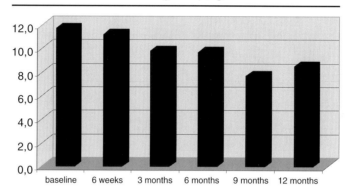

PDT treatment was performed according to the Visudyne protocol.

The intravenous infusion of 6 mg/m^2 body surface area of verteporfin, was followed by irradiation, 15 minutes after the start of sensitizer administration, with light at 689 nm delivered by an ocular photoactivation diode and laser-linked slit lamp (Coherent Inc., Palo Alto, CA) at an intensity of 600 mW/cm^2 over 83 seconds. The spot size was determined after measuring the greatest linear dimension of the entire lesion and additionally adding 1000 μm. Retreatment was performed when we noted any leakage in the late phase angiograms at the three months check-ups.

14 eyes of 13 Patients were included with an average age of 67.8 years (ranging from 54 to 92 years) 10 patients (11 eyes) were female and 3 patients were male. The mean observation time was about 22 months ranging from 18 to 27 months. The patients received 1 to 3 treatments, in the 1st year (3 eyes once, 6 eyes twice, 5 eyes three times).

Results

The Table 1 shows a diagram of the mean values of decimal distance acuity. At baseline the mean distance acuity was 0,19 (ranging from 0,1 to 0,5) and improved to 0,22 (ranging from 0,05 to 0,63) after 6 weeks and 0,26 (ranging from 0,06 to 1,0) after 1 year. 7% of the eyes showed an increase of more than 3 lines or 3 lines and 43% of less then 3 lines but more than 1 line. 29% remained unchanged and 21% had a decrease of distance acuity of more than 1 line but less than three lines.

The mean reading acuity, tested with Jäger Charts, was Jg 11,7 (ranging from Jg2 to no reading acuity = Jg17) at baseline and Jg 8,2 (ranging from Jg1 to Jg15) after 1 year (the result are presented in Table 2). There was an almost linear improvement of the mean values of reading acuity in the 1ˢᵗ year. The reading acuity increased in 71,4% (from 1 up to 10 levels), remained unchanged in 21,4% and decreased in 7,1%.

The changes of central visual field can be best analyzed by following the mean defect changes. There was stabilization of the mean values of the mean defect rather than an improvement. The mean values of the mean defect were 14,65 dB (from 4,2 dB to 28,6 dB) at baseline and 13,16 (from 5,3 to 23,8) after one year. There was an improvement of the central visual field in 71,4%. At baseline in 71,4% the size of the absolute and relative scotomas was within 5 degrees. In Fig. 1 a patient's greyscales and defect curves are presented. Although there was an increase of the absolute scotoma there was an improvement of distance acuity and mean defect because of the decrease of the relative scotoma and a shift of the scotoma to the right side due to eccentric fixation [15–17].

With OCT we see in Fig. 2 a superficial lying membrane in front of the pigment epithelium at baseline examination and a smaller and less prominent zone of higher reflectivity after successful PDT (3 treatments) [18–20]. The retinal thickness decreased in this case from 344 μm to 276 μm, measured at corresponding locations near the membrane due to the decrease of retinal edema [21, 22]. The mean values of the retinal thickness near the membrane decreased from 335,86 μm at baseline to 264,43 μm after 1 year. 78,6% of the eyes showed a decrease of retinal thickness.

The mean values of the maximal potential of the B-wave in the multifocal ERG [23–26] increased from mean 103,25 nV/deg² (from 64,7 to 178) at baseline to 112,9 nV/deg² (from 64,5 to 254) after one year. 64,28% of the eyes showed an improvement of the mERG. There was a stabilisation of the maximal potential of the B-wave in the first 6 months, after this time the values increased. You see a patient's example in Fig. 3. In the Fluorescein Angiography (FA) all membranes were classic without any occult parts. The greatest linear diameter of the lesion decreased from mean 2,4 mm (ranging from 0,9 mm to 4,9 mm) to 1,9 mm (ranging from 0,6 mm to 4,2 mm) after 6 weeks and 2,0 (ranging from 1,0 mm to 3,8 mm) after 12 months; the best results were measured after 6 weeks. In 71,4% there was a decrease of the greatest diameter of the lesion. In Fig. 4 we present the Angiograms of the patient: PN male, 73 years old, one single treatment. There is an obvious decrease of leakage visible especially in the late phase angiograms.

In comparison with the VIP study, the mean age of our patients was higher (67,8 vs 51 in the VIP study) the membranes larger (2500 μm vs 1900 μm in the VIP study) 85% of the membranes in the VIP study and 100% in our study were classic without any occult parts. The mean baseline distance acuity was 0,31 in the VIP study and 0,19 in our study (the distance acuity in VIP study was tested in 2 m distance). In the VIP study mean 3,4 treatments were applied, and mean 2,4 treatments were applied to our patients.

As far as distance acuity is concerned a moderate decrease (up to three lines) occurred in 25% in the VIP study and in 21% in our study, in 13% there was a decrease of more than 3 lines in the VIP study, but none of our patients lost more than 3 lines. 30% in the VIP study and 29% in our study remained unchanged. 26% of the patients in the VIP study showed an increase of less than 3 lines, the group with moderate increase was very large in our study (43%). Reading acuity an central visual field were not part of the study regimen of the VIP study.

Conclusion

Not only the distance acuity but also the reading acuity and central visual field could be improved in more than 70%. The greatest diameter of the lesion in the FA and the retinal thickness measured in the OCT could be reduced in more than 70%. The maximal

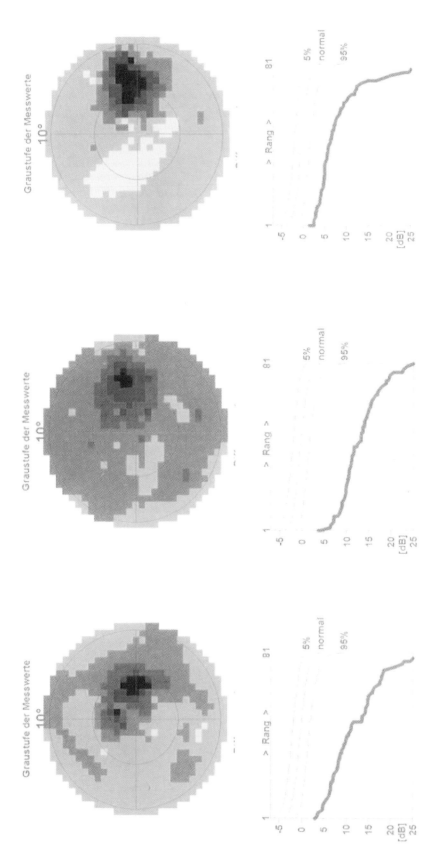

Fig. 1. Shows greyscales and defect curves of patient WM, female, 59 years old: the mean defect was 11,8dB at baseline 12,9 after 6 weeks and 8,1 after 12 months (lower values of mean defect mean improvement of the visual field). The distance acuity increased from 0,1 at baseline to 0,12 after 6 weeks and 0,25 after 12 months. Although there was an increase of the absolut scotoma there was an improvement of distance acuity and mean defect because of the decrease of the relative scotoma and a shift of the scotoma to the right side due to eccentric fixation

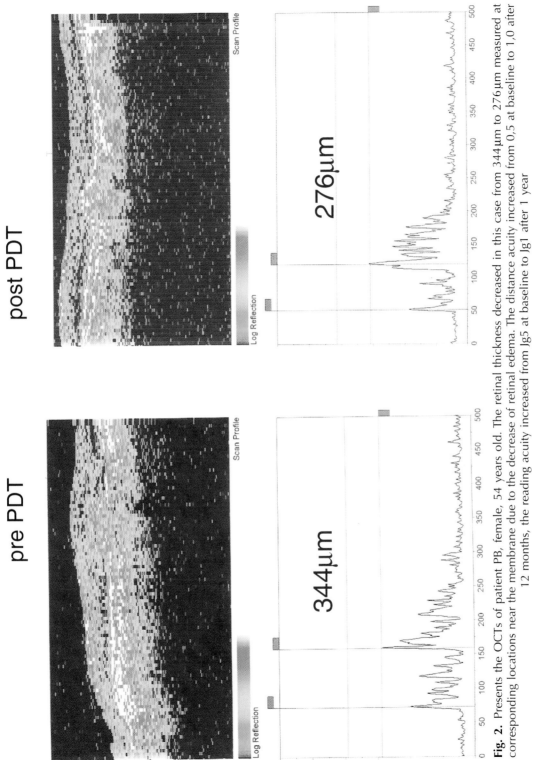

Fig. 2. Presents the OCTs of patient PB, female, 54 years old. The retinal thickness decreased in this case from 344 μm to 276 μm measured at corresponding locations near the membrane due to the decrease of retinal edema. The distance acuity increased from 0,5 at baseline to 1,0 after 12 months, the reading acuity increased from Jg5 at baseline to Jg1 after 1 year

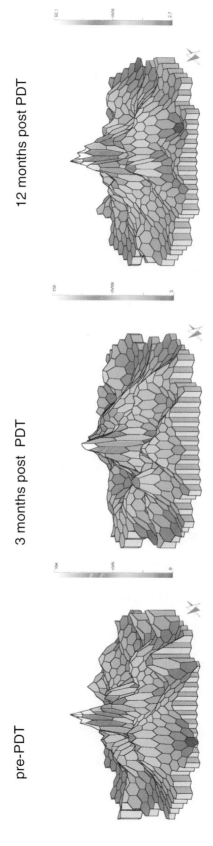

Fig. 3. Shows the mERG of patient WM. The maximal potential of the B-wave increased from 94,2 nV/deg² at baseline to 125,0 nV/deg² after 6 weeks and 126 nV/deg² after 12 months

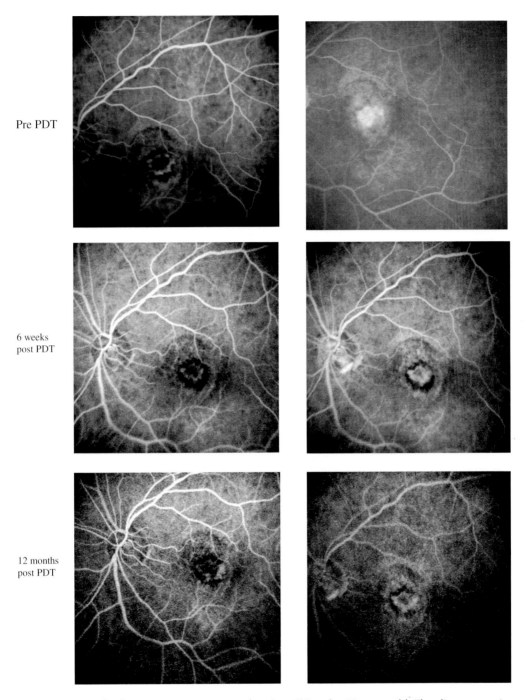

Fig. 4. Presents the fluorescein angiograms of patient PN male, 73 years old. The distance acuity increased from 0,16 at baseline to 0,2 after 6 weeks and 0,5 after 12 months, the reading acuity increased from Jg16 to Jg12 and Jg10 after 12 months. The early phase angiograms show only slightly differences but there is obviously less leakage in the late phase angiograms after 6 weeks and 12 months

potential of the B-wave could be improved in 62,3%. Although PDT is very effective in high myopic eyes most of theses patients remain visually impaired [27].

Here are some characteristics of our patients:100% classic membranes, the mean values of the greatest diameter of the lesion were rather small. The location of the membranes was more superficial than in AMD cases. In 70% the size of the absolute and relative scotoma were within 5 degrees (rather small). 35% of the patients were not yet 60 years old.

References

1. Krumpaszky HG, Haas A, Klauss V, Selbmann HK (1997) New blindness incidents in Wurttemberg-Hohenzollern. Ophthalmologe 94(3):234–6
2. Curtin BJ, Karlin DB (1971) Axial length measurements and fundus changes of the myopic eye. Am J Ophthalmol 1(1 Part 1):42–53
3. Curtin BJ (1979) Physiologic vs pathologic myopia: genetics vs environment. Ophthalmology 86(5):681–91
4. Tabandeh H, Flynn HW Jr, Scott IU, Lewis ML, Rosenfeld PJ, Rodriguez F, Rodriguez A, Singerman LJ, Schiffman J (1999) Visual acuity outcomes of patients 50 years of age and older with high myopia and untreated choroidal neovascularization. Ophthalmology 106(11): 2063–7
5. Avila MP, Weiter JJ, Jalkh AE, Trempe CL, Pruett RC, Schepens CL (1984) Natural history of choroidal neovascularization in degenerative myopia. Ophthalmology 91(12):1573–81
6. Soubrane G, Pison J, Bornert P, Perrenoud F, Coscas G (1986) Subretinal neovessels in degenerative myopia: results of photocoagulation. Bull Soc Ophtalmol Fr 86(3):269–72
7. Macular Photocoagulation Study Group (1991) Subfoveal neovascular lesions in age-related macular degeneration. Guidelines for evaluation and treatment in the macular photocoagulation study. Arch Ophthalmol 109(9):1242–57
8. Verteporfin in Photodynamic Therapy (VIP) Study Group (2001) Photodynamic therapy of subfoveal choroidal neovascularization in pathologic myopia with verteporfin. 1-year results of a randomized clinical trial–VIP report no. 1. Ophthalmology 108(5):841–52
9. Treatment of Age-Related Macular Degeneration with Photodynamic Therapy (TAP) Study Group (1999) Photodynamic therapy of subfoveal choroidal neovascularization in age-related macular degeneration with verteporfin: one-year results of 2 randomized clinical trials–TAP report. Arch Ophthalmol 117(10):1329–45
10. Hotchkiss ML, Fine SL (1981) Pathologic myopia and choroidal neovascularization. Am J Ophthalmol 91(2):177–83
11. Secretan M, Kuhn D, Soubrane G, Coscas G (1997) Long-term visual outcome of choroidal neovascularization in pathologic myopia: natural history and laser treatment. Eur J Ophthalmol 7(4):307–16
12. Ferris Fld, Kassoff A, Bresnick Gh, et al (1982) New visual acuity charts for clinical research. Am J Ophthalmol 94: 91–6
13. Jaakkola A, Vesti E, Immonen I (1998) Correlation between Octopus perimetry and fluorescein angiography after strontium-90 plaque brachytherapy for subfoveal exudative age related macular degeneration. Br J Ophthalmol 82(7):763–8
14. Ito A, Kawabata H, Fujimoto N, Adachi-Usami E (2001) Effect of myopia on frequency-doubling perimetry. Invest Ophthalmol Vis Sci 42(5):1107–10
15. Sunness JS, Applegate CA, Haselwood D, Rubin GS (1996) Fixation patterns and reading rates in eyes with central scotomas from advanced atrophic age-related macular degeneration and Stargardt disease. Ophthalmology 103(9):1458–66
16. Trauzettel-Klosinski S, Tornow RP (1996) Fixation behavior and reading ability in macular Scotoma Neuro-ophthalmology 16(4):241–53
17. Guez JE, Le Gargasson JF, Rigaudiere F, O'Regan JK (1993) Is there a systematic location for the pseudo-fovea in patients with central scotoma? Vision Res 33(9):1271–9
18. Hee MR, Baumal CR, Puliafito CA, Duker JS, Reichel E, Wilkins JR, Coker JG, Schuman JS, Swanson EA, Fujimoto JG (1996) Optical coherence tomography of age-related macular degeneration and choroidal neovascularization. Ophthalmology 103(8):1260–70

19. Hee MR, Izatt JA, Swanson EA, Huang D, Schuman JS, Lin CP, Puliafito CA, Fujimoto JG (1995) Optical coherence tomography of the human retina. Arch Ophthalmol 113(3):325–32
20. Hee MR, Puliafito CA, Wong C, Duker JS, Reichel E, Rutledge B, Schuman JS, Swanson EA, Fujimoto JG (1995) Quantitative assessment of macular edema with optical coherence tomography. Arch Ophthalmol 113(8):1019–29
21. Puliafito CA, Hee MR, Lin CP, Reichel E, Schuman JS, Duker JS, Izatt JA, Swanson EA, Fujimoto JG (1995) Imaging of macular diseases with optical coherence tomography. Ophthalmology 102(2):217–29
22. Zolf R, Glacet-Bernard A, Benhamou N, Mimoun G, Coscas G, Soubrane G (2002) Imaging analysis with optical coherence tomography: relevance for submacular surgery in high myopia and in multifocal choroiditis. Retina 22(2):192–201
23. Jurklies B, Weismann M, Husing J, Sutter EE, Bornfeld N (2002) Monitoring retinal function in neovascular maculopathy using multifocal electroretinography – early and long-term correlation with clinical findings. Graefes Arch Clin Exp Ophthalmol 240(4):244–64
24. Kawabata H, Adachi-Usami E (1997) Multifocal electroretinogram in myopia. Invest Ophthalmol Vis Sci 38(13):2844–51
25. Seeliger MW, Jurklies B, Kellner U, Palmowski A, Bach M, Kretschmann U (2001) Multifocal electroretinography (mfERG). Ophthalmologe 98(11):1112–27
26. Terasaki H, Miyake Y, Niwa T, Ito Y, Suzuki T, Kikuchi M, Kondo M (2002) Focal macular electroretinograms before and after removal of choroidal neovascular lesions. Invest Ophthalmol Vis Sci 43(5):1540–5
27. Thölen A, Bernasconi P, Fierz A, Messmer E (2001) Lesefähigkeit nach photodynamischer Therapie (PDT) für altersabhängige Makuladegeneration und für hohe Myopie. Der Ophthalmologe [Suppl1]

Correspondence: Ilse Krebs, M.D., Department of Ophthalmology, The Ludwig Boltzmann Institute of Retinology and Biomicroscopic Laser Surgery, Rudolf Foundation Hospital, Juchgasse 25, A-1030 Vienna, Austria.

Interim analysis of the MIRA-1 – multicenter double masked placebo controlled trial of rheopheresis in dry age-related macular degeneration (AMD) with soft drusen

Part of the Framework of Clinical Studies and Investigations to Prove Safety and Efficacy of Rheopheresis as a Novel Treatment Option for AMD

R. Klingel[1] for the MIRA-1 Study Group

[1] Apheresis Research Institute, Cologne, Germany

The MIRA-1 Study Group is comprised of the following members:

Writing Committee and Principal Ophthalmologic Investigators:
David Boyer, M.D., (Retina Vitreous Associates, Beverly Hills, Ca); David Brown, M.D., (Eye Centers of Florida, Ft. Myers, Fl); Richard Davis, M.D., (OccuLogix Corporation); Ronald Danis, M.D., (Retina & Vitreous Service, Indiana University, Indianapolis, IN); Dana Deupree, M.D., (St. Luke's Cataract and Laser Institute, Tarpon Springs, Fl); Alexander Eaton, M.D., (Eye Centers of Florida, Ft. Myers, Fl), Bert Glaser, M.D., (Glaser-Murphy retina Treatment Center, Towson, MD); Reinhard Klingel, M.D., Ph.D., (Apheresis Research Institute, Cologne, Germany); Robert Gale Martin, M.D., and Greg Mincey, M.D., (Carolina Eye Associates, Southern Pines, NC), Dan Montzka, M.D., (St. Luke's Cataract and Laser Institute, Tarpon Springs, Fl); Robert Murphy, M.D., (Glaser-Murphy retina Treatment Center, Towson, MD); Joseph Olk, M.D., (The Retina Center of St. Louis County, St. Louis, MO), Donald R. Sanders, M.D., Ph.D., (Center for Clinical Research, Elmhurst, IL), Mano Swartz, M.D., (University of Utah, Moran Eye Center, Salt Lake City, UT), Jose Pulido, M.D., (Department of Ophthalmology and Visual Sciences UIC Eye Center University of Illinois, Chicago, IL).

Principal Investigators at Rheopheresis Therapy Units (Nephrology/Apheresis):
Mark Aarons, M.D., (Pinehurst Nephrology Associates); Theresa Boyd, M.D., (BRT Labs); Philip DeChristopher, M.D., (University of Illinois, Chicago); Lawrence Dewberry, M.D., (Palm Harbor Nephrology Associates); Leo McCarthy, M.D., (Indiana University, Indianapolis); John Mellas, M.D., (Renex Dialysis Clinic); Samuel Pepkowitz, M.D., (Cedars-Sinai Medical Center); Gary Rabetoy, M.D., (University of Utah); Joel VanSickler, M.D., (Southwest Florida Regional Medical Center).

UCLA Jules Stein Fundus Photography Reading Unit:
Michael Cornish, M.D., Gary Holland, M.D., David Saraf, M.D. and Susan Ransome.

Medical BioStatistics and Data Management:
ProMedica International: Ginger Clasby, Pat Ticknor, Shannon Stoddard, Angel Rey, M.D., Melodee Sellers, Laura Callahan.
BioStat International: Maureen Lyden, MS.

Study Design, Analysis and Additional Support:
Burkhart and Associates: John Burkhart, Ph.D.
Center for Clinical Research: Yolanda Gonzalez and David Hotopp
Pepper Test Scoring: Erica Watkins and Gayle Watson, Ph.D.
LabCorp Clinical Trials Department: Dan Herlihy, Cathleen Prokesch, Nick Niles, and Teri
    Olimpaito.

Abstract

Rheopheresis is a safe and effective modality of therapeutic apheresis to treat micro-circulatory disorders. Elimination of a defined spectrum of high molecular weight proteins from human plasma including pathophysiologically relevant risk factors for AMD such as fibrinogen, LDL-cholesterol, α2-macroglobulin, fibronectin, and von-Willebrand factor results in the reduction of blood and plasma viscosity as well as erythrocyte and thrombocyte aggregation. Pulses of lowering blood and plasma viscosity performed as series of Rheopheresis treatments lead to rapid changes of blood flow, with the potential induction of sustained improvement of microcirculation, and recovery of retinal function. Change of the activity of promotors of the natural course of AMD development and progression might represent the mechanism of sustained improvement of microcirculation, i.e. recovery of retinal function. To evaluate safety and efficacy of Rheopheresis for the treatment of dry AMD with soft drusen in the MIRA-1 trial 150 patients are to be randomized in a 2:1 ratio to receive 8 Rheopheresis or 8 sham apheresis treatments over 10 weeks and followed for one year. Investigational sites include 9 study centers and an additional reading center in the US. Qualified patients have dry AMD with multiple large soft drusen, VAC of 0.16–0.625, and for homogeneity of patient groups defined serum levels of selected high-molecular weight plasma proteins. The interim analysis included 43 subjects. In primary eyes the mean ETDRS-line difference at 12 months post baseline between treated and control group was 1.6 lines (p = 0.0011, repeated measures analysis). The difference was significant throughout the first post-treatment year. Subgroup analysis indicated that eyes with baseline VAC worse than 20/40 derived the greatest treatment benefit at one year with mean difference of 3.0 ETDRS-lines compared to placebo (p = 0.001). No severe treatment related adverse events occurred. In conclusion the interim analysis of the MIRA-1 trial demonstrated statistically significant and clinically relevant effects of Rheopheresis on VAC when compared to placebo controls for the 12-month study interval. The framework of completed and still ongoing controlled clinical trials in combination with post certification studies including the *RheoNet*-registry represents a comprehensive quality management approach for this novel interdisciplinary therapy for AMD. A hypothesis based upon current knowledge of pathogenic mechanisms of the development and progression of AMD can be conclusively linked with the putative mechanism of action of Rheopheresis for AMD. A recommendation for high-risk AMD-patients was defined. Based on the positive results of the MIRA-1 interim analysis 8 Rheopheresis treatments are currently recommended as the initial treatment series.

Introduction

Age-related macular degeneration (AMD) is the leading cause of severe, irreversible loss of vision and legal blindness in people older than 65 years in the Western world. In Germany in the year 2000 absolute prevalence of patients between 43 and 86 years with findings of wet AMD was about 430.000, the equivalent prevalence of legally blind AMD patients was about 20.000, accounting for 15–32% of all cases of blindness in Germany

[1]. In AMD, progressive damage to the macula results in loss of central vision and affects a person´s ability to read, recognize faces, or drive. AMD can be classified into early and late stages, and occurs in two forms: the non-exudative form (dry AMD) and the exudative form (wet AMD). Clinical manifestations appear as drusen, atrophy of the retinal pigment epithelium (RPE) and choriocapillaris, i.e. dry AMD. RPE detachment, and choroidal neo-vascularizations (CNV) are characteristic for wet AMD. Patients with wet AMD account for about 25% of total AMD patients [2]. About 80% of severe vision loss caused by AMD is due to the wet form. Patients with only drusen in one or both eyes typically do not have much loss of vision, but they have an increased risk for progression to the late form of the disease and resultant loss of visual acuity (VAC) [3]. Risk factors for that development include number, size and confluence of drusen and abnormal pigmental clumping [3, 4]. Patients with bilateral soft drusen have a 12.4% risk to develop exudative AMD within 10 years [5]. Patients with exudative AMD in one eye and soft drusen in the fellow eye represent a high-risk group to become legally blind [4]. In summary large numbers of hard drusen predict the incidence of soft drusen and pigmentary abnormalities and that the presence of the latter lesions significantly increases the risk for the development of geographic atrophy and exudative macular degeneration [6].

Pathogenic mechanisms of AMD – putative links to therapeutic apheresis

The pathogenesis of AMD is not yet fully understood, but a hypothetical sequence of pathogenic events is consistent with known data. Models for AMD pathogenesis include RPE and Bruch's membrane senescence, genetic defects, oxidative insults, ocular perfusion abnormalities, and local inflammatory processes [2, 7]. Also functional deterioration of astrocytes in the outer retina have to be discussed as a consequence of changes in retinal microcirculation [8]. Cholesterol, fibrinogen, and α2-macroglobulin have been established as risk factors for AMD in epidemiological studies [9, 10, 11]. In a controlled cross sectional study patients with dry and wet AMD showed significantly elevated mean levels of vascular endothelial growth factor (VEGF, $p = 0.019$), plasma viscosity ($p < 0.001$), fibrinogen ($p < 0.001$), and von-Willebrand factor (vWF, $p < 0.001$) compared to healthy controls [12]. These results confirm an association between markers of angiogenesis (VEGF), hemorheology (fibrinogen, plasma viscosity), and endothelial dysfunction (vWF) with the pathogenesis of AMD. Molecules associated with local inflammatory processes like IgG, IgA, IgE, C1q, C3 were abundantly detected in subretinal membranes [13].

In the vascular model of Friedman it is hypothesized that lipid deposition in sclera and Bruch's membrane, a stratified extracellular matrix situated between the RPE and choriocapillaris, leads to scleral stiffening and impaired choroidal perfusion, which in turn could adversely affect metabolic transport function of the RPE [14]. The impaired RPE cannot metabolize and transport material shed from the photoreceptors, leading to accumulation of metabolic debris and drusen. This pathogenic model is in accordance with a huge body of findings demonstrated by fluorescein and indocyanine green angiographic methods, laser Doppler flowmetry, and color Doppler imaging [2]. Both choroidal blood flow and choroidal blood volume were about 29% lower in subjects aged 46–76 years compared to subjects aged 15–45 years probably related to a decrease in density and diameter of the choriocapillaris with increasing age [15, 16]. In patients with dry AMD and large soft drusen choroidal blood flow and choroidal blood volume were again 37%, 33% respectively lower then in age-matched control subjects. The presence of tissue ischemia and hypoxia in dry AMD may trigger the development of angiogenesis with progression to wet AMD (Fig. 1) [15, 16]. In patients with bilateral AMD pulsatile ocular

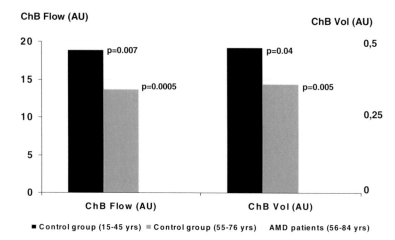

Fig. 1. The effect of aging and AMD on retinal blood flow. The figure shows relative choroidal blood flow (ChB Flow) and volume (ChB Vol) in arbitrary units (AU) in control subjects aged 15–45 years, 55–76 years respectively and AMD patients (56–84 years). Both ChB Flow and ChB Vol were about 29% lower in subjects aged 46–76 years compared to subjects aged 15–45 years. In patients with dry AMD and large soft drusen ChB Flow and ChB Vol were again 37%, 33% respectively lower then in age-matched control subjects [modified from 15, 16]

blood flow in eyes with drusen was lower than their fellow eyes with neovascular lesions [17]. These results confirm the clinical risk assessment of soft drusen mentioned above.

Cellular functions of RPE depend upon oxygen concentration [18]. Phagocytosis is a major function of RPE cells and is essential to maintain homeostasis of the micro-environment in the eye. Blood flow can have a direct functional relationship with tissue cells via shear stress. Decreased blood flow could result in decreased RPE phagocytosis by insufficient tissue oxygenation, and reduced induction of TGF-ß in the vessel wall via reduced shear stress [18, 19, 20]. The senescent RPE accumulates metabolic debris as remnants of incomplete degradation from phagocytosed rod and cone membranes. Progressive engorgement of these RPE cells leads to drusen formation with subsequent progressive dysfunction of the remaining RPE. With aging the capacity of Bruch's membrane to facilitate macromolecular exchange between the choroidal and the RPE compartments becomes reduced, representing an important aspect of retinal microcirculation [21, 22]. Bruch's membrane thickened with drusen then could facilitate the development of CNV [2].

The macular region including the fovea is an avascular zone, much thinner than the rest of the retina, and receives nourishment by diffusion from the surrounding vasculature and choriocapillaris. Diffusional transport capacities across the Bruch's-choroid complex decline with aging [23]. Angiogenic and antiangiogenic factors in the retina coordinate vascular flow and regeneration with the corresponding metabolic requirements of the retina. Most important are vascular endothelial growth factor (VEGF) and pigment epithelium derived factor (PEDF), both regulated by tissue oxygenation [22]. Expression of VEGF is induced by hypoxia, thus promoting neovascularization, PEDF is induced by increase of oxygen, thus inhibiting neovascularization.

The integrity of the vessel wall under quiescent conditions as well as its appropriate responsiveness under conditions of stimulation, inflammation or vascular injury is controlled by a number of adhesive interactions. Two major adhesive proteins relevant for haemostatic mechanisms co-localized in the extracellular matrix (ECM) of the vessel wall have to be mentioned: von Willebrand factor and vitronectin [24]. By immunohistochemistry and RT-PCR analysis it was shown that vitronectin is a major constituent of human drusen, and that it is expressed by local RPE cells [7]. More common ECM components such as laminin, fibronectin, collagens, and proteoglycans were not detected, indicating, that drusen-associated vitronectin is the result of selective accumulation. Vitronectin is present in high concentrations in plasma and is also common in ECM. Functionally it is related to processes of thrombosis, fibrinolysis, inflammation, and cellular adhesion. Self-association of vitronectin results in the formation of multimeric species of the protein [25]. The balance between monomeric and multimeric forms of vitronectin is important for pathophysiologically relevant changes of ECM sites and fibrinolytic state in plasma [26]. The binding and deposition of vitronectin to Bruch's membrane could compromise the exchange of metabolites between the choriocapillaris and the RPE, eventually leading to RPE and photoreceptor cell dysfunction and degeneration. RPE cells or byproducts of abnormal RPE and/or photoreceptor cell metabolism could serve as nucleation sites for the deposition for proteins such as vitronectin. In a mouse model a vitronectin receptor antagonist could reduce neovascularization in dose-dependent fashion, indicating that vitronectin deposition might be finally a contributing factor of neovascularization [27]. Recent studies implicate inflammation and complement mediated attack as early events in drusen biogenesis. It is likely that RPE cell debris entrapped between the RPE monolayer and Bruch's membrane serves as a chronic inflammatory stimulus and a potential nucleation site for drusen formation [7, 28]. Thus, the process of drusen biogenesis may be envisaged as a secondary manifestation of primary RPE pathology that is exacerbated by consequences of local inflammatory processes.

Therapeutic options for AMD

In the majority of AMD patients the therapeutic situation is very unsatisfactory, especially for patients with dry AMD [2, 3]. High-dose supplementation with vitamins C and E, beta carotene, and zinc was recently shown to have some benefit after a 5 year follow-up [29]. Even not all patients with wet AMD are eligible for the following treatment options targeting the different forms of CNV: laser therapy including standard laser photocoagulation, transpupillary thermotherapy (TTT), and photodynamic therapy (PDT), external beam irradiation, and surgical procedures like removal of neovascular membranes or macular rotation. 42% of patients after treatment with PDT showed a letter score loss in the study eye of at least 15 from baseline at the 3 year examination [30]. Laser photocoagulation and TTT are currently tested for dry AMD. However, reports on the occurrence of increased incidence of neovascular lesions after laser photocoagulation or TTT could indicate that both approaches might turn out to be unfavourable for the subsequent course of AMD [31, 32, 33, 34]. From a pathophysiological point of view, regarding angiogenic growth factors both treatment modalities seem to induce VEGF rather than PEDF. In conclusion from the current situation, successful therapy for more subgroups of patients with AMD is urgently needed.

Rheopheresis

Rheopheresis is a safe and effective application of membrane differential filtration (MDF) which was specifically designed) for extracorporeal hemorheotherapy (Fig. 2a,b) [35]. The elimination of an exactly defined spectrum of high-molecular weight proteins including fibrinogen, α2-macroglobulin, LDL-cholesterol, fibronectin, and von-Willebrand-factor results in the reduction of blood and plasma viscosity, erythrocyte and thrombocyte aggregation, and improves erythrocyte flexibility. Pulses of lowering blood and plasma viscosity lead to rapid changes of blood flow, subsequently inducing sustained improvement of microcirculation, which in the eye means recovery of retinal function. In this context microcirculation stands for the complete interactive network between

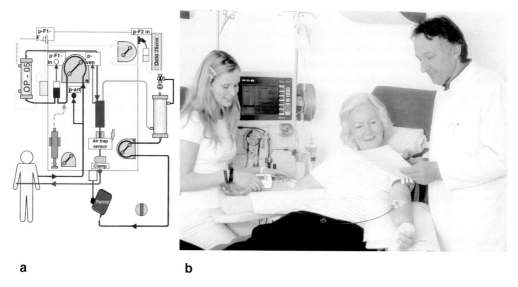

Fig. 2. The principle of Rheopheresis (membrane differential filtration with the specifically designed Rheofilter) in a schematic drawing (**a**) and treatment of an AMD patient in a modern apheresis center (**b**) are shown

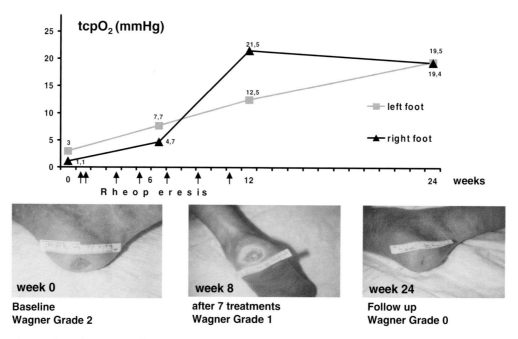

Fig. 3. Rheopheresis accelerated wound healing of foot ulcers of ischemic diabetic foot syndrome and was associated with an improvement of Wagner stage and a pronounced increase in tcpO₂. Values of tcpO₂ remained stable and enhanced for the 3 months follow-up period [modified from 36]

retinal pigment epithelium, choriocapillaris, extracellular matrix, and blood components. In a pilot trial with 8 patients Rheopheresis accelerated wound healing of foot ulcers of ischemic diabetic foot syndrome and was associated with an improvement of Wagner stage and a pronounced increase in tcpO₂ (Fig. 3) [36]. Values of tcpO₂ remained stable

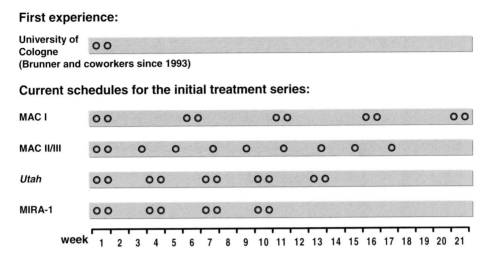

Fig. 4. Schedules for the initial treatment series of Rheopheresis for AMD investigated in clinical trials: First experiences at the University of Cologne were made with two treatments within 1 week. MAC-I is the controlled trial at the University of Cologne, Germany [38], Utah-trial was conducted at the University of Salt Lake City, USA, MAC-II at the University of Frankfurt, Germany, and MIRA-1

and enhanced for the 3 months follow-up period. As an adjunct therapeutic option Rheopheresis may preserve a functional lower extremity, delay amputation or reduce the extent of amputation. Values of $tcpO_2$ were still above baseline levels at the 3-month follow-up examination, suggesting a sustained, beneficial effect on tissue oxygenation, which is closely related to tissue function. The achievement of clinically relevant wound healing in 4 out of 8 patients was encouraging. In another pilot trial in patients with diabetic retinopathy, visual function was reported to improve after a series of MDF-treatments [37].

Rheopheresis for AMD – clinical trials

Two prospective, controlled, and randomized clinical trials for the treatment of AMD patients with Rheopheresis have been completed, two are ongoing with modified treatment schedules (Fig. 4) [38, 39]. In the study of the University of Cologne 40 patients were included. 20 patients received 10 Rheopheresis treatments over a period of 21 weeks. The control group was followed without treatment. Eyes of patients in the therapy and control group both showed CNV in 9/20 eyes, and soft drusen in 11/20 eyes. Comparing initial and final VAC in Rheopheresis and control patients a mean difference of 1.6 EDTRS lines was detected after the treatment series, which was statistically significant with $p < 0.01$ [38]. Patients with soft drusen and no CNV had the best therapy results. Electrophysiologic investigation of the retina showed significant improvement of photopic a-wave and the flicker electroretinogram, equivalent to functional improvement of the central photoreceptor complex. Improvement of the pulsatile ocular blood flow and shortening of the arteriovenous passage time in patients with AMD after Rheopheresis treatments was demonstrated earlier (Fig. 5) [40, 41].

30 patients with dry AMD and soft drusen were included in a three-armed, sham-controlled, randomized clinical trial conducted at the University of Utah, Salt Lake City. With 10 Rheopheresis treatments 40% of patients showed improvement in at least 3 out of the following 4 parameters to assess visual function: ≥2.5 ETDRS lines best spectacle

a Mean change in visual acuity

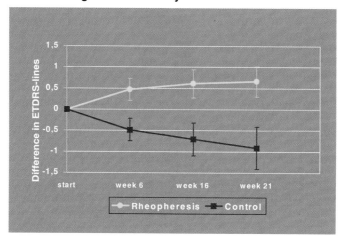

b Pulsatile ocular blood flow

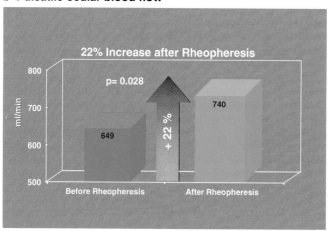

Fig. 5. Parameters which were investigated in clinical trials and demonstrated the positive effect of Rheopheresis in AMD patients: (**a**) mean change of visual acuity (ETDRS-lines) over time, (**b**) increase of pulsatile ocular blood flow, (**c**) decrease of arteriovenous passage time, (**d**) electrophysiological parameters of retinal function, i.e. photopic a-wave and 30 Hz flicker ERG [modified from 38, 40, 41]

corrected visual acuity (BCVAC) in the study eye, ≥2.5 ETDRS lines in the partner eye, 20% improvement of reading ability in the Pepper visual skills for reading test, and 20% improvement of quality of life tested by the VF14 [39]. In a case series including 10 AMD patients with high-risk AMD and soft drusen improvement of visual acuity essentially identical to the Cologne trial could be confirmed [42]. In fluorescein angiography reduction of soft drusen in number and size was associated with improvement of VAC. However, morphological changes in the retina are not well correlated with VAC also in the natural course of AMD, and should be not considered as the treatment goal [43].

The MIRA-1 interim analysis

MIRA-1 is a 12-months randomized, prospective, multi-center, double-masked, placebo-controlled, FDA clinical trial designed to compare Rheopheresis treatment against

c Arterio-venous passage time

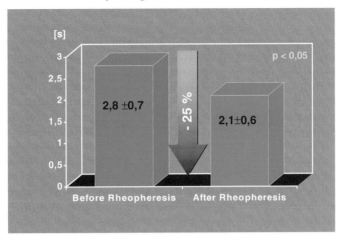

d Electrophysiology

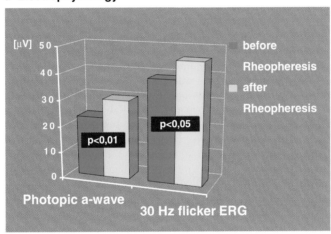

Fig. 5. *Continued*

placebo-control treatment in 150 patients with intermediate to late-stage (AREDS Grade 3 to 4, BCVA between 20/32 and 20/125 inclusive), high-risk (≥10 large soft drusen), dry AMD who also demonstrated defined serum levels of select hemorheologic macromolecules in their blood to achieve optimal homogeneity of the study groups. The complete list of inclusion criteria is shown in Table 1. Patients are to be randomized in a 2:1 ratio to receive 8 Rheopheresis or 8 sham-apheresis treatments over 10 weeks and followed for one year. It is important to note that patients in both the Rheopheresis treatment group as well as the placebo-control group of the current trial were both provided with the same daily vitamin supplementation formula, and they were prohibited from using other vitamin supplements so that differential supplementation use would not be a confounding variable. The MIRA-1 protocol provided for daily oral intake of the following: vitamin C 400 mg (four-times RDA), 200 IU of vitamin E (6 times RDA), 40 mg zinc (2.5 times RDA), and 3000 IU of beta carotene (1.8 times RDA). Although these levels were considered suprathreshold at the time of the initiation of the trial, they represent only about half of those levels used in the AREDS study.

Table 1. Inclusion and exclusion criteria of the MIRA-1 trial

Inclusion Criteria:

Patients of any race between the ages of 50 and 85 years inclusive.

Patients must weigh >/=110 lbs (50 kg).

Study eye must have a diagnosis of non-exudative "dry" ARMD with soft, semi soft, and or confluent drusen with an equivalent surface area of approximately 31,000 micron^2.

Study eye must have a best-corrected visual acuity using the ETDRS chart between 20/32 and 20/125 inclusive.

Geographic atrophy is allowed as long as it is less than 3 disc diameters within 3000 nm of the foveal center.

Serous pigment epithelial detachment is allowed as long as no clearly identifiable neovascularization is present. (No such patient was included in the interim analysis)

Patients must have elevated baseline concentrations of 2 of the following 3 rheologic factors: a total serum cholesterol level of ≥ 200 mg/dl, a fibrinogen level of ≥ 300 mg/dl, or a serum immunoglobulin A (IGA) level ≥ 200 mg/dl, as determined at the qualifying evaluation.

Patients must have a score of no more than 75 on the VFQ-25 Visual Functioning Questionnaire.

Study eye must not have conditions that limit the view of the fundus.

Patients must have normal prothombin (PT) and prothomboplastin (PTT) clotting times with the exception of patients who are stable on long-term coumadin.

Patients must have adequate bilateral antecubital venous access.

Patient taking lipid-lowering medication at the beginning of the treatment phase must agree to continue to take them throughout the treatment phase using their current regimen.

Patients must be available for minimum study duration of approximately 12 months.

Patients must be highly motivated, alert, oriented, mentally competent and able to understand and comply with the requirements of the study.

Patients must agree to discontinue their previous vitamin regimen and to substitute their regimen with a uniform supplement regiment provided by the study, OcularRx (Science-Based Health, Corde Madera, CA). This was done to ensure that every patient in the study ingested the same supplement regimen.

Exclusion criteria:

Study eye with concomitant retinal or choroidal disorder other than AMD.

Study eye with significant central lens opacities.

Study eye with a diagnosis of exudative "wet" AMD.

Study eye with other ocular diseases.

Patients who are in poor general health.

Patients with a hematocrit <35%, evidence of active bleeding or a platelet count <100,000 k/ul.

Patients with significant cardiac problems.

Patients with uncontrolled hypertension.

Patients with recent history of cerebral vascular disease.

Patients with severe hepatic failure, or uncontrolled diabetes.

Patients with a history of HIV infection, AIDS, hepatitis or other immunosuppressive disorders.

Patients who are allergic to fluorescein sodium and to indocyanine green

Patients unwilling to adhere to visit or examination schedules.

Patients with a known history of alcoholism, drug abuse, or any other condition that would limit validity of consent.

In the interim-analysis repeated measures analysis of the initial goup of 43 randomized, intent-to-treat patients (28 Rheopheresis treatment and 15 placebo-control patients) with preangiogenic dry AMD after a follow-up period of 12 months (n = 36) was performed. The MIRA-1 study had a double masking procedure. All patients were covered with an opaque shroud from the neck down prior to initiating each treatment in order to mask them from observing their treatment. Additionally, their arms were covered with drapes throughout the process. A partition was positioned in front of the blood pump and plasma therapy system so that the patient could not view the system. The pump was activated regardless of treatment arm assignment so that in each case the patient heard the background noise of the powered machine. Subjects randomized to the Placebo arm of the Study received masked needle sticks in both arms without connection to the tubing circuit. Placebo patients then underwent a 2-hour charade – complete with frequent machine alarms and IV positioning checks. Ophthalmologic investigators were masked since treatments were performed at separate locations and the treatment personnel were prohibited from discussing treatment arm assignments with the ophthalmic investigators, neither did the physicians have access to the study treatment envelope, treatment forms or the randomization log, which were locked in separate areas.

The primary efficacy endpoint for the Study and this interim analysis was prospectively identified as the comparison of mean change in LogMAR BCVA in the designated primary (study) eyes cohort comparing the Rheopheresis treatment group with the placebo-control group. Secondary efficacy outcomes included proportions of eyes with ≥2 lines (10 letters) or ≥3-line (15 letters) loss or gain of best-corrected ETDRS acuity. In addition, the proportion of cases with baseline ETDRS BCVA worse than 20/40 that achieved 20/40 or better acuity post-treatment, was also determined because of the functional significance of 20/40 vision as a legal threshold criterion for maintaining a valid driver's license. The study's endpoints, i.e. mean changes in ETDRS (LogMAR) visual acuity from baseline to the available post-treatment interval visits, were compared using 2-group ANOVA with repeated measures analysis with unstructured covariance using SAS/STAT Software. Both the group effect (treatment vs. placebo efficacy) and time effect (determines if LogMAR acuity changes observed between Rheopheresis treatment and placebo-control change or are constant during the course of the study) were tested.

The baseline characteristics of the Rheopheresis treatment and placebo-control groups with regard to age, gender, and mean baseline LogMAR acuity were not significantly different in the Rheopheresis treatment and placebo-control groups. The mean visual acuity was 20/47 for the Rheopheresis treated group and 20/49 for the placebo-control group (p = 0.81). With the exception of baseline serum uric acid level, which was significantly higher in the Rheopheresis treatment group than in the placebo-control group (5.24 mg/dl treatment vs. 4.26 mg/dl placebo, p = 0.01), there were no significant differences at baseline between the Rheopheresis treatment and placebo-control groups in any other of the 62 blood parameters tested. Nine mean baseline laboratory values were elevated in both the Rheopheresis treatment and placebo-control group (i.e. fibrinogen, international normalization ratio (INR), prothrombin time (PT), serum intra-cellular adhesion molecule-1 (sICAM-1), total cholesterol, VLDL cholesterol, LDL cholesterol, serum osmolality and whole blood viscosity). No severe treatment related adverse events occurred. In the primary eye cohort, the 12-month post-baseline mean LogMAR line difference between Rheopheresis treatment and placebo-control groups was 1.6 lines (group effect p = 0.0011) (Fig. 6a). The time effect was not significant (p = 0.2560), indicating a "therapeutic plateau" i.e. there was no significant change in the therapeutic benefit of the Rheopheresis treatment group relative to the placebo-control group over the 12-month course of the trial. Similar findings were consistently observed in both the all qualifying eyes cohort (p = 0.0053 and p = 0.2570), and the all eyes cohort (p = 0.002 and p = 0.4093) as well. The Rheopheresis treatment group consistently had a greater proportion of cases with line improvements at each post-baseline interval, compared against the placebo-control group regardless of which threshold criterion (≥1.5 lines, ≥2 lines, ≥2.5 lines or ≥3 lines) for BCVA improvement was used (Fig. 7a). At 9 and 12 months post-baseline, 12% to 13% of the Rheopheresis treatment eyes had a ≥3-line improvement in BCVA respectively, compared to 0% and 0% of the eyes in the Placebo-Control group. Similarly, the Rheopheresis treatment group consistently had a smaller proportion of cases

160   R. Klingel

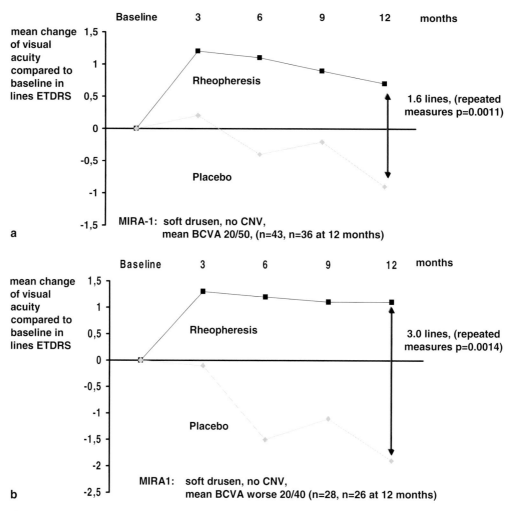

Fig. 6. Interim-results of the controlled, randomized MIRA-1 US multicenter trial evaluating the efficacy of Rheopheresis for the treatment of dry AMD with soft drusen. Mean change in visual acuity (No. of ETDRS-lines) from baseline to the examination at each specified time is depicted. The treatment group received 8 Rheopheresis treatments, the control group received a placebo sham apheresis. Repeated measures interim analysis including 43 patients showed a statistically significant difference between both groups at the 12 months follow-up. (**a**) Results of all primary study eyes, (**b**) results of primary study eyes with BCVAC worse than 20/40

with BCVA line losses at each post-baseline interval compared with the placebo-control group (Fig. 8a). At 12 months post-baseline, only 4.0% of the Rheopheresis treatment eyes had a ≥3-line loss of BCVA compared to 18.2% of the eyes in the placebo-control group.

In the subset of patients with baseline LogMAR BCVA of worse than 20/40, the mean 12-month post-baseline LogMAR line difference between Rheopheresis treatment and placebo-control groups was 3.0 lines (15 letters) (Fig. 6b). The group effect demonstrated a p-value of 0.0014 and the time effect was again not significant (p = 0.2928), indicating that there was no significant change in therapeutic effect of the Rheopheresis treatment group relative to the placebo-control group over the 12-month course of the trial. The mean line difference between the two groups tends to increase over time largely due to progressive loss of BCVA in the placebo-control eyes, while the improvement in BCVA

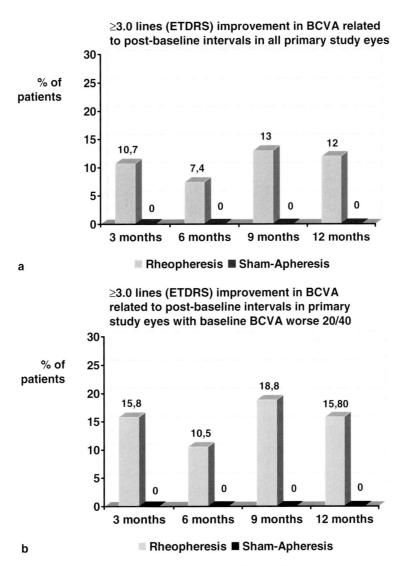

Fig. 7. Interim-results of the controlled, randomized MIRA-1 US multicenter trial evaluating the efficacy of Rheopheresis for the treatment of dry AMD with soft drusen. Improvement of ≥3.0 lines ETDRS in BCVA related to post-baseline intervals is shown. (**a**) Results of all primary study eyes, (**b**) results of primary study eyes with BCVAC worse than 20/40

in the Rheopheresis treated eyes remained essentially constant. Again, the group effect and time effect outcomes were consistent in both the all-qualifying eyes (p = 0.0122 and p = 0.2747) and the all eyes (p = 0.0050 and p = 0.3565) cohorts as well. In the subset of cases with baseline LogMAR BCVA worse than 20/40, the Rheopheresis treatment group consistently had a greater proportion of cases with ETDRS line improvements at each post-baseline visit compared to the placebo-control group (Fig. 7b). In fact, none of the placebo-control cases had a ≥3-line improvement in vision at any post-baseline interval, compared to 18.8%, and 15.8% of the Rheopheresis Treatment patients achieving this level of improvement at 9 months and 12 months post-baseline respectively. With respect to vision loss, the Rheopheresis treatment subgroup consistently had a smaller proportion of cases with ETDRS line losses at each post-baseline interval compared to the

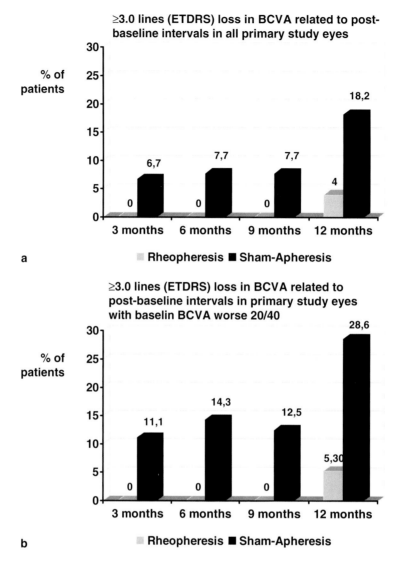

Fig. 8. Interim-results of the controlled, randomized MIRA-1 US multicenter trial evaluating the efficacy of Rheopheresis for the treatment of dry AMD with soft drusen. Loss of ≥3.0 lines ETDRS in BCVA related to post-baseline intervals is shown. (**a**) Results of all primary study eyes, (**b**) results of primary study eyes with BCVAC worse than 20/40

placebo-control group (Fig. 8b). At 12 months post-baseline, only 5.3% of Rheopheresis treated cases demonstrated a ≥3-line loss of BCVA compared to 28.6% of placebo-control patients. In the subgroup of Rheopheresis treated eyes with baseline LogMAR acuity worse than 20/40, 57.9% improved to 20/40 or better at the 12-month post-baseline interval compared to only 14.3% of the placebo-control group. The proportions of cases demonstrating visual improvements or losses were similar in the all qualifying eyes and the all eyes cohorts.

Clinical data from German Rheopheresis Competence Centers

In a recent reference controlled RheoNet-registry analysis 27 eyes with dry AMD and soft drusen of 18 Patients were evaluated after completion of the initial treatment series in clinical practice. The initial BCVAC was 0.1–0.8. Patients were treated based on oph-thalmological findings only, there was no selection by plasma parameters. In total 160 Rheopheresis treatments were performed in cooperation with 5 Rheopheresis competence centers. BCVAC was assessed with ETDRS-charts at baseline and after the treatment series. Patients received in mean 8.8 treatments within 18.3 weeks. Rheopheresis was safe and well tolerated. Compared to baseline ETDRS BCVAC 37% of eyes had a ≥2-line, 44% a 1-line improvement. 15% of patients did not change in VAC, 4% had a 1-line, 0% a ≥2-line loss. The mean change in VAC was 1.26 ETDRS-lines. In comparison, interim results of the MIRA-1 study revealed 3 months post baseline in 28.6% of treated eyes an improve-ment of ≥2-lines compared to only 6.7% of the eyes in the placebo group. The mean line change was 1.2 at that time. This reference controlled registry analysis is in good accor-dance with the results of 3 controlled clinical trials and demonstrates the potential of Rheopheresis as a novel treatment for patients with dry AMD and soft drusen (Fig. 8). From the University of Cologne results of 20 patients were reported after long-term treat-ment, demonstrating that the therapeutic effect of the initial treatment series can be main-tained upto 4 years [44]. Eyes suffering from dry AMD had a mean improvement of visual acuity of 1.9 EDTRS lines after 24 months, 1.2 lines after 36 months, and 0.8 lines after 48 months. After a mean period of 12 months follow-up 2–4 booster treatments could be considered depending upon the individual course [44]. However, these long-term results must be confirmed with larger patient numbers. In summary these data are already appro-priate to fulfill *class I* – requirements of the categories of evidence-based-medicine.

Quality management and safety issues: the RheoNet-registry

As the backbone of quality management the RheoNet-registry was established collecting Rheopheresis safety and efficacy parameters. All methods of extracorporeal blood purifi-cation can potentially cause adverse reactions and side effects, which all are well known due to the huge worldwide experience with hemodialysis, plasma exchange, immunoad-sorption, and LDL-apheresis. Hypotension, allergic reactions due to blood membrane interactions, hemolysis, or events associated with anticoagulation have to be mentioned. Anticoagulation for Rheopheresis can be performed with standard and low molecular weight heparin or citric acid. Safety of MDF was analyzed including data from 1702 ambulatory MDF-LDL-apheresis treatments of 52 patients [45]. In 98% of MDF-treatments no adverse reactions occurred. In 2% hypotensive episodes were observed, no severe adverse events occurred [45]. It must be emphasized that patients with the indication of LDL-apheresis mostly suffer from symptomatic coronary artery disease, often with the history of myocardial infarction and cardiovascular surgery. Therefore these patients have a significantly higher risk profile for an extracorporeal treatment, than the average AMD patient. In a trial of Rheopheresis in 10 patients with acute ischemic stroke also no severe adverse events were reported [46]. In the controlled trial of the University of Cologne 20 patients with a mean age of 72 years received a total of 200 Rheopheresis treatments [38]. Hypotension was observed in 6%, hemolysis in 2.5% of treatments. A current RheoNet-registry analysis was performed in December 2002 on the basis of 2021 Rheo-pheresis treatments in 322 patients, including 207 patients with AMD. Mean age was 66 years (72 years for AMD patients), Table 2. All adverse events (AE) or side effects, which were caused or associated with Rheopheresis treatments were registered as reported by the German Rheopheresis competence centers. AE were catagorized as "reported" (AE-r), or as subgroup "reported and with the need of intervention, temporary break or discontinuation of the treatments" (AE-rI). In 4.65% of treatments AE were reported, but only in 1.19% AE needed intervention, temporary break or discontinuation of the treat-ment. With 0.89% transient hypotension was the most frequent AE of category AE-rI,

Table 2. RheoNet-registry report on adverse events and vascular access problems of 2021 Rheopheresis treatments performed before December 2, 2002 in German Rheopheresis competence centers including 322 patients with a mean age of 66 years (207 AMD patients, mean age 72 years)

	Total reported adverse events/side effects (AE-r)		Reported adverse events/side effects with need of intervention, temporary break or discontinuation (AE-rI)	
	absolute number	%	absolute number	%
Hypotension	42	2.08	18	0.89
Hematoma/bleeding	16	0.79	0	0.00
Edema	2	0.10	0	0.00
Dizziness	12	0.59	0	0.00
Eye flickering	2	0.10	0	0.00
Traces of blood in plasma circuit/suspicion of hemolysis (asymptomatic)	4	0.20	3	0.15
Chilling	11	0.54	1	0.05
Fever	1	0.05	1	0.05
Leukocytosis	1	0.05	0	0.00
Retinal bleeding	1	0.05	0	0.00
Headache	1	0.05	0	0.00
Severe intolerability/tetany like symptoms	1	0.05	1	0.05
Total	94	4.65	24	1.19
	Total reported vascular access problems of 2021 Rheopheresis treatments		Reported vascular access problems with need of intervention, temporary break or discontinuation	
Vascular access problems (puncture or flow)	146	7.22	29	1.43

followed by 0.15% of treatments with detection of traces of blood in the plasma circuit. Hypotension could be controlled in all cases by infusion of saline. No clinical signs of hemolysis were observed. AMD in general has an increased risk of retinal hemorrhage. Only one case of retinal bleeding was reported in an AMD patient 1 day after a Rheopheresis treatment, which caused no irreversible visual impairment. To minimize the bleeding risk citric acid anticoagulation could be used alternative to heparin. Problems with the vascular access (puncture or flow) were reported in 7.22% of treatments, only 1.43% were category AE-rI. Only 1 severe AE-rI (0.05%) was reported in a female patient with sudden deafness, who presented clinical signs equivalent to a severe tetanic reaction, which completely resolved within 24 hours after Rheopheresis. Based on interdisciplinary cooperation between ophthalmologists and nephrologists Rheopheresis can be regarded as a very safe ambulatory treatment for elderly patients with AMD.

Rheopheresis for AMD – mechanism of action

Extracorporeal plasma therapy was not yet used in ophthalmology and therefore requires explanation not only with respect to methodology, but also regarding the mechanism of action. As explained before AMD at cellular and molecular levels is at least in part a microcirculatory disorder of the retina. Therefore it seems to be reasonable to use Rheopheresis, which can successfully treat diseases with impaired microcirculation [35]. It is important for the understanding of the therapeutic potential of Rheopheresis, that the single pulses of plasma protein elimination with associated reduction of plasma viscosity can result in sustained improvements of microcirculation. This of course is a hypothesis, but it is confirmed by available clinical data for AMD, ischemic diabetic foot syndrome, and fibrinogen/LDL-apheresis for sudden deafness [36, 38, 47]. Rheopheresis directly targets risk factors and pathophysiologically relevant factors of AMD by lowering plasma viscosity, and eliminating fibrinogen, cholesterol, von-Willebrand factor, α2-macroglobulin, and probably multimeric vitronectin. However, these plasma parameters should be regarded as epidemiological risk factors, and not predictive for the individual therapeutic response. A functional reserve exists in the retina affected by AMD, which is determined by the individual pattern of reversible and irreversible morphologic changes of the retina. AMD spontaneously has a chronic progressive course. Irreversible functional and morphologic changes increase over time. The capacity of the individual functional reserve cannot be assessed by any diagnostic procedure. Goal of the Rheopheresis treatment is to restore and activate or stabilize the functional reserve of the retina. The regenerative potential of retinal pigment epithelium is well documented in vitro as well as in vivo. But as visual function in general the regenerative potential is highly depending upon microenvironmental conditions, i.e. the degree of morphologic retinal changes and the microcirculatory impairment at cellular and molecular levels. RPE phagocytic function is regulated by tissue oxygen concentration [19]. Rheopheresis treatment results in sustained improvement of tissue oxygenation induced by the repeated therapy pulses, as recently confirmed in a pilot trial in patients with ischemic diabetic foot syndrome [36]. In AMD Rheopheresis could improve RPE phagocytic function directly by the increase of tissue oxygenation, and additionally via shear stress mediated induction of TGF-ß [18, 19, 20]. One of the latest pathogenic pathways described in AMD is the equilibrium shift between the angiogenic growth factor opponents VEGF and PEDF promoting angiogenesis [48]. Rheopheresis could correct this imbalance in favor of inhibition of angiogenesis, resulting in the amelioration of the natural progressive course of AMD. The hypothesis that Rheopheresis might re-balance the angiogenic growth factor systems of VEGF and PEDF is clinically supported by the finding, that also diabetic retinopathy improved from Rheopheresis treatment [37]. In conclusion, repetitive pulses of plasma protein elimination seam to be capable to change the activity of promotors of the natural course of AMD development and progression. If ophthalmological science has completely elucidated AMD pathogenesis, it will be possible to explain the exact mechanism of action of Rheopheresis for AMD.

Indication for Rheopheresis in high-risk AMD-patients

Due to the spreading knowledge about the potential of Rheopheresis numerous AMD-patients wished to become treated unrelated to controlled clinical trials. In total more than 300 patients with AMD have received extracorporeal hemorheotherapy at the University of Cologne and essentially confirmed the study results in clinical practice (Brunner et al., personal communication). Therefore, a recommendation for high-risk AMD-patients was defined and included in the Apheresis-Guidelines of the German Society for Clinical nephrology, to guarantee that Rheopheresis would be exclusively used for AMD-patients within tight limitations of an interdisciplinary quality management approach [49]. This recommendation for clinical practice will be continuously updated by data from ongoing clinical trials and analysis of the RheoNet-registry to develop complete evidence-

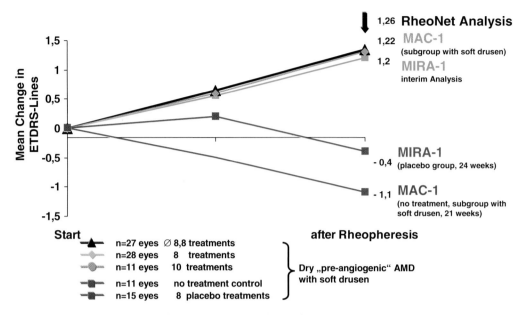

Fig. 9. Reference-controlled RheoNet-registry analysis of 27 eyes with dry AMD and soft drusen. Mean change in visual acuity after the Rheopheresis treatment series in these eyes is compared to corresponding treatment and control groups from the MAC-I trial and interim results of the MIRA-1 trial

based guidelines. The following conditions should be demonstrated to consider Rheopheresis for an individual AMD-patient in clinical practice: (1) bilateral AMD, (2) soft drusen in the better eye, (3) BSCVA 0.1–0.63 of the better eye, (4) exclusion of CNV in the better eye, and (5) Rheopheresis should be complementary and not competitive to other possible therapeutic options for this AMD-patient. Two schedules for 8–10 Rheopheresis treatments were used in the past and seemed to be equally effective. Target for a single treatment is 100% plasma volume. Schedule 1 consists of two Rheopheresis treatments per week, followed by 4-week (MAC-I trial) or 2-week intervals (MIRA-1 trial). Schedule 2 consists of two Rheopheresis treatments in the first week, followed by single treatments every two weeks [42]. Based on the positive results of the MIRA-1-interim-analysis 8 single treatments are currently recommended as the initial treatment series.

Reimbursement issues

Prerequisites exist for acceptance in the medical community, international aproval and reimbursement of novel therapies. Safety and efficacy must be assessed by criteria of evidencive-based-medicine to ensure that selection and other common sources of bias are minimized. Gold standard for the systematic review of health care is a double-blinded, randomized placebo-controlled clinical trial following Good Clinical Practice guidelines (ICH-GCP) with a publication according to the revised Consort-statement. Within the European community aspects of approval and permission are under law of the European community. But the health care budget must be available in the national health care system, which directs the final decision on reimbursement to national law. Rheopheresis for AMD was first investigated in Germany, therefore the German situation will be considered in the following in more detail. Organisation of the German health care system is currently determined by seperation into ambulatory (out-patient) care and in-hospital care. Related to income statutory health insurance is mandatory, currently covering app. 88% of the German population, the voluntary health insurance system covers approximately 9%. Reimbursement within the statutory health insurance by federal social law depends on the regulations of the National Association of Statutory Health Insurance Physicians (NASHIP). After that decision reimbursement budgets are mainly negotiated between health care authorities and health insurance carriers. Currently lipid-apheresis is the only indication of therapeutic apheresis with regular reimbursement. Reimbursement for Rheopheresis currently depends upon individual application for a single patient. With respect to recent decisions of the German supreme court for social law there is a dilemma. Without a positive decision of NASHIP statutory health insurance carriers are not permitted to reimburse new therapies. On the other hand the supreme court defined exceptions. If the patient suffers from a morbid condition, which is life threatening or results in a sustained deterioration of quality of life reimbursement is permitted. No alternative treatment must be is available and according to available evidence there must be a reasonable expectation for successful therapy. These strained relations characterize the current status of Rheopheresis for AMD in Germany. As a consequence Rheopheresis for AMD is only available for self-paying patients or after successful individual application for reimbursement, which represent pure economic non-medical conditions.

Conclusion

In the majority of AMD patients the therapeutic situation is very unsatisfactory, especially for patients with dry AMD. Rheopheresis is a safe and effective modality of therapeutic apheresis to treat microcirculatory disorders, and represents a novel therapeutic approach for patients with dry AMD. A series of Rheopheresis treatments with effective pulses of decreased plasma viscosity and elimination of microcirculatory relevant high-molecular weight proteins can induce sustained improvement of the progressive natural course of AMD. The implementation of Rheopheresis into clinical practice is guided by the requirements of evidence-based medicine. However, limitations under the financial constraints of public health care sytems increase. The RheoNet-registry and the development and continuous update of therapy guidelines provide an appropriate framework for the quality management of the interdisciplinary cooperation between ophthalmologists with apheresis specialists, namely nephrologists. A hypothesis based upon current knowledge of pathogenic mechanisms of the development and progression of AMD can be conclusively linked with the putative mechanism of action of Rheopheresis for AMD. The final results of the MIRA-1 trial will allow the exact definition for the indication of Rheopheresis in patients with dry AMD.

References

1. Pfau N, Kupsch S, Kern AO, Beske F (2000) Epidemiology and socioeconomic importance of blindness and severe vision loss in Germany (Publication in German). Schriftenreihe des IGSF – Institut für Gesundheits-System-Forschung 84:1–161
2. Ciulla TA, Harris A, Martin BJ (2001) Ocular perfusion and age-related macular degeneration. Acta Ophthalmol Scand 79:108–15
3. Fine SL, Berger JW, Maguire MG, Ho AC (2000) Age-related macular degeneration. N Engl J Med 342:483–92
4. Sarraf D, Gin T, Yu F, Brannon A, Owens SL, Bird AC (1999) Long-term drusen study. Retina 19:513–19

5. Lanchoney DM, Maguire MG, Fine SL (1998) A model of the incidence and consequences of choroidal neovascularization secondary to age-related macular degeneration. Comparative effects of current treatment and potential prophylaxis on visual outcomes in high-risk patients. Arch Ophthalmol 116:1045–52

6. Klein R, Klein BEK, Tomany SC, Meuer SM, Huang GH (2002) Ten-year incidence and progression of age-related maculopathy. Ophthalmol 109:1767–79

7. Hageman GS, Luthert PJ, Chong NHV, Johnson LV, Anderson DH, Mullins RF (2001) An integrated hypothesis that considers drusen as biomarkers of immune-mediated processes at the RPE-Bruch's membrane interface in aging and age-related macular degeneration. Prog Ret Eye Res 20:705–32

8. Ramirez JM, Ramirez AI, Salazar JJ, de Hoz R, Trivino A (2001) Changes of astrocytes in retinal aging and age-related macular degeneration. Exp Eye Res 73:601–15

9. Eye Disease Case-Control Study Group (1992) Risk factors for neovascular age-related macular degeneration. Arch Ophthalmol 110:1701–8

10. Smith W, Mitchell P, Leeder SR, Wang JJ (1998) Plasma fibrinogen levels, other cardiovascular risk factors, and age-related maculopathy. Arch Ophthalmol 116:583, 587

11. Vingerling JR, Dielemans I, Bots ML, Homan A, Grobbee DEL, de Jong PTVM (1995) Age-related macular degeneration is associated with atherosclerosis. Am J Epidemiol 142:404–9

12. Lip PL, Blann AD, Hope-Ross M, Gibson JM, Lip GYH (2001) Age-related macular degeneration is associated with increased vascular endothelial growth factor, hemorheology, and endothelial dysfunction. Ophthalmol 108:705–10

13. Baudouin C, Peyman GA, Fredj-Reygrobellet D, Gordon WC, Lapalus P, Gastaud P, Bazan NG (1992) Immunohistochemical study of subretinal membranes in age-related macular degeneration. Jpn J Ophthalmol 36:443–51

14. Friedman E (1997) A hemodynamic model of the pathogenesis of age-related macular degeneration. Am J Ophthalmol 124:677–82

15. Grunwald J, Hariprasad S, DuPont J (1998) Effect of aging on foveolar choroidal circulation. Arch Ophthalmol 116:150–4

16. Grunwald J, Hariprasad S, DuPont J, Maguire M, Fine S, Brucker A, Maguire A, Ho A (1998) Foveolar choroidal blood flow in age-related macular degeneration. Invest Ophthalmol Vis Sci 39:385–90

17. Chen SJ, Cheng CY, Lee AF, Lee FL, Chou JCK, Hsu WM, Liu JH (2001) Pulsatile ocular blood flow in asymmetric exudative age related macular degeneration. Br J Ophthalmol 85:1411–15

18. Tamai M, Mizuno K, Chader GJ (1982) In vitro studies on shedding and phagocytosis of rod outer segments in the rat retina: effect of oxygen concentration. Invest Ophthalmol 22:439–48

19. Sheu SJ, Sakamoto T, Osusky R, Wang HM, Ogden TE, Ryan SJ, Hinton DR, Gopalakrishna R (1994) Transforming growth factor-ß regulates human retinal pigment epithelial cell phagocytosis by influencing a protein kinase C-dependent pathway. Graefe's Arch Clin Exp Ophthalmol 234:695–701

20. Ueba H, Kawakami M, Yaginuma T (1997) Shear stress as an inhibitor of vascular smooth muscle cell proliferation. Role of transforming growth factor beta 1 and tissue-type plasminogen activator. Arterioscler Thromb Vasc Biol 17:1512–16

21. Moore DJ, Clover GM (2001) The effect of age on the macromolecular permeability of human Bruch's membrane. Invest Ophthalmol Vis Sci 42:2970–5

22. King GL, Suzuma K (2000) Pigment-epithelium-derived factor – a key coordinator of retinal neuronal and vascular functions. N Engl J Med 342:349–51

23. Hussain AA, Rowe L, Marshall J (2002) Age-related alterations in the diffusional transport of amino acids across the human Bruch's-choroid complex. J Opt Soc Am A Opt Image Sci Vis 19:166–72

24. Preissner KT, Pötsch B (1995) Vessel wall-dependent metabolic pathways of the adhesive proteins von-Willebrand factor and vitronectin. Histol Histopathol 10:239–51

25. Stockmann A, Hess S, Declerck P, Timpl R, Preissner KT (1993) Multimeric vitronectin. J Biol Chem 268:22874–82

26. Kost C, Benner K, Stockmann A, Linder D, Preissner KT (1996) Limited plasmin proteolysis of vitronectin – characterization of the adhesion protein as morpho-regulatory and angiostatin-binding factor. Eur J Biochem 236:682–8

27. Hammes HP, Brownlee M, Jonczyk A, Sutter A, Preissner KT (1996) Subcutaneous injection of a cyclic peptide antagonist of vitronectin receptor-type integrins inhibits retinal neovascularization. Nature Medicine 2:529–33

28. Johnson LV, Leitner WP, Staples MK, Anderson DH (2001) Complement activation and inflammatory processes in drusen formation and age related macular degeneration. Exp Eye Res 73:887–96

29. Age-Related Eye Disease Study Research Group (2001) A randomized, placebo-controled, clinical trial of high-dose supplementation with vitamins C and E, beta carotene, and zinc for age-related macular degeneration and vision loss. Arch Ophthalmol 119:1417–36

30. Treatment of Age-Related Macular Degeneration with Photodynamic Therapy (TAP) Study Group (2002) Verteporfin therapy for subfoveal choroidal neovascularization in age-related macular degeneration. Three-year results of an open-label extension of 2 randomized clinical trials – TAP report no.5. Arch Ophthalmol 120:1307–14

31. Currie ZI, Rennie IG, Talbot JF (2000) Retinal vascular changes associated with transpupillary thermotherapy for choroidal melanomas. Retina 20:620–6

32. Guymer RH, Hageman GS, Bird AC (2001) Influence of laser photocoagulation on choroidal capillary cytoarchitecture. Br J Ophthalmol 85:40–6

33. Kaga T, Fonseca RA, Dantas MA, Spaide RF (2001) Transient appearance of classic choroidal neovascularization after transpupillary thermotherapy for occult choroidal neovascularization. Retina 21:172–3

34. Kaiser RS, Berger JW, Maguire MG, Ho AC, Javornik NB (2001) Laser burn intensity and the risk for choroidal neovascularization in the CNVPT fellow eye study. Arch Ophthalmol 119:826–32

35. Klingel R, Fassbender C, Faßbender T, Erdtracht B (2000) Rheopheresis – rheologic, functional and structural aspects. Therapeutic Apheresis 4:348–57

36. Klingel R, Mumme C, Faßbender T, Himmelsbach F, Altes U, Lotz J, Pohlmann T, Beyer J, Küstner E (2003) Rheopheresis in patients with ischemic diabetic foot syndrome – results of an open label prospective pilot trial. Therapeutic Apheresis and Dialysis 7:444–55

37. Lüke C, Widder RA, Soudavar F, Walter P, Brunner R, Borberg H (2001) Improvement of macular function by membrane differential filtration in diabetic retinopathy. J Clin Apheresis 16:23–8

38. Brunner R, Widder RA, Walter P, Lüke C, Godehardt E, Bartz-Schmidt K-U, Heimann K, Borberg H (2000) Influence of membrane differential filtration on the natural course of age-related macular degeneration – a randomized trial. Retina 20:483–91

39. Swartz M, Rabetoy G (1999) Treatment of non-exudative age-related macular degeneration using membrane differential filtration apheresis. Invest Ophthalmol Vis Sci 40:319 (abstract)

40. Brunner R, Widder RA, Fischer RA, Walter P, Bartz-Schmidt K-U, Heimann K (1996) Clinical efficacy of haemorheological treatment using plasma exchange, selective adsorption and membrane differential filtration in maculopathy, retinal vein occlusion and uveal effusion syndrome. Transfus Sci 17:493–8

41. Soudavar F, Widder RA, Brunner R, Walter P, Bartz-Schmitz KU, Borberg H, Heimann K (1998) Changes of retinal haemodynamics after elimination of high molecular weight proteins and lipids in patients with age-related macular degeneration. Invest Ophthalmol Vis Sci 39:386 (abstract)

42. Fell A, Engelmann K, Richard G, Fassbender C, Wahls W, Klingel R (2002) Rheopheresis – a sytemic approach to therapy of age-related macular degeneration. Ophthalmologe 99:780–4

43. Abdelsalam A, Del Priore L, Zarbin MA (1998) Drusen in age-related macular degeneration: pathogenesis, natural course, and laser photocoagulation-induced regression. Surv Ophthalmol 44:1–29

44. Widder RA, Farvili E, Reis RGJ, Lüke C, Walter P, Kirchhof B, Borberg H, Brunner R (2002) The treatment of age-related macular degeneration (ARMD) with extracorporeal treatment procedures. A follow-up of four years. Invest Ophthalmol Vis Sci 43:2906 (abstract)

45. Godehardt E, Messner H, Wallstab UH (1993) Extracorporeal LDL cholesterol elimination by membrane differential filtration. In: Gotto AM, Mancini M, Richter WO, Schwandt P (eds) Treatment of severe dyslipoproteinemia in the prevention of coronary heart disease. 4:208–12

46. Berrouschot J, Barthel H, Scheel C, Köster J, Schneider D (1998) Extracorporeal membrane differential filtration – a new and safe method to optimize hemorheology in acute ischemic stroke. Acta Neurol Scand 97:126–30

47. Suckfüll M for the Hearing Loss Study Group (2002) Fibrinogen and LDL-apheresis in treatment of sudden hearing loss: a randomized multicentre trial. Lancet 360:1811–17
48. Ohno-Matsui K, Morita I, Tombran-Tink J, Mrazek D, Onodera M, Uetama T, Hayano M, Murota SI, Mochizuki M (2001) Novel mechanism for age-related macular degeneration: an equilibrium shift between the angiogenesis factors VEGF and PEDF. J Cell Physiol 189:323–33
49. Mann H, Bosch Th, Braun N, Fassbinder W, Klingel R, Klinkmann J, Lonnemann G, Querfeld U, Ramlow W, Schettler V (2002) Apheresis-standard of the German society for clinical nephrology. Mitteilungen der Deutschen Arbeitsgemeinschaft für Klinische Nephrologie XXXI/2002: 103–38 (Article in German)

Correspondence: Reinhard Klingel, MD, PhD, Apheresis Research Institute, Stadtwaldguertel 77, D-50935 Cologne, Germany, E-mail: afi@apheresis-research.de

Vitreous pathobiology and pharmacologic vitreolysis

J. Sebag

Professor of Clinical Ophthalmology,
Doheny Eye Institute,
University of Southern California,
Los Angeles, California, USA

I. Introduction

Once regarded as a vestigial organ, vitreous is now considered an important ocular structure, at least with respect to several pathologic conditions of the posterior segment [1, 2]. In the normal state, vitreous is a clear and solid gel (Fig. 1) that is firmly adherent to the retina, especially in youth. This remarkable tissue is, in essence, an extended extracellular matrix, composed largely of water with a very small amount of structural macromolecules.

II. Vitreous anatomy

A. Vitreous body

Vitreous is a viscoelastic extracellular matrix that fills the center of the eye. Although composed primarily (98%) of water, vitreous normally exists in a gel state as a result of the intricate organization of its macromolecular components [2, 3]. Hyaluronan (HA) imparts viscoelasticity while the structural *frame* is provided by collagen, primarily type II but also type IX, and a hybrid of types V/XI [4]. As shown in Fig. 2, the type IX collagen is situated on the surface of the fibril, making it easier for this component to interact with other vitreous molecules, thereby playing an important role in maintaining the gel state.

B. Vitreo-retinal interface

The peripheral vitreous, known as the vitreous cortex, consists of densely packed fibrils with collagen (types II, IX, and a hybrid of types V/XI) and a high concentration of HA. In youth, the posterior vitreous cortex is firmly adherent to the internal limiting lamina (ILL) of the retina. The ILL, which is actually the basal lamina of retinal Mueller cells, is composed of type IV collagen closely associated with glycoproteins. While the exact nature of vitreoretinal adhesion is not known, it most probably results from the biophysical properties of the extracellular matrix molecules found at this interface [5].

III. Aging, anomalous PVD, and vitreo-retinal diseases

During aging, there is weakening of vitreo-retinal adhesion [1, 2], probably due to the effect of free radicals generated by incident light and reactive oxygen species from retinal cell metabolism, in addition to endogenous enzyme effects. Liquefaction of the gel may also be due to light as well as the action of proteolytic enzymes and endogenous metal-

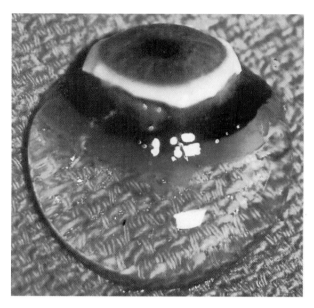

Fig. 1. Vitreous dissected of the sclera, choroid, and retina in a 9-month old child is a solid gel in spite of being situated on a surgical towel in room air

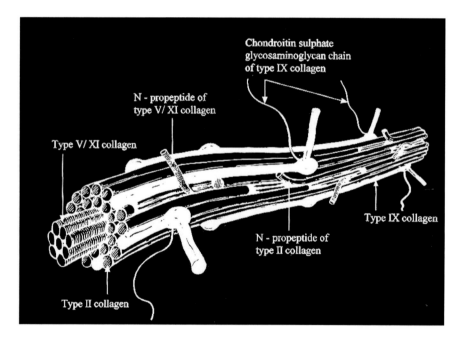

Fig. 2. Schematic diagram of human vitreous collagen fibril (d'après Bishop). Various proteogly-cans, glycoproteins, and other molecules might also play a role in the organization of the two major structural macromolecules into a three-dimensional network [4] that achieves the physiologic vitreous functions of media clarity and shock-absorption [1]

loproteinases. Concurrent weakening of the vitreo-retinal interface and gel liquefaction results in innocuous posterior vitreous detachment (PVD). Liquefaction without concurrent vitreoretinal dehiscence results in *Anomalous PVD,* sometimes with splitting of the

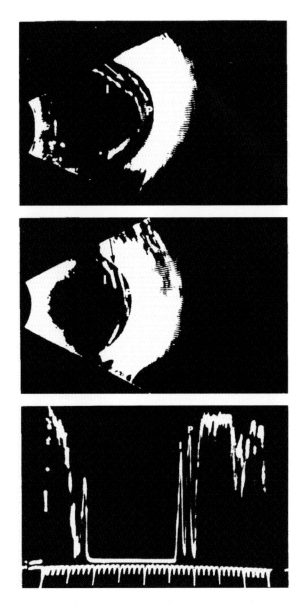

Fig. 3. B-scan ultrasonography of posterior vitreoschisis (courtesy of Dr. Ron Green, Doheny Eye Institute, Los Angeles, California)

posterior vitreous cortex, known as vitreoschisis (Fig. 3), exerting abnormal traction upon the retina.

The particular consequences of this traction depend upon where traction is exerted. In the periphery, retinal tears and detachments result due to unusual vitreo-retinal adhesion from cystic retinal tufts (Fig. 4) or verruca (Fig. 5).

At the macula there can be vitreo-macular traction syndrome, macular holes, or macular pucker.

In Proliferative Diabetic Vitreo-Retinopathy new blood vessels grow into the overlying posterior vitreous cortex (Fig. 6).

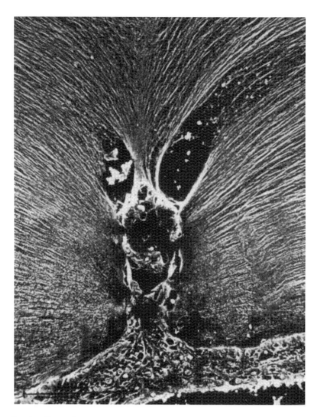

Fig. 4. Cystic retinal tuft. The tuft is a cystoid formation of fibers, similar to those of the nerve fiber layer, and cells, similar to those found in the inner plexiform layer of the retina. The tuft is connected to the internal limiting lamina of the retina. This scanning electron micrograph shows the insertion of the vitreous collagen fibers on the tuft's apical surface. Their orientation changes toward the tuft's surface (courtesy of Dr. Stephan Dunker and Professor Juergen Faulborn)

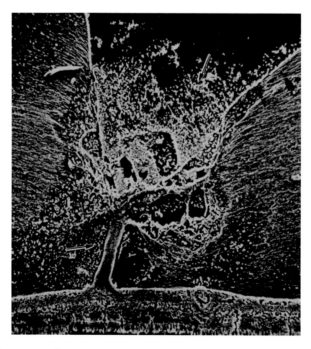

Fig. 5. Verruca. The verruca has a structure similar to that of a tree. Its "roots" are embedded in the inner layers of the retina. Cellular elements resembling cells of the inner plexiform layer can be seen near the retinal surface. The "trunk" of this structure extends from the retina to the middle parts of the vitreous cortex. The "branches" of the verruca are intertwined with interrupted vitreous collagen fibers. Local condensation of collagen fibers exists as well as local collagen destruction (arrows) and interruption of the internal limiting lamina of the retina. [reprinted with permission from Dunker S, Glinz J, Faulborn J: Morphologic studies of the peripheral vitreoretinal interface in humans reveal structures implicated in the pathogenesis of retinal tears. Retina 17:124–130, 1997.]

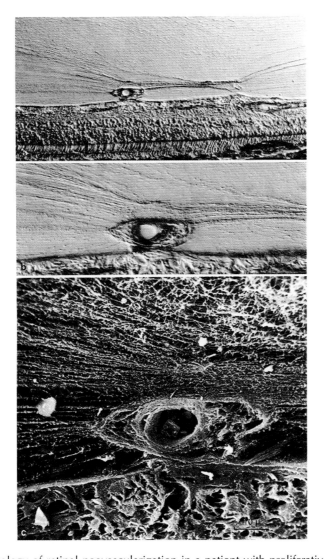

Fig. 6. Histopathology of retinal neovascularization in a patient with proliferative diabetic vitreo-retinopathy demonstrates that the new vessels grow out of the retinal plane into the overlying posterior vitreous cortex. Prominent vitreous fibers insert into the new vessels and can transmit tractional forces induced by diabetic vitreopathy. Such traction can be important in the pathogenesis of vitreous hemorrhage and traction retinal detachment. [Reprinted with permission from Faulborn J, Bowald S: Microproliferations in proliferative diabetic retinopathy and their relation to the vitreous. Graef Arch Clin Exp Ophthalmol 223:130, 1985.]

As a result of alterations induced by diabetic vitreopathy [6] (Fig. 7) there is Anomalous PVD (liquefaction without vitreo-retinal dehiscence) and untoward traction upon the optic disc and retina. This can stimulate new blood vessels to grow even more aggressively, can tear the new blood vessels to induce vitreous hemorrhage, often into vitreoschisis cavities (Fig. 8) and/or can pull on the retina resulting in traction retinal detachment. There can also be effects on the macula causing macular edema that is largely unresponsive to laser photocoagulation.

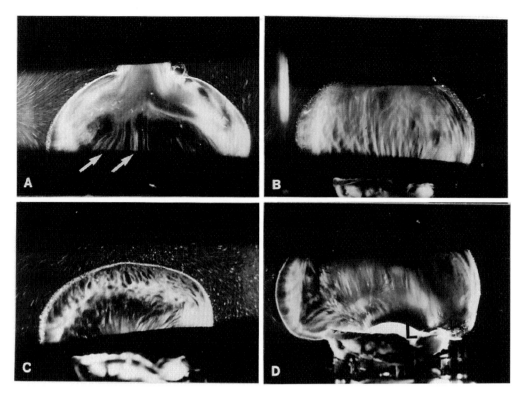

Fig. 7. A Right eye of a 9 year old girl with a five year history of type I diabetes shows extrusion of central vitreous through the posterior vitreous cortex into the retro-cortical (pre-retinal)space. The subcortical vitreous appears very dense and scatters light intensely. Centrally, there are vitreous fibers (arrows) with an antero-posterior orientation and adjacent areas of liquefaction. **B** Central vitreous in the left eye of the patient in 7A shows prominent fibers that resemble those seen in non-diabetic adults (Figs. 4, 5). **C** Peripheral vitreous of same specimen as 7B shows fibers inserting into the vitreous cortex with adjacent collections of liquid vitreous. **D** Anterior vitreous of same specimen as 7B shows fiber insertion into the vitreous base about the lens (L). [Reprinted with permission from Sebag J: Abnormalities of human vitreous structure in diabetes. Graef Arch Clin Exp Ophthalmol 231:257, 1993.]

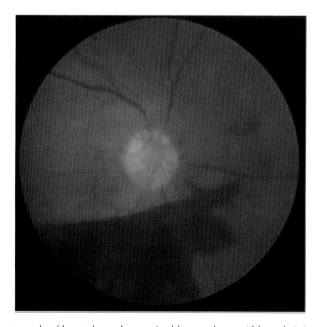

Fig. 8. Fundus photograph of boat-shaped preretinal hemorrhage. Although it is possible the blood is located between the vitreous and retina, it is more likely loculated between the inner and outer walls of a vitreoschisis cavity

IV. Rationale for pharmacologic vitreolysis

To date, surgical instrumentation and techniques have primarily been designed to separate vitreous from the retina and remove it from the eye. While often quite effective, these interventions are not always successful. Furthermore, as they are costly and highly invasive, they are rarely performed as prophylaxis. Thus, less invasive and more effective means are needed to improve surgical outcomes and enable preventative therapies. Pharmacologic adjuncts to surgery could improve today's results and also provide new ways to avoid surgery in the future.

V. Pharmacologic vitreolysis

Coined [7] in 1998, this term refers to the use of exogenous (to the vitreous) agents to alter the biochemical and biophysical states of the macromolecules responsible for maintaining vitreous structure and vitreo-retinal adhesion. The goals of Pharmacologic Vitreolysis are thus to induce liquefaction of the gel and promote dehiscence of the vitreous from the retina. It is important to note that the success of Pharmacologic Vitreolysis depends upon inducing these two processes simultaneously, or at least insuring that liquefaction does not progress without sufficient vitreo-retinal dehiscence. Uncoupling these two processes, particularly by inducing liquefaction without weakening vitreo-retinal adherence, may worsen matters significantly by provoking rather than preventing or ameliorating Anomalous PVD and its untoward sequelae; i.e. vitreo-papillopathies, vitreo-maculopathies, and peripheral retinal traction.

There have been a variety of approaches attempted to date. Albeit unsuccessfully, Hyaluronidase was employed as early as 1949 and Collagenase in 1973. Table 1 outlines the approaches that are currently being developed. The different pharmacologic agents can be broadly grouped as enzymatic and non-enzymatic. Within the enzymatic group there are substrate-specific agents and non-specific agents.

Early observations of the effects of blood on vitreous laid the groundwork for approaches based upon extracting active agents from blood for Pharmacologic Vitreolysis. *Plasmin* is a non-specific protease that can be isolated from the patient's own serum for use at surgery. It has been tested in rabbits [8] and several small series of pediatric and adult patients undergoing vitrectomy by Drs. Mike Trese, George Williams, and colleagues. This agent is primarily advocated as an adjunct to vitreo-retinal surgery. A phase II clinical trial of autologous plasmin agent is currently being organized in the United States. There are also other, so-called "exogenous", sources of plasmin. Studies [9] have shown that effective intravitreal levels of plasmin can be generated by injecting tissue plasminogen activator (tPA) and breaking down the blood-vitreous barrier with cryopexy or laser photocoagulation. Other studies [10] have used combinations of plasminogen and urokinase.

Table 1. Pharmacologic vitreolysis

I. Enzymatic Vitreolysis
A. Non-Specific
1. Plasmin
2. Dispase
B. Substrate-Specific
1. Chondroitinase
2. Hyaluronidase
3. Collagenase
II. Non-Enzymatic Vitreolysis

Another relatively non-specific protease currently under investigation is **Dispase**. The first investigations [11] used Dispase to induce PVD in enucleated porcine and human cadaver eyes, noting no untoward effects upon retinal histology and ultrastructure. Subsequent studies [12] were successful in using this agent *in vivo* to remove cortical vitreous during vitreous surgery in the pig. Since Dispase has proteolytic activity against type IV collagen and fibronectin, there is some concern that the ILL of the retina might be adversely affected by this agent. Yet, the histologic studies [11] in porcine and human cadaver eyes found that only the lamina rara externa of the ILL was affected, with lesser effects upon the lamina densa. The subsequent animal studies found that this agent did not alter the ERG *in vivo*, and no neuroretinal ultrastructural abnormalities were detected *post-mortem* [12].

A substrate-specific enzyme that has been in development for a number of years by Drs. Greg Hageman and Steve Russell is **Chondroitinase**. This agent lyses chondroitin sulfate, a molecule that may be important in the maintenance of both the gel state of vitreous [13], as well as vitreo-retinal adhesion; hence, there has been considerable interest in the use of this agent. Indeed, studies [14] have purportedly shown that when used as an adjunct to vitreous surgery, Chondroitinase facilitates the removal of premacular membranes. Several years ago, a phase I trial using this agent during vitreous surgery in patients was completed in the United States, yet the results still await publication. In this trial, patients with macular holes and others with proliferative diabetic vitreo-retinopathy were treated with Chondroitinase during vitreous surgery, with no untoward effects. Yet, phase II studies of efficacy have yet to be undertaken.

In addition to facilitating vitreo-retinal surgery as currently performed, Pharmacologic Vitreolysis could possibly replace vitrectomy, as was proposed with **Hyaluronidase** to clear vitreous hemorrhage without vitrectomy. However, in the Phase III FDA trial undertaken in the United States, this drug was not found to be effective. This may be due to the fact that the trial included patients with both type I and type II diabetes. In the former group the patients are younger and more likely to have an attached vitreous without a weakened vitreo-retinal interface. Thus, although the enzyme may have decreased the viscosity of vitreous gel and facilitated the outflow of red blood cells, the persistent attachment of the posterior vitreous cortex to the retina and to any neovascular complexes arising from the retina and optic disk would cause recurrent vitreous hemorrhage, and possibly retinal detachment. Indeed, there has been some discussion of using this agent to induce posterior vitreous detachment in patients with non-proliferative diabetic retinopathy, since liquefaction of the vitreous body and detachment of the posterior vitreous cortex away from the retina prior to the onset of new vessel growth into the vitreo-retinal interface (see below) will have a far better prognosis than if the vitreous were still attached to the However, Hyaluronidase is not likely to induce vitreo-retinal separation and PVD, at least on theoretical grounds. Indeed, studies [15] in experimental animal models have shown contradictory results in this regard, with the most recent studies [16] finding no such effect. On the other hand, combining Hyaluronidase with SF6 has purportedly induced PVD in the rabbit, as has been described with plasmin and SF6 [17]. It is plausible that the expanding gas, and not the enzyme, is responsible for these effects, since many years ago Lincoff and Machemer reported similar effects with expanding gas alone.

A. Ideal solutions for pharmacologic vitreolysis

It is important to note that in the Dispase studies, there was no evidence of vitreous liquefaction. This underscores the concept that few, if any, single agents can achieve both of the desired components of effective Pharmacologic Vitreolysis; i.e. liquefaction of the gel and vitreo-retinal dehiscence. Dispase causes dehiscence but not liquefaction.

Hyaluronidase liquefies vitreous gel but without gas probably does not induce PVD. Chondroitinase may do both but the depolymerization of HA and chondroitin sulfate only results in a reduction of vitreous gel wet weight and not gel destruction [18]. Collagenases would probably be needed to achieve such effects. Indeed, vitreous molecular morphology is so complex and there are so many different changes that occur with aging and various diseases, that the future will probably see the use of a mixture of agents whose relative concentrations will need to be adjusted in consideration of the patient's age, disease, and the desired effect. Ideally this would begin by inducing vitreo-retinal dehiscence, and then be followed by liquefaction of the gel vitreous [19].

References

1. Sebag J (1989) The vitreous – structure, function, and pathobiology. New York: Springer
2. Sebag J (1998) Vitreous – from biochemistry to clinical relevance. In: Tasman W, Jaeger EA (eds) Duane's foundations of clinical ophthalmology. Philadelphia: Lippincott Williams & Wilkins, Vol 1, Ch 16
3. Sebag J (1998) Macromolecular structure of vitreous. In: Chirila TV (ed) Polymer science and the eye. Prog Polym Sci 23:415–46
4. Bishop PN (2000) Structural macromolecules and supramolecular organization of the vitreous gel. Progr in Retinal Eye Res 19:323–44
5. Sebag J, Hageman GS (2000) Interfaces. Eur J Ophthalmol 10:1–3
6. Sebag J (1996) Diabetic vitreopathy (Guest Editorial). Ophthalmology 103:205–6
7. Sebag J (1998) Pharmacologic vitreolysis. Retina 18:1–3
8. Verstraeten T, Chapman C, Hartzer M, Winkler BS, Trese MT, Williams GA (1993) Pharmacologic induction of PVD in the rabbit. Arch Ophthalmol 111:849
9. Hesse L, Nebeling B, Schroeder B, Heller G, Kroll P (2000) Induction of posterior vitreous detachment in rabbits by intravitreal injection of tissue plasminogen activator following cryopexy. Exp Eye Res 70:31–9
10. Unal M, Peyman GA (2000) The efficacy of plasminogen-urokinase combination in inducing posterior vitreous detachment. Retina 20:69–75
11. Tezel TH, Del Priore LV, Kaplan HJ (1998) Posterior vitreous detachment with dispase. Retina 18:17–5
12. Oliviera LB, Tatebayashi M, Mahmoud TH, et al (2001) Dispase facilitates posterior vitreous detachment during vitrectomy in young pigs. Retina 21:324–31
13. Hageman GS, Johnson LV (1984) Lectin-binding glycoproteins in the vertebrate vitreous body and inner limiting membrane-tissue localization and biochemical characterization. J Cell Biol 99:179a
14. Hageman GS, Russell SR (1997) Chondroitinase-mediated disinsertion of the primate vitreous body. Invest Ophthalmol Vis Sci 38(ARVO):S662
15. Harooni M, McMillan T, Refojo M (1998) Efficacy and safety of enzymatic posterior vitreous detachment by intravitreal injection of hyaluronidase. Retina 18:16
16. Hikichi T, Masanori K, Yoshida A (2000) Intravitreal injection of hyaluronidase cannot induce posterior vitreous detachment in the rabbit. Retina 20:195–8
17. Hikichi T, Yanagiya N, Kado M, Akiba J, Yoshida A (1999) Posterior vitreous detachment induced by injection of plasmin and sulfur hexafluoride in the rabbit vitreous. Retina 19:55–8
18. Bishop PN, McLeod D, Reardon A (1999) Effects of hyaluronan lyase, hyaluronidase, and chondroitin ABC lyase on mammalian vitreous gel. Invest Ophthalmol Vis Sci 40:2173–8
19. Sebag J (2002) Is pharmacologic vitreolysis brewing? Retina 22:1–3

Correspondence: J. Sebag, MD, FACS, FRCOphth., VMR Institute, 7677 Center Avenue, Huntington Beach, CA 92647, USA.

Diffuse diabetic macular edema: results after intravitreal triamcinolone acetonide*

I. Kreissig, J. Jonas, and R. F. Degenring

Department of Ophthalmology, Faculty of Clinical Medicine Mannheim, Ruprecht Karls-University Heidelberg, Germany

Abstract

Purpose: To evaluate the clinical outcome of an intravitreal injection of triamcinolone acetonide as treatment of diffuse diabetic macular edema.

Materials and methods: The prospective, interventional, clinical case series study included 20 patients (26 eyes) who received an intravitreal injection of 20 mg to 25 mg of triamcinolone acetonide as treatment of diffuse diabetic macular edema. The injection was done under topical anesthesia and sterile conditions in the operating room. Mean follow-up ranged at 6.64 ± 6.10 months. The study group was compared with a control group of 16 patients who underwent macular grid laser coagulations.

Results: In the study group, visual acuity increased significantly ($p < 0.001$) from 0.12 ± 0.08 at baseline to a maximum of 0.19 ± 0.14 during the follow-up. Seventeen (81%) of 21 eyes with a follow-up of more than 1 month gained in visual acuity. In the control group, visual acuity did not change significantly. In the study group, intraocular pressure increased significantly ($p < 0.001$) from 16.9 ± 2.5 mm Hg to a mean maximal value of 21.3 ± 4.7 mm Hg, and decreased significantly ($p = 0.028$) to 17.7 ± 4.7 mm Hg at the end of the study. This occurred parallel to the disappearance of the crystals in the vitreous. Intraocular pressure could be controlled with topical antiglaucomatous drops.

Conclusion: Intravitreal injection of 20 mg to 25 mg triamcinolone acetonide might increase visual acuity in patients with clinically significant diffuse diabetic macular edema.

Introduction

Diabetic macular edema had been treated so far by focal laser coagulation applied to leaks in the retina. But this is not feasible when there is a diffuse macular edema [1]. As alternative a vitrectomy with peeling of the internal limiting membrane had been suggested by Hillal Lewis and systemic cortisone by Deutman. Yet despite all, the discussion on an optimal treatment of diffuse diabetic macular edema is still ongoing.

The following study was done to evaluate whether an intravitreal injection of high-dosed crystalline cortisone, i.e. triamcinolone acetonide, will reduce the macular edema and thus increase visual acuity.

---

*Read at the 2nd International Conference on Vitreoretinal Diseases in Vienna/Austria, September 8, 2002.

Patients

The study included 20 diabetic patients or 26 eyes which had had a loss of vision for at least 1 year and in which visual acuity had remained decreased for at least 3 months due to diffuse macular edema. Each eye had received an intravitreal injection of crystalline triamcinolone acetonide.

The mean age of the patients was 66.9 ± 8.9 years, the refractive error +0.4 ± 1.62 diopters, 8 eyes were pseudophakic and 18 phakic in which the degree of lens opacification was determined. The grading was done at the slit lamp by a scale ranging from "0", a very clear lens, to "5", a very pronounced lens opacification.

The visual acuity was determined by the Snellen chart. Mean visual acuity was 0.12 ± 0.08. Prior to inclusion in the study a grid laser coagulation of the macula was done in 9 eyes. A peripheral and focal macular laser coagulation, if performed, was done 6 months prior to inclusion in the remaining 17 eyes. Fluorescein angiography demonstrated a diffuse macular edema. The follow-up ranged between 1 week and 18 months, the mean was 6.64 ± 6.10 months.

The patients of the study were compared with 16 patients of a control group, who also had a diffuse diabetic macular edema, but were not treated with an intravitreal injection of crystalline cortisone. The control group matched in respect to age, gender, refractive error, and preoperative visual acuity. The mean age of the control group was 70.54 ± 4.70 years, the refractive error +0.58 ± 1.31 diopters, visual acuity 0.16 ± 0.08. In all 16 patients a grid laser coagulation of the macula was done prior to inclusion in the study. The mean follow-up was 7.04 ± 3.51 months. In every patient fluorescein angiography demonstrated a diffuse macular edema.

Method

Preparation and intravitreal injection of triamcinolone acetonide

The entire ampulla of 1 ml containing 40 mg of triamcinolone acetonide (in Germany as Volon A or in USA as Kenalog) is shaken and a volume of 0.62 ml or 20 to 25/40 mg is extracted and filled into a tuberculine syringe which has a volume of 1 ml. After that a millipore filter is inserted on top of the syringe and the solution pressed through the millipore filter. This removes the supernatant (solvent agent) and keeps the triamcinolone acetonide crystals in the syringe. Now the tuberculine syringe is filled up to 1 ml with Ringer's solution. This procedure is repeated twice. At the end, the tuberculine syringe is just containing the triamcinolone acetonide crystals and now the syringe is re-filled up to 0.2 ml with Ringer's solution.

The supernatant is to be removed, because some studies had suggested that the solvent might be toxic to the intraocular tissues and cause an inflammatory reaction [2, 3]. Since during the preparation of the triamcinolone injection a bacterial contamination might occur, this has to be done under sterile conditions in the operating room or the solution for injection should be prepared by the pharmacy department under sterile conditions in their laboratory.

As well under sterile conditions the eye is prepared and draped; the injection itself is performed as any intraocular surgery. The injection is done under topical anesthesia and the 0.2 ml of Ringer's solution, containing 20 mg to 25 mg of triamcinolone acetonide, is injected into the vitreous through a 27 gauge needle through conjunctiva at the pars plana. After the injection, the patient is asked to sit up and to keep an upright position for at least 2 hours to prevent the cortisone crystals from settling into the macular area.

Results

Visual acuity

In the triamcinolone group, visual acuity had increased significantly with a p-value of <0.001; it had increased from 0.12 ± 0.08 at baseline to a maximum of 0.19 ± 0.14 at 10 to 16 weeks. If only the eyes with a minimum follow-up of 1 month are analyzed, the mean maximal visual acuity was 0.18. Paranthetically, 17 of 21 eyes or 81%, with a minimal follow-up of 1 month, demonstrated an increase in visual acuity. When comparing the visual acuity at baseline of the study with the visual acuity determined at various intervals during the entire follow-up, the increase in visual acuity was statistically significant at 6 weeks (p = 0.003) and 10 weeks (p = 0.014), at 5 months (p = 0.028) and 6 months (p = 0.018) after the injection. Towards the end of the follow-up at 3 to 6 months, the triamcinolone acetonide crystals had resolved and disappeared completely from the vitreous cavity.

Fluorescein-angiograms

In the 21 patients for whom fluorescein angiograms pre- and post-treatment were available, fluorescein leakage had decreased significantly with a p-value of <0.001 from a mean of $32.3 \pm 13.6 \, mm^2$ at baseline of the study to a minimum of $26.8 \pm 15.3 \, mm^2$ at 2 to 4 months after the injection of triamcinolone. Evaluated in a subjective and masked fashion, the post-injection angiograms of all 21 eyes demonstrated less fluorescein leakage.

In the control group, visual acuity did not change significantly during the follow-up of 7 months and it ranged at the end of the follow-up at 0.15 ± 0.17 which did not differ significantly (p = 0.35) from 0.16 ± 0.08 at the baseline of the study.

Intraocular pressure

In the study group, intraocular pressure increased significantly with a p-value of <0.001 from a mean of $16.9 \pm 2.5 \, mm \, Hg$ at baseline to a mean maximal value of $21.3 \pm 4.7 \, mm \, Hg$ during follow-up. It decreased again significantly (p = 0.028) to $17.7 \pm 3.6 \, mm \, Hg$ at 5 months after the injection. The intraocular pressures taken at the end of the follow-up period, did not differ significantly (p = 0.31) from the ones at baseline of the study. During the entire study period intraocular pressure was higher than 21 mm Hg in 9 of the 26 study eyes or in 34.6%. But in these 9 eyes, intraocular pressure could be controlled by topical antiglaucomatous medication, such as, Timolole drops twice per day. A glaucomatous damage of the optic nerve was not detected by biomorphometry of the optic nerve head.

Complications

Under the described regimen, in none of the 26 diabetic eyes treated, cortisone crystals had settled at the macular region. Instead, the crystals were located preretinally within the vitreous cortex at 6 o'clock. They did not interfere with visual acuity. In none of the eyes included in the triamcinolone study group, postoperative infectious endophthalmitis or proliferative vitreoretinopathy had developed. In none of the study eyes, a progression of diabetic retinopathy was observed. In the 18 phakic eyes, the degree of lens opacification had slightly increased, however, not significantly. In none of the study eyes a cataract operation was done during the follow-up.

Conclusion

In the presented study with a prospective, non-randomized comparative study design, an intravitreal injection of triamcinolone acetonide of 20 mg to 25 mg into an eye with diffuse diabetic macular edema resulted in a significant increase in visual acuity combined with a significant decrease of fluorescein leakage in the angiogram compared to the baseline of the study during the mean follow-up of 6.6 months. When comparing the baseline values of visual acuity with the visual acuity at 6 and 12 months after the injection of triamcinolone acetonide, the post-injection visual acuity was still slightly higher than before the injection. In 17 of 21 diabetic eyes treated, with a follow-up of 1 month, visual acuity had increased after the injection of triamcinolone acetonide, whereas in the control group visual acuity had not changed significantly.

Major side-effects of intraocular triamcinolone, such as, an untreatable high increase of intraocular pressure or a toxic effect on the retina and optic nerve, were not observed.

However, additional questions have to be answered, such as, the dosage of the triamcinolone acetonide injection: 25 mg [4–9] versus 4 mg [10] or the frequency and interval of a re-injection [11]. Future randomized studies with a larger number of patients have to address these questions and to determine whether an intravitreal injection of triamcinolone acetonide can provide an additional option in the treatment of diffuse diabetic macular edema.

References

1. Early Treatment Diabetic Retinopathy Study research group (1985) Photocoagulation for diabetic macular edema. Early Diabetic Retinopathy Study report number 1. Arch Ophthalmol 103:1796–806
2. Hida T, Chandler D, Arena JE, Machemer R (1986) Experimental and clinical observations of the intraocular toxicity of commercial corticosteroid preparations. Am J Ophthalmol 101:190–5
3. McCuen BW, Bessler M, Tano Y, et al (1981) The lack of toxicity of intravitreally administered triamcinolone acetonide. Am J Ophthalmol 91:785–8
4. Jonas JB, Hayler JK, Panda-Jonas S (2000) Intravitreal injection of crystalline cortisone as adjunctive treatment of proliferative vitreoretinopathy. Br J Ophthalmol 84:1064–7
5. Jonas JB, Hayler JK, Söfker A, Panda-Jonas S (2001) Intravitreal injection of crystalline cortisone as adjunctive treatment of proliferative diabetic retinopathy. Am J Ophthalmol 131:468–71
6. Jonas JB, Kreissig I, Söfker A, Degenring R (2003) Intravitreal injection of triamcinolone for diffuse diabetic edema. Arch Ophthalmol 121:57–61
7. Jonas JB, Kreissig I, Degenring R (2003) Intraocular pressure after intravitreal injection of triamcinolone acetonide. Br J Ophthalmol 87:24–7
8. Kreissig I, Degenring R, Jonas JB (2002) Intravitreal triamcinolone acetonide as treatment of central retinal vein occlusion. Ophthalmic Research 34:162
9. Jonas JB, Kreissig I, Hugger P, Sander G, Panda-Jonas S, Degenring R (2003) Intravitreal triamcinolone acetonide for exudative age related macular degeneration. Br J Ophthalmol 87:462–8
10. Challa JK, Gillies MC, Penfold PL, et al (1998) Exudative macular degeneration and intravitreal triamcinolone: 18 months follow-up. Aust N Z J Ophthalmol 26:277–81
11. Jonas JB, Kreissig I, Degenring R (2002) Repeated intravitreal injections of triamcinolone acetonide as treatment of progressive exudative age-related macular degeneration. Graefes Arch Clin Exp Ophthalmol 240:872–3

Correspondence: Ingrid Kreissig, MD, Department of Ophthalmology, Faculty of Clinical Medicine, Mannheim, Germany.

Optical coherence tomography titrated photocoagulation in diabetic clinically significant macular edema

T. Das, G. Simanjuntak, and K. Sumasri

L V Prasad Eye Institute, L V Prasad Marg, Banjara Hills Hyderabad, India

Clinically significant macular edema (CSME) is the commonest cause of legal blindness in diabetic patients. It is known to occur more often in adult onset diabetics [1]. The Early Treatment of Diabetic Retinopathy Study (ETDRS) defines the CSME to have at least one of the three characteristics: (1) macular edema within 500μ of the center of fovea; (2) hard exudates within 500μ of the center of fovea with associated retinal edema; (3) retinal edema of one disc diameter, a part of which is within one disc diameter of the center of macula [2]. The ETDRS has amply demonstrated that macular laser photocoagulation reduces macular edema, and thus stabilizes or improves the central visual acuity [3]. In the ETDRS study the diagnosis of CSME was made on the basis of stereo fundus photographs and fluorescein angiography. The fluorescein angiography (FA) identified two forms of macular edema-focal and diffuse [4]. Both types of macular edema respond to laser photocoagulation, though the focal edema respond better than diffuse edema [2]. It has been opined that FA is not mandatory for diagnosis of CSME, and that stereoscopic evaluation by slit lamp biomicroscopy could be enough to treat and monitor the effect of treatment in many instances. However, it is known that the degree of macular edema, and not the amount of fluorescein dye leakage determines the extent of visual loss. Hence objective and reproducible measurement of macular edema could be an important determinant in management of CSME.

The optical coherence tomography (OCT) provides such a tool. The OCT is a non-contact non-invasive micron resolution imaging modality that obtains cross sectional images of the retina. It is effective in documenting various pathologies of posterior segment [5].

Good agreement seems to exist between subjective reading of stereo fundus photographs, and objective retinal thickness measurement of OCT [6]. Three patterns of macular edema are described in OCT [7]. They are spongy edema, cystoid edema and serous detachment types. The macular thickness in diabetic eyes reportedly is more than the non-diabetic eyes even before the maculopathy sets in [8]. Possibly this can be used for early detection of diabetic maculopathy. It has been suggested that foveal thickness above 180μ measured by OCT can a useful index for early detection of macular edema [9].

We conducted a pilot study to determine the usefulness of the OCT in laser treatment of diabetic macular edema. The study was designed to answer the following questions:

1. Is there a good correlation between FA and OCT for assessment of CSME?
2. Can OCT replace FA for treatment and follow-up of patients with CSME?

The study was not designed to compare the stereo fundus photographs or biomicroscopic evaluation of CSME with the OCT measurements.

Materials and methods

The study included 37 eyes of 22 consecutive patients with non-insulin dependent diabetes mellitus (NIIDM) seen in the Kanuri Santhamma Retina Vitreous Center, L V Prasad Eye Institute, Hyderabad, India. The inclusion criteria were: (1) adult NIIDM patients, (2) biomicroscopic and FA diagnosis of CSME, and (3) willingness to participate in the study and maintain a regular follow-up for 6 months. The main exclusion criteria were (a) juvenile Type I diabetes, (b) known allergy to Na Fl dye, (3) pregnancy, (4) clinical and angiographic diagnosis of proliferative diabetic retinopathy or macular ischemia, and (5) absence of consent. Two patients did not have follow-up for a period of 6 months, and were thus excluded. In the final analysis 35 eyes of 20 patients were included.

Examination. The ocular examinations included a detailed history of diabetes (duration and control), nature of the visual symptoms, slit lamp examination of the anterior segment of eye, applanation tonometry, and a dilated fundus examination including both biomicroscopy and indirect ophthalmoscopy. Following the clinical confirmation of diabetic maculopathy, all patients received color fundus photography (Zeiss, Germany), fluorescein angiography (FA) (Zeiss, Germany) and optical coherence tomography (OCT) (Zeiss, Germany). The pupil in both eyes were dilated with 1% tropicamide and 1% cyclopentolate solution applied two times at an interval of 15 minutes to ensure at least 5 mm dilatation of the pupil before fundus photography, FA and OCT.

Fundus photography: Thirty-degree color fundus photograph of the posterior pole was taken before FA and OCT.

Fluorescein angiography: Intravenous injection of 3 ml 20% Sodium fluorescein dye, was given and fundus photographs taken at recommended intervals. All the angiogram were done using a 30 degree field. Retinal edema in fluorescein angiogram was defined as the increasing hyperfluorescence around the fovea center with or without identifiable microaneurysm.

Optical coherence tomography: The macular thickness was measured using the fast macular scan program and the retinal map program in OCT-3. The fast macular scan program simultaneously projects six lines onto the macula. Retinal map (vertical and horizontal) gives the average macular thickness in 5 locations-fovea, and the four cardinal directions (superior, inferior, nasal, and temoral) around the fovea. These regions are distributed in 3 zones – 1 mm, 2.22 mm, and 3.45 mm around the center of fixation. Should the center of fixation is the fovea, then the distribution of retinal thickness is shown in the fovea and 8 cardinal locations in 1 mm (around the fovea), 2.22 mm (superior, inferior, temporal, nasal) and 3.45 mm (superior, inferior, temporal, nasal) around the fovea. The thickness of these areas are color coded and the absolute value printed thus eliminating any subjective bias of the examiner. The thicker areas are shown in hot colors including white and the thinner areas in cold colors including black. In general green color represents a normal thickness of the retina. The retinal edema was defined as thickness greater than 200μ.

Both FA and OCT pictures were printed in high-resolution Kodak printing paper. They were analyzed by two independent reviewers (FA by GS, and OCT by KS). So as to match with the area of interest with the OCT, three circles of 1 mm, 2.2 mm, and 3.45 mm diameter were drawn around the center of fovea in the FA print outs. The center of fovea was identified as the center of the foveal avascular zone (FAZ) in the angiogram. The three circles were drawn using the soft ware of the Zeiss fundus camera system. The angioram with the circles drawn in the macula was superimposed on the identical 30 degree color fundus photograph obtained in the same system. Thus 9 areas in each eye were examined. These are the center of fovea, and the superior, inferior, temporal, and nasal quadrants in 2220μ and 3450μ around the fovea center.

The CSME was defined as per the ETDRS criteria using the FA picture [4]. But the zones of retinal thickening was extended up to 3450μ around the fovea center so as to match the OCT zones.

Laser photocoagulation, after obtaining informed consent, was done as per the standard guidelines [10] using 532 nm laser (Zeiss). The patients were reexamined every 2 months for a period of 6 months. In each re-examination visit, a detailed ocular examination was repeated including FA and OCT. Repeat laser photocoagulation was offered, and done after another informed consent, if needed. Decision for repeat laser photocoagulation was based on the retinal thickness of the OCT in the inner circle of 1000μ around the fovea center. Should there be thickened retina beyond this zone, laser was not offered and the patients was requested for a close follow-up.

The FA reader was masked from other results of ocular examinations including OCT. The OCT reader was masked to the laser treatment and visual results; however, since the fundus photographs was taken by the same individual this masking was only partial. The masking was undone at the time of final analysis. The analysis consisted of correlating the fundus photograph, FA and the OCT. While comparing the latter two, all the 9 zones between the three circles were analyzed.

FA was considered the gold standard, and OCT was compared with the FA. Three situations were considered that can arise in FA-OCT comparison. They are: (1) a positive FA and positive OCT, (2) a positive FA and negative OCT, and (3) a negative FA and positive OCT. They were called *Positive-Positive*, *Positive-Negative*, and *Negative-Positive* respectively where the first segment of the phrase represented the FA and the second segment of the phrase represented the OCT.

Results

Demography

The study consisted of 19 male and one female patient. The average age was 55.8 years (range 41–72 years). Both eyes were involved in 15 patients and one involved in 5 patients. All the patients had type 2 diabetes.

FA and OCT correlation

There was good agreement in 31 eyes where both FA and OCT detected macular edema. There was disagreement in 4 eyes. In one patient (2 eyes) there was FA edema, but no OCT edema in both eyes; in one patient (2 eyes) there was OCT edema, but no FA edema. In the later patient there was incorrect base line measurement in retinal map, and precise measurement of the retinal edema was not possible. Thus *Positive-Positive* (FA positive and OCT positive) was seen in 31 (88.6%) eyes. *Positive-Negative* (FA positive and OCT negative) was seen in 2 (5.7%) eyes. *Negative-Positive* (FA negative and OCT positive) was seen in 2 (5.7%) eye.

In general, there was good agreement of FA and OCT in severe macular edema. The OCT was superior to FA in mild macular edema, and interpretation was rather difficult when the scan line passed through confluent hard exudates.

Three case reports illustrating these the three common situations are briefly described. The first case also demonstrates OCT-titrated laser photocoagulation response.

Case reports

Positive-positive and OCT-titrated response (Fig. 1)

68 year old man with type 2 diabetic for 22 years, one eye (other eye gross reduction of vision due to exudates at the fovea) and earlier treated for diabetic macular edema

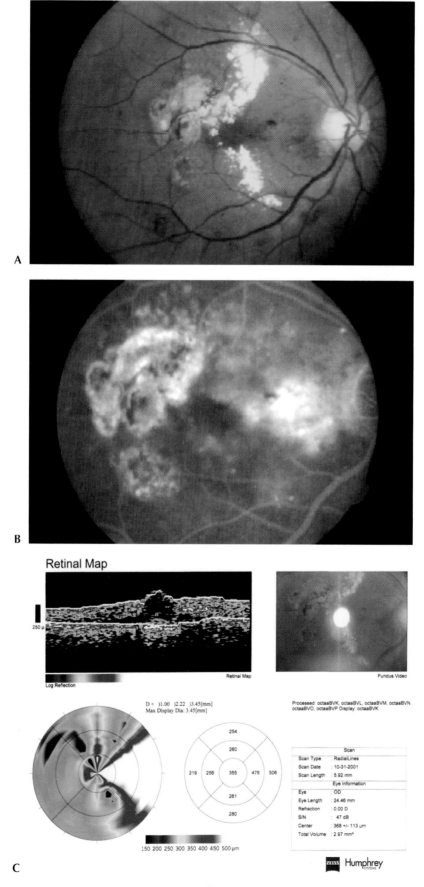

Fig. 1.

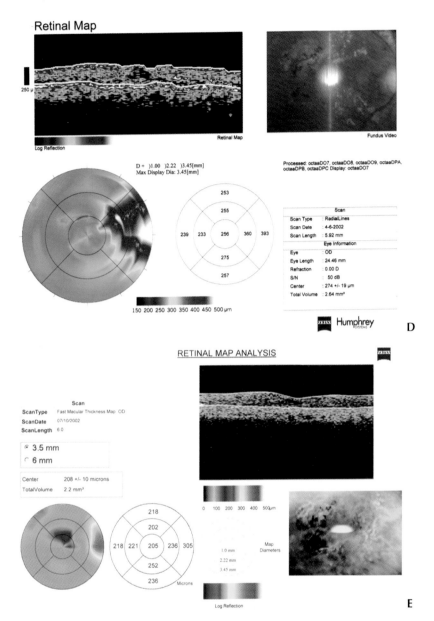

Fig. 1. **A** Pre treatment color fundus photograph. Note the exudates in the posterior pole. Previous laser photocoagulation marks are seen temporally. CSME is not appreciated, though the patient complaints of recent reduction of vision. (20/30, N12). **B** Corresponding fluorescein angiography shows retinal edema in the nasal pre treatment fluorescein angiography. Note edema in the nasal to the fovea. **C** Corresponding optical coherence tomography confirms the nasal macular edema in all zones. The retinal edema superiorly is a reflection of the confluent hard exudates superiorly. **D** Post treatment optical coherence tomography following first treatment. There was reduction of the macular edema in all the zones – 27.9%, 24.7%, and 22.3% in the inner, intermediate nasal and outer nasal quadrants respectively. **E** Post treatment coherence optical coherence tomography following second treatment. There was further reduction of macular edema. The macular edema reduced by 42.2%, 50.6%, and 39.7% in the inner, intermediate nasal, and outer nasal quadrants respectively. The visual acuity improved to 20/20, N6

returned with complaints of recent reduction of vision. The right (better) eye had visual acuity 20/30, N12. Fundus examination showed presence of hard exudates temporal to fovea with previous photocoagulation marks; the fluorescein angiograph demonstrated presence of diffuse macular edema nasal to fovea. In the optical coherence tomograph the edema measured 256 μ within the inner circle, 478 μ at the nasal intermediate (2.22 mm) zone and 506 μ at the nasal outer (3.45 mm) zone. He received two sittings of macular photocoagulation in interval of 4 months. At 3 months following the last laser treatment the vision improved to 20/20, N6. There was reduction of macular edema at all the zones- 27.9% (355 μ to 256 μ) in the inner zone, 24.7% (478 μ to 306 μ) in the nasal intermediate zone, and 22.3% (506 μ to 393 μ) in the nasal outer zone following the first laser treatment. This edema further reduced by 42.2% (355 μ to 205 μ) in the inner zone, by 50.6% (478 μ to 236 μ) in the nasal intermediate zone, and by 39.7% (506 μ to 305 μ) in the nasal outer zone following the second treatment. At the last follow up examination, the center of fovea measured 173 μ and the visual acuity had returned to 20/20, N6.

Positive-negative (Fig. 2)

50 year old man with 10 year old type 2 diabetes had visual acuity of 20/20, N6 both eyes fundus examination showed superficial retinal hemorrhages and hard exudates in the posterior pole. The fluorescein angiogram both eyes demonstrated edema surrounding and encroaching upon fovea. The optical coherence tomogram in either eye did not show any retinal edema. The average thickness of the inner zone in right eye was 191 μ and fovea 148 μ; the average thickness of the inner zone in the left eye was 183 μ and the fovea 160 μ. The surrounding intermediate and outer zones in both eyes measured between 199 μ–254 μ though the color code was maintained at green. Based on the OCT evaluation, laser photocoagulation was not offered. In subsequent follow up examinations at 4 and 6 months there was no change in visual acuity or fundus status. The diabetes mellitus remained well controlled.

Negative-positive (Fig. 3)

56 year old with 10 year history of type 2 diabetes presented with visual acuity of 20/40, N8 and 20/60, N12. The fundus examination showed presence of hard exudates at the macula, the left eye more confluent. The fluorescein angiography showed leaking microaneurysms far from the fovea; since the retinal edema was not with in 1000 μ of the fovea, either eye did not have clinically significant macular edema as per the ETDRS definition of CSME. The optical coherence tomogram provided an erroneous reference line value when the scan line passed through the hard exudates.

Discussion

Clinically significant macular edema is one of the principal causes of moderate to severe reduction of vision in diabetic individuals with retinopathy. The reduction of vision is dependent on the extent and type of macular edema. Stereo fundus photography, fluorescein angiography and slit lamp biomicroscopy are the advocated techniques of evaluating the diabetic macular edema. Stereo fundus photography is the professed technique. It needs expertise and competence of the ophthalmic technician or photographer for good photography. The evaluation is purely subjective.

Fluorescein angiography demonstrates presence and extent of leaking microaneurysms. Since they are the one closely associated with macular edema in diabetics,

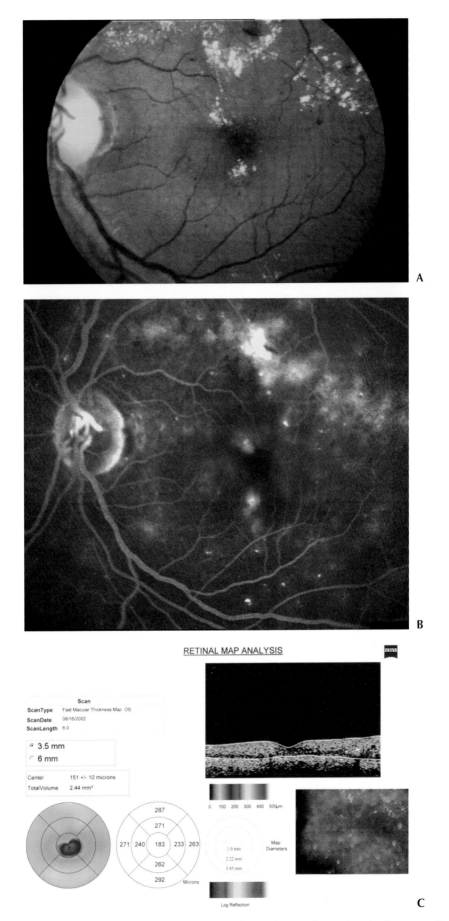

Fig. 2. **A** Left eye color fundus photograph. The exudates close to fovea, but the larger confluent ones are far from the macula. **B** Left eye fluorescein angiography. There is edema in the macular area. **C** Left eye optical coherence tomography. The OCT does not show macular edema within 1000 μ of the center of fovea. The average macular thickness in the inner zone of 1000 μ is 183 μ. There is no retinal edema up to 3.45 mm from the center of macula

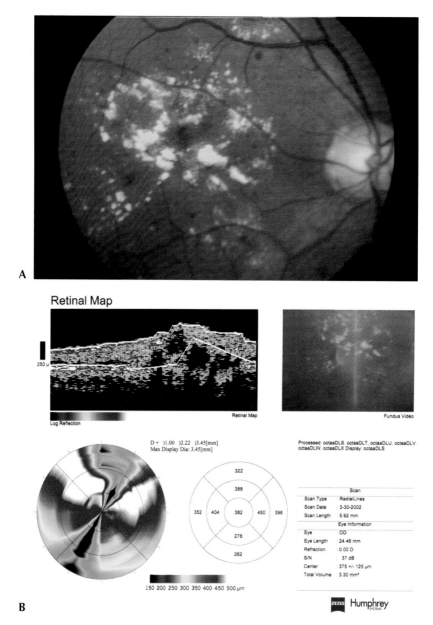

Fig. 3. A Right eye color fundus photograph. Note the exudates in the macular area. **B** Right eye optical coherence tomography. The high reflection from the exudates gives a wrong baseline curve making erroneous value for retinal thickness measurement

the angiography is usually considered the gold standard. Additionally, the angiography also delineates the microaneurysms and differentiates the leaking from the non-leaking one, and thus helps in laser photocoagulation. Fluorescein angiography is semi quantitative in nature, and obviously more objective than stereo fundus photograph. It is often argued that the CSME can be diagnosed by slit lamp biomicroscopy alone, thus making other photographic procedures such as stereo fundus photography and fluorescein angiography redundant. However, it can not be denied that the technique is subject to serious inter and intra observer variability.

The OCT on the other hand is both objective and reproducible. The technical training is not very exerting, and once the scan line passes through the retinal area of interest, the incorporated soft ware automatically measures the retinal thickness. The current soft ware also shows the distribution of the retinal thickness at 9 areas of interest in the posterior pole. The areas include the fovea (1000 μm around the center of foveola), and the four cardinal directions-superior, inferior, nasal and temporal at 2200 μm and 3450 μm from the foveola. Evidences are now accumulating to suggest that in many instances of diabetic maculopathy the OCT alone can be used to treat and monitor laser therapy in CSME. A good correlation between stereo fundus photography and OCT is reported [6]. The OCT probably demonstrates the macular edema preceding the clinical appearance of retinopathy [8]. The OCT also demonstrates reduction of retinal edema following laser treatment in diabetic maculopathy [11].

The macular edema is the main event in diabetic maculopathy and is responsible for reduction of vision. Laser photocoagulation reduces the macular edema and reduction in edema improves the vision. Hence tools that measures the macular edema objectively is better suited for initiating and monitoring the laser treatment. Fluorescein angiography and stereo fundus photography are more objective than slit lamp biomicroscopy. Following photocoagulation the fluorescein dye leakage is known to reduce, so also the macular edema as measured by OCT. It has been suggested that macular edema is better correlated with the state of vision in diabetic maculopathy, and not the extent of dye leakage. This was evidenced in both eyes of one patient in our study group. In this patient despite the presence of fluorescein dye leakage in the macula, the vision was 20/20 in both eyes, and the average macular thickness in the inner zone (1000 μm) was normal (182 and 193 μm).

This is, however, not to deny the known advantages of fluorescein angiography or strereo fundus photography. FA is capable of detecting ischemic maculopathy; the OCT can not. Poor vision disproportionate to the clinical signs of maculopathy, and poor visual evoked potential (VEP) are other two clinical and objectively measurable parameters of ischemic maculopathy. The OCT can, however, distinguish the retinal exudates. Since fundus examination will always precede an OCT examination, one has to interpret the OCT readings cautiously.

The FA has the capacity to differentiate an early or subtle proliferative diabetic retinopathy (PDR) from non proliferative diabetic retinopathy (NPDR) with or without maculopathy. The other clinical sign of increasing retinal ischemia secondary to diabetes are retinal arterial narrowing. Stereo fundus photography and biomicroscopy are the most convincing way of looking for the macular exudates and their location. The exudates appear as highly reflective localized structures. Should the exudates are confluent and confined to a small area in the posterior pole, the reflections from the exudates interfere with the reference line for accurate mapping of the retinal thickness. The retina appear thicker in OCT, while it is not apparently so in the stereo fundus photography or stereo biomicroscopy. This is one of the reasons for *Negative-Positive* image.

The treatment strategy will grossly differ in both ischemic macula and PDR that the OCT can not distinguish. In ischemic maculopathy one will not consider photocoagulation at all, and pan retinal photocoagulation is the treatemnt of choice in PDR with macular photocoagulation in concurrent presence of maculopathy. OCT is not designed to identify retinal ischemia. The OCT, however, can distinguish the retinal exudates. Since fundus examination will always precede an OCT examination, one has to interpret the OCT readings cautiously.

In this study it was noted that there was good agreement between FA and OCT in severe macular edema. In mild macular edema the retinal map provided better results, and the FA was better understood when the OCT was also used. Perhaps the OCT detectable macular edema precedes the angiographic edema [9]. There was considerable difficulty of OCT interpretation in presence of moderate to severe retinal exudates.

In our opinion at the current state of knowledge, the OCT should be clubbed with other two modalities of ascertaining the macular edema – the stereo fundus photography, and angiography. We also believe that after the base line evaluation with photography (or biomicroscopy) and angiography, OCT alone can be used for follow-up and further titration of treatment. The advantages include: (1) avoid an invasive procedure such as fluorescein angiography, and (2) the OCT can be done in patients with known allergy or contraindications to Na Fl dye. It can be concluded that at the current state of knowledge, the fundus photography, FA and OCT are all complementary for diagnosis and treatment of diabetic macular edema. Fundus photography is good to demonstrate and delineate the retinal exudates. FA is useful for study of leaking microaneurysms, and macular ischemia. OCT is a superior mode for the objective assessment of retinal edema.

Following successful macular laser photocoagulation, the retinal edema regresses earlier than photographic reduction of the retinal exudates. While fluorescein angiography can also demonstrate the reduction of dye leakage (read subjectively), the OCT can objectively demonstrate reduction of macular thickness both in the center of macula and the immediate surrounding zones. Hence it is prudent to use the OCT in conjunction with fundus photography and fluorescein angiography for treatment and follow-up evaluation of diabetic macular edema.

References

1. Moss SE, Klein R, Klein BEK (1988) The incidence of vision loss in a diabetic population. Ophthalmology 95:1340–8
2. Early Treatment Diabetic Retinopathy Study Research Group (1985) ETDRS report 1: Photocoagulation for diabetic macular edema. Arch Ophthalmol 103:1796–1806
3. Early Treatment Diabetic Retinopathy Study Research Group (1987) ETDRS Report: 4. Photocoagulation for diabetic macular edema. Int Ophthalmol Clin 27:254–64
4. Bresnick GH (1983) Diabetic maculopathy: a critical review highlighting difuse macular edema. Ophthalmology 90:1301–17
5. Puliafito CA, Hee MR, Schuman J, Fujimoto JG (1996) Optical coherence tomography of ocular diseases. Thorofare, Slack Inc
6. Strom C, Sander B, Larsen N, Larsen M (2002) Diabetic macular edema assessed with optical coherence tomography and stereo fundus photography. Invest Ophthalmol Vis Sci 43:241–5
7. Otani T, Kishi S, Maruyama Y (1999) Patterns of diabetic macular edema with optical coherence tomography. Am J Ophthalmol 127:688–93
8. Schaudig UH, Glaefke C, Scholz F, Richard G (2000) Optical coherence tomography for retinal thickness measurement in diabetic patients without clinically significant macular edema. Ophthalmic Surg Lasers 31:182–6
9. Sanchez-Tocino H, Alvarez-Vidal A, Maldonado MJ, Moreno-Montanes M, Garcia-Layana A (2002) Retinal thickness study with optical coherence tomography in patients with diabetes. Invest Ophthalmol Vis Sci 43:1588–94
10. Early Treateement Diabetic Retinopathy Study Group (1995) Focal photocoagulation treatment of diabetic macular edema: relationship of treatment effect top fluorescein angiographic and other retinal characteristics at baseline. ETDRS report No.19. Arch Ophthalmol 113:1144–5
11. Rivellese M, George A, Sulkes D, Reichel E, Puliafito C (2000) Optical coherence tomography after laser photocoagulation for clinically significant macular edema. Ophthalmol Surg Lasers 31:192–7

Correspondence: Taraprasad Das, MD, FRCS, L V Prasad Eye Institute, L V Prasas Marg, Banjara Hills, Hyderabad 500 034, India, E-Mail: tpd@lvpei.org

Long-term visual results after vitrectomy in diabetic macular edema

G. Kieselbach[1], F. Kralinger[2], M. Pedri[1], J. Troger[1], and M. T. Kralinger[1]

[1] Ophthalmic Clinic, University Innsbruck, Austria
[2] Trauma Surgery Clinic, University Innsbruck, Austria

Introduction

Since the introduction of lasercoagulation, therapy of diabetic macular edema, which is the most frequent cause for loss of vision in diabetic patients, had become possible. The accumulation of intraretinal fluid due to hyperpermeability of the retinal vasculature may lead to focal, diffuse and cystoid edema [1].

The Early Treatment Diabetic Retinopathy Study findings have demonstrated that focal laser coagulation reduces the risk of moderate visual loss by at least of 50% [2]. Still the prognosis for diabetic patients with macular edema in regard to visual acuity is poor. Especially cystoid and diffuse edemas often fail to respond to laser treatment while in case of focal edema at least a stabilization in visual acuity can be achieved for a limited time [2, 3, 4, 5].

Various clinical trials have been undertaken to investigate into new treatment modalities for diabetic macular edema. On the assumption that the relief of vitreal traction might lead to a decrease of a macular edema the first surgical attempts with vitrectomy were undertaken.

In a series of ten patients, Lewis et al. studied the effect of vitrectomy on diabetic macular edema associated with macular traction. The visual acuity improved in six out of ten patients [6]. Harbour et al. [7] evaluated the surgical results in patients with a thickened and taut posterior hyaloid membrane in combination with diabetic macular edema and stated that early surgical intervention may result in better visual outcome. But further investigation showed that not only macular edemas in combination with tractional forces either induced by the vitreous or by a thickened inner limiting membrane benefited from vitrectomy. The workgroups of Ikeda, Tachi, Pendergast, Gandorfer, Otani and La Heij demonstrated that diffuse macular edema without a thick posterior hyaloid responded to a surgical intervention and that the resorption of the edema was facilitated after vitrectomy [8–13].

In sum, there is evidence that vitrectomy is useful in treating macular edema in diabetic patients. But to our knowledge, the benefit of vitrectomy for a follow-up period longer than 28 months has not been reported yet. In the present retrospective study our aim was to investigate the long-term efficacy of vitrectomy on diabetic macular edema. The follow-up period ranged from 12 to 120 months with a mean of 54.7 months.

Methods

We reviewed the clinical records of 66 patients who had undergone vitrectomy for diabetic macular edema at the University Clinic of Ophthalmology in Innsbruck between 1992 and 2000. Lasercoagulation had been administered in accordance with the ETDRS treatment guidelines for diabetic macular edema. All eyes received NSAID for at least 8 weeks after laser treatment. In case the edema did not respond to lasercoagulation the eyes received surgical treatment.

Pars plana vitrectomy was performed in retrobulbar anesthesia with 2% scandicain and hyalase in 69 eyes of 66 patients. In 14 eyes (20.6%) extracapsular cataract extraction with phacoemulsification and intraocular lens implantation into the capsular bag was performed simultaneously. A standard three-port vitrectomy was performed and posterior vitreal detachment was induced (when necessary) by suction with the fluid – needle after removal of the anterior and central vitreous. In 51 eyes (73.9%) the inner limiting membrane (ILM) in the macular area was peeled. Fluid/air or gas exchange was carried out before closure of the sclerostomies and subconjunctival application of gentamicin. Topical corticosteroids and NSAIDs were applied after surgery. During chart review, the following preoperative data were obtained of each patient: age, gender, follow-up, the lens status, best-corrected Snellen visual acuity, the type and duration of diabetes, insulin-dependence and tension. Slit-lamp biomicroscopy was performed with a 78-diopter lens or in special cases with a fundus contact lens to determine the extent and pattern of the macular edema, the presence and quantity of hard exudates and whether the vitreous was still attached. Fluorescein angiography was only obtained in cases where no judgment of the macula on the basis of funduscopy only was feasible.

Postoperative data included the best-corrected visual acuities at standardized follow-up time points. Follow up time ranged between 12 and 120 months.

For statistical analysis visual acuities were converted to logMAR equivalents. The percent change in best-corrected visual acuity was determined for evaluation whether surgery resulted in a better visual outcome. The calculation was accomplished with the following formula: percent change = ([final visual acuity-preoperative visual acuity]/final visual acuity) × 100. Preoperative and postoperative visual acuities were compared with the Wilcoxon signed rank test. Multiple linear regression was used to analyze the association between final visual outcome and preoperative clinical parameters including preoperative visual acuity. P values of less than 0.05 were considered to indicate statistical significance. SPSS statistical software was used for statistical analysis.

Results

The study comprised 69 consecutive eyes of 66 patients undergoing vitrectomy for diabetic macular edema. Thirty-one of our patients were male and 38 patients were female. The ages ranged between 19 and 85 with a mean of 53.6 ± 17.9 years. Mean duration of diabetes was 14.93 ± 8.32 years and in 34.8% of cases a type I disease was diagnosed versus 65.2% cases with type II disease. Ninety-three percent of our patients had an insulin-dependent diabetes mellitus (IDDM).

In 58 (84.1%) of the eyes lasercoagulation for macular edema according to the EDTRS guidelines was carried out before vitrectomy. Cystoid macular edema was present in 25 (36.2%) of the eyes. Hard exudates were observed in 58.6% of the cases and in 16.2% these exudates formed plaques. A posterior chamber lens was present in 13.2% while all the residual eyes were phakic at the time of surgery. The follow-up ranged from 12 to 120 months with 54.7 months mean. In fifty-seven percent of the patients follow-up was accomplished until 3 years. At 6 years 35% of the baseline patients could be examined and at 10 years still 19% could be tested. Nine (13.2%) eyes had a posterior chamber lens at time of vitrectomy whereas cataract extraction was accomplished at time of vitrectomy in 14 (20.6%) and in the follow-up period in 15 (22.1%) of the eyes. Thirty eyes (44.1%) remained phakic.

The mean preoperative best-corrected visual acuity improved from 20/320 to 20/80 at the time of best postoperative best-corrected visual acuity (P < 0.0001, Wilcoxon signed rank test). At the time of final examination the best-corrected final visual acuity was 20/160 (P < 0.001, Wilcoxon signed rank test). The mean increase in Snellen lines was 2.7 ± 7.9 in regard to the final visual acuity and 5.9 ± 6.0 in regard to the best postoperative visual acuity. The median change in best-corrected visual acuity was improved by 33.7% at the final follow-up examination.

In 78.4% of the eyes the macular edema was resolved at final visit, while it improved in 11.8% and persisted in 9.8% of our patients. Only in 7.8% a cystoid macular edema was still present in the postoperative follow-up. Moderate amounts of hard exsudates could be detected in 29.6% of all eyes versus no hard exsudates in 66.7%. Plaques of hard exsudates could be seen in only two eyes.

For prognostic perspective we analyzed whether the type and duration of diabetes mellitus, insulin-dependence, sex, age, lens status, time of cataract extraction, cystic changes, ILM peeling, hard exudates, plaques of hard exudates, soft exudates and laser treatment before vitrectomy were associated with the final visual outcome. Linear regression analyses demonstrated a statistically significant correlation for laser treatment before vitrectomy (p = 0.007). The eyes that had received focal or grid lasercoagulation prior to vitrectomy had a better visual outcome compared to eyes with no laser photocoagulation in the macular area. A statistic trend (p = 0.09) for the presence of hard exudates was found implicating that in case no hard exudates were present at time of vitrectomy the final visual acuity tended to be better. On the other hand the amount of hard exudates did not seem to play a role since no correlation was identified either for the presence of multiple hard exuadates or the presence of plaque-like hard exudates.

Discussion

Although the efficacy of vitrectomy for diabetic macular edema for short- and intermediate-term follow up has been reported, the long-term outcome for these cases has not been described yet. Initially the reduction of the edema in response to vitrectomy was related to the relief of tractional forces induced by the vitreous or related membranes [6, 7]. Recent studies confirmed a decrease of edema even in case of no preexisting tractional forces around the macula and also in case of posterior vitreous detachment (PVD) [8–13]. Yamamoto and coworkers also demonstrated that vitrectomy is effective in reducing macula edema even if no epimacular membrane is present [14].

Our results confirm that vitrectomy is effective in stabilization of the visual acuity independent of whether the ILM is removed or not since no correlation between eyes with peeling of ILM and eyes without peeling in respect to the final visual outcome was found in our data. The missing correlation does not indicate that peeling is not advantageous because of a normal learning curve to remove the ILM within the last years. Only if the ILM is not visible or breaking in small pieces so that the peeling may cause injury at the macula the ILM removal will not be carried out yet. Perhaps the theory that ILM removal is not so important can be supported by experimental data that suggest various mechanisms responsible for the resorption of an edema following vitrectomy. Surgical extraction of the vitreous initiates the relief of retinal hypoxia due to the possibility of oxygen transport via fluid currents in the vitreous cavity that additionally enable oxygen exchange between well-perfused and ischemic areas. The increase in oxygen supply induces a constriction of the arterioles and thereby initiates a decrease of the hydrostatic pressure. This reformation of the physiologic balance in hydrostatic and oncotic pressure leads to a reflux of extracellular fluid into the vessels and thereby to the resolution of the edema [15]. Another assumption is that vitrectomy leads to a removal – at least temporarily – of growth factors and enzymes from the eyes that are known to play a role in the pathophysiology of macular edemas. For instance the vascular endothelial growth

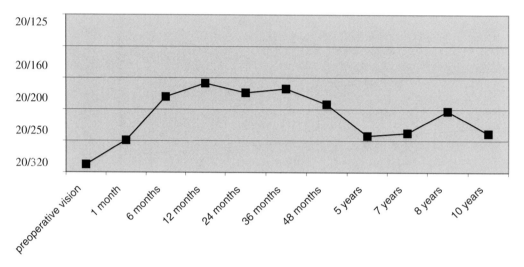

Fig. 1. Mean values of visual acuity

factor (VEGF) has been shown to evoke two mechanisms that have an influence on macular edema. First, it increases the permeability of the retinal vasculature via mediation of protein kinase C and second, it decreases the levels of occludin, a protein that is necessary for ensuring tight junctions [16, 17]. Another factor influencing the tight junctions has been found in histamine that acts by reducing the expression of ZO-1 [18].

Whatever the resolution mechanism may be found out finally at the presence the clinical findings indicate that vitrectomy is beneficial in cases of diabetic macular edema.

In 90.2 % of our patients vitrectomy resulted in decreasing the macular edema and in 78.4% we saw a total resorption of the edema. Furthermore our results indicate a stabilizing effect for extended periods since our data comprise a follow up until a maximum of 10 years (Fig. 1). There was a strong correlation of the final visual acuity and laser treatment before vitrectomy in our patients. Macular edema therapy was strictly administered in accordance with the EDTRS guidelines. The 11 eyes (15.9%) that have not been lasered before vitrectomy were eyes with a very poor baseline visual acuity with large exsudative areas and large ischemic zones, which was the reason why no laser photocoagulation had been performed in the first place. In these cases a restoration of the visual acuity cannot possibly be achieved like in eyes with no capillary drop-out. On the other hand laser photocoagulation prior to vitrectomy may have a protective and stabilizing effect on the macular perfusion and therefore result in better visual outcome after surgery.

A trend of statistic correlation was found in respect to hard exudates implicating that in case no hard exuadates are present before vitrectomy the final visual acuity tends to be higher (p = 0.09).

In regard to the time of lens extraction and the final visual acuity no correlation could be found via regression analyses in our patients. Cataract surgery has been reported to have an influence on the macular situation in controversial ways: first a preexisting macular edema may deteriorate after surgery and second a primary not exsudative macula can become exudative (Irvine-Gass Syndrome) [19, 20]. The introduction of extracapsular small incision techniques and phacoemulsification has decreased the incidence of Irvine-Gass Syndrome to 1.7% [21]. Pseudophakia or cataract extraction at the time of vitrectomy proved to be advantageous for posterior compartment surgery in so far that it enables a complete removal of the vitreous and radical lasertherapy of the anterior retina.

Despite the limitations of a retrospective investigation our findings support previous studies concluding that patients who do not respond to laser treatment may benefit from vitrectomy with or without peeling of the ILM. As far as we are aware the number of eyes in our study was higher and the period of follow-up was longer compared to previous studies. Yet, our data are also solely based on a retrospective and not-controlled case series. Therefore a prospective, controlled and randomized trial is required to back up the findings indicating that vitrectomy in persisting macular edema is really beneficial.

References

1. Klein R, Klein BE, Moss SE, et al (1984) The Wisconsin epidemiologic study of diabetic retinopathy. IV. Diabetic macular edema. Ophthalmology 91:1464–74
2. Photocoagulation for diabetic macular edema (1985) Early Treatment Diabetic Retinopathy Study report number 1. Early Treatment Diabetic Retinopathy Study research group. Arch Ophthalmol 103:1796–806
3. Bresnick GH (1986) Diabetic macular edema. A review. Ophthalmology 93:989–97
4. Olk RJ (1986) Modified grid argon (blue-green) laser photocoagulation for diffuse diabetic macular edema. Ophthalmology 93:938–50
5. Blankenship GW (1979) Diabetic macular edema and argon laser photocoagulation: a prospective randomized study. Ophthalmology 86:69–78
6. Lewis H, Abrams GW, Blumenkranz MS, Campo RV (1992) Vitrectomy for diabetic macular traction and edema associated with posterior hyaloidal traction. Ophthalmology 99:753–9
7. Harbour JW, Smiddy WE, Flynn HW Jr, Rubsamen PE (1996) Vitrectomy for diabetic macular edema associated with a thickened and taut posterior hyaloid membrane. Am J Ophthalmol 121:405–13
8. Ikeda T, Sato K, Katano T, Hayashi Y (2000) Improved visual acuity following pars plana vitrectomy for diabetic cystoid macular edema and detached posterior hyaloid. Retina 20:220–2
9. Tachi N, Ogino N (1996) Vitrectomy for diffuse macular edema in cases of diabetic retinopathy. Am J Ophthalmol 122:258–60
10. Gandorfer A, Messmer EM, Ulbig MW, Kampik A (2000) Resolution of diabetic macular edema after surgical removal of the posterior hyaloid and the inner limiting membrane. Retina 20:126–33
11. Pendergast SD, Hassan TS, Williams GA, et al (2000) Vitrectomy for diffuse diabetic macular edema associated with a taut premacular posterior hyaloid. Am J Ophthalmol 130:178–86
12. La Heij EC, Hendrikse F, Kessels AG, Derhaag PJ (2001) Vitrectomy results in diabetic macular oedema without evident vitreomacular traction. Graefes Arch Clin Exp Ophthalmol 239:264–70
13. Otani T, Kishi S (2002) A controlled study of vitrectomy for diabetic macular edema. Am J Ophthalmol 134:214–9
14. Yamamoto T, Akabane N, Takeuchi S (2001) Vitrectomy for diabetic macular edema: the role of posterior vitreous detachment and epimacular membrane. Am J Ophthalmol 132:369–77
15. Stefansson E (2001) The therapeutic effects of retinal laser treatment and vitrectomy. A theory based on oxygen and vascular physiology. Acta Ophthalmol Scand 79:435–40
16. Antonetti DA, Barber AJ, Khin S, et al (1998) Vascular permeability in experimental diabetes is associated with reduced endothelial occludin content: vascular endothelial growth factor decreases occludin in retinal endothelial cells. Penn State Retina Research Group. Diabetes 47:1953–9
17. Aiello LP, Bursell SE, Clermont A, et al (1997) Vascular endothelial growth factor-induced retinal permeability is mediated by protein kinase C in vivo and suppressed by an orally effective beta-isoform-selective inhibitor. Diabetes 46:1473–80
18. Gardner TW, Lesher T, Khin S, et al (1996) Histamine reduces ZO-1 tight-junction protein expression in cultured retinal microvascular endothelial cells. Biochem J 320 (Pt 3):717–21
19. Dowler JG, Sehmi KS, Hykin PG, Hamilton AM (1999) The natural history of macular edema after cataract surgery in diabetes. Ophthalmology 106:663–8
20. Ikeda T, Sato K, Katano T, Hayashi Y (1999) Vitrectomy for cystoid macular oedema with attached posterior hyaloid membrane in patients with diabetes. Br J Ophthalmol 83:12–14

21. Wright PL, Wilkinson CP, Balyeat HD, et al (1988) Angiographic cystoid macular edema after posterior chamber lens implantation. Arch Ophthalmol 106:740–4

Correspondence: Gerhard Kieselbach, MD, Associate Professor, University of Innsbruck, Department of Ophthalmology, Anichstrasse 35, A-6020 Innsbruck, Austria, E-mail: gerhard.kieselbach@uibk.ac.at

Vitrectomy in eyes with diabetic macular edema

U. Stolba, I. Krebs, S. Binder, B. Neumaier, S. Brunner,
and T. Anaoko-Mensah

Department of Ophthalmology, Rudolf Foundation Hospital, Ludwig Boltzmann Institute for
Retinology and Biomicroscopical Laser Surgery, Vienna, Austria

Introduction

Macular edema is the leading cause of visual impairment in patients with diabetic retinopathy [1, 2]. The mechanism of diffuse macular edema includes leckage from the abnormal retinal capillaries and microaneurysms [1] and tractional forces at the vitreo-retinal interface [3].

Grid-pattern laser coagulation has been the standard treatment for clinical significant diffuse edema showing a resolution of the edema in 68–94% of the eyes [4–6]. However, the functional results were limited.

The role of the vitreomacular interface has been implicated in the pathogenesis since Nasrallah found a lower incidence of posterior vitreous detachment in eyes with diabetic macular edema compared to eyes without edema [7]. Previous studies have reported favourable anatomic and functional results after vitrectomy and removal of the posterior hyloid [8–14]. However, Hikichi also found a spontaneous resolution of the edema in 55% of eyes with postieror vitreous separation and in 25% of eyes without or with incomplete posterior vitreous detachment [15].

Based of these outcomes we initiated a randomized clinical trial on patients with diffuse macular edema comparing the functional results after pars plana vitrectomy with those after grid-laser treatment.

Material and methods

46 eyes of 40 patients are enrolled into the study. 34 eyes of 30 patients with an age between 38 and 74 years have passed the 6 months control which is presented here.

All patients have a history of diabetic maculopathy with diffuse edema for more than 6 months. In all eyes a grid laser treatment has been performed at least 4 months prior to the enrollment. We included only eyes where the posterior hyloid was attached echographically or where a preretinal membrane was present in the OCT. We excluded eyes with a lens opacification more than NO3NC3C3P3 according to the LOCS III charts, eyes with massive subfoveal hard exudates, ischemic maculopathy or cystoid macular edema, as well as eyes with signs of proliferative changes.

The eyes were randomized initially into an operation group (Group I: 16 eyes) and a control group (Group II: 18 eyes).

Surgery was performed as a standard vitrectomy with removal of the posterior hyloid followed by ICG staining and peeling of the inner limiting membrane. In patients at an age over 65 years surgery was combined with a phacoemulsification and posterior chamber lens implantation.

Initially and one, three, and six months postoperatively we evaluated the visual acuity for far (ETDRS charts) and for near (Jäger charts). Improvements and deteriorations were

Table 1. Results ETDRS

		1 m p.o.	3 m p.o.	6 m p.o.
⬆	Group I	11 (69%)	3 (19%)	3 (19%)
	Group II	5 (27.5%)	1 (5.5%)	3 (16.5%)
=	Group I	2 (12.5%)	11 (69%)	13 (81%)
	Group II	10 (55.5%)	10 (55.5%)	9 (50%)
⬇	Group I	3 (19%)*	2 (12.5%)	0 (0%)
	Group II	3 (16.5%)	7 (39%)	6 (33%)

*) 1 eye with p. o. hem.

defined as changes of a least 10 optotypes or 2 lines respectively. OCT measurements were performed to evaluate the height of the edema. A decrease or increase was determined as a change of at least 10% of the preceeding value.

Results

Clinical results

Surgery was uneventful in all cases. Postoperatively a vitreous hemorrhage occurred in one eye which resolved spontaneously after 4 weeks.

Biomicroscopically the edema has disappeared 1 month postoperatively in the operation group in 10 out of 16 eyes (62.5%) compared to 3 out of 18 eyes (16.6%) in the control group.

ETDRS results (Table 1)

One month after surgery 69% (11 of 16) of the operated eyes were improved in comparison to 27.5% (5 of 18) of the controlled eyes. 12.5% (2 of 16) as against 55.5% (10 of 18) were unchanged. In the later observation period the majority of the eyes in both groups were stable (50–81%) but there were always more improved eyes in the operation group (19% as against 5.5 to 16.5%) and much more deteriorated eyes in the control group (33 to 39% as against 0 to 12.5%).

An evaluation of the initial and the 6 months outcomes showes that 50% of the operated eyes (8 of 16) in comparison to 22% (4 of 18) of the control cases have a better visual acuity for far at this time.

Reading acuity results (Table 2)

At the month one examination 37% (6 of 16) of the eyes in the operation group showed an improved acuity for near compared to 16.5% (3 of 18) of the control cases. In the later follow up period most of the eyes remained unchanged in both groups (67 to 81%). There was only 1 eye (6%) which deteriorated in the operation group after 3 months but 4 eyes (25%) improved at this time in this group. In the control group one eye (5.5%) respectively improved after 3 and 6 months but more eyes deteriorated (2 to 3) during the same time.

An evaluation of the initial and the 6 months outcomes showes that 8 times more patients result in a better acuity for near (44% as against 5.5%) in the operation group.

Table 2. Results acuity for near

		1 m p.o.	3 m p.o.	6 m p.o.
⬆	Group I	6 (37%)	4 (25%)	1 (6%)
	Group II	3 (16.5%)	1 (5.5%)	1 (5.5%)
=	Group I		11 (69%)	15 (94%)
	Group II		14 (78%)	15 (83.5%)
⬇	Group I	1 (6%)*	1 (6%)	0 (0%)
	Group II	1 (5.5%)	3 (16.5%)	2 (11%)

*)1 eye with p.o. hem.

Table 3. Results OCT

		1 m p.o.	3 m p.o.	6 m p.o.
⬇	Group I	9 (56.5%)	3 (19%)	3 (19%)
	Group II	3 (16.5%)	2 (11%)	0 (0%)
=	Group I	7 (44%)	13 (81%)	11 (69%)
	Group II	10 (55.5%)	12 (67%)	13 (72.5%)
⬆	Group I	0 (0%)	0 (0%)	2 (12.5%)
	Group II	5 (27.5%)	4 (22%)	5 (27.5%)

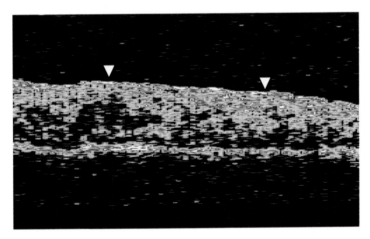

Fig. 1. Patient MP – preoperative OCT showing a macular edema (maximal thickness 606 μ). On the surface a thickened posterior hyloid characterized by a high reflectivity is present (white arrows)

Optical coherence tomography results (Table 3)

According to the clinical findings 56.5% (9 of 16) of the operated eyes showed a decrease in the height of the edema (Figs. 1, 2) compared to 16.5% (3 of 18) of the controlled eyes. During follow up there were only two eyes (12.5%) in the operation group where the edema increased after 6 months. In contrast, we found 22 to 27.5% of eyes in the control group with an increase of the edema up to 6 months.

A comparison of the 6 months results shows that 56.5% of the operated cases as against 22% of the controlled ones had a minor height of the edema in the OCT.

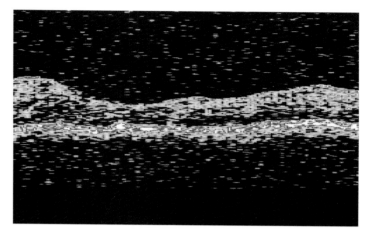

Fig. 2. Patient MP – 1 month after surgery with a distinct decrease of the edema (maximal thickness 200 μ)

Discussion

The various mechanisms of the development of diabetic macular edema requires different approaches in the management. Whereas grid laser treatment is adequate to reduce leackage from abnormal retinal capillaries [4–6] it may be insufficient when tractional forces at the vitreoretinal interface are present. The posterior hyloid was found to be attached more often in eyes with diabetic macular edema [15] and spontaneous resolution is possible after separation. However, improvements are also described without treatment . A statistically significant difference between grid laser coagulation and the natural course was only found up to two years [16].

The background of our randomized study was to find out inhowfar a pars plana vitrectomy with peeling of the internal limiting membrane improves the visual function of patients with persistent macular edema compared to non-operated controls.

Our results demonstrate a 69% success rate after surgery which is in the middle of a wide range from 38% [13] to 91% [12]. The deviation of the outcomes is explained by the small series and different methods in evaluating the functional results and baseline characteristics. A good correlation is found between the number of the finally improved eyes after 6 months in our study (50%) and the studies of Otani [14] and Tachi [10] with success rates of 57% and 53% respectively.

The highest success rate (91%) is reached by Gandorfer [12] who combined vitrectomy with ILM-peeling. The removal of this membrane which offers a scaffold for proliferating astrocytes may almost completely release all tractional forces on the macula. However, there is no prospective, randomized trial which proofs the benefit of peeling the inner limiting membrane.

There is an agreement that the best results are obtained in the earl observation period [9, 12] whereas the number of improved eyes dropped to 19% after 3 and 6 months in our series (Table 1). There were only 2 eyes (12.5%) in the operation group which deteriorated after surgery without any obvious reason and one eye with a temporary postoperative vitreous hemorrhage.

The results in the control group were significantly worse. Although 27.5% of the eyes showed an increased vision after 1 month at least 50% of the eyes remained unchanged and up to 39% deteriorated during the study. A comparison of the initial and final values shows that the patients in the operation group have a 2 to 2.5 times higher chance for an improvement.

Correlating to these findings OCT measurements showed a decrease of the retinal thickness in 56.5% of the operated eyes in contrast to 16.5% of the control eyes (Table 3). There was a good accordance between improved visual acuity and decrease of the edema in both groups. Interestingly Otani reported a tomographical disappearance of the edema in 100% of the cases but a visual improvement in only 57% which he attributes to the accumulation of subfoveal exudate during absorption of the macular edema and the preoperative macular function [12, 17]. This could explain why it was not possible to improve the visual acuity for near by vitrectomy to the same extent as the ETDRS vision in our series. However, there was also a distinct better outcome in the operation group (37%) one month after surgery than in the control group (16.5%). We found 2 to 8 times more patients in the operation group with a better reading vision than initially determined.

In conclusion, a randomized study was recommended in prior reports to evaluate the advantages of vitreoretinal surgery in eyes with diffuse macular edema. The preliminary results reveal a significant better outcome of the visual acuities for far and near with a distinct reduction of the retinal thickness in the operated eyes. The most distinct increase of the functional level is reached one month after surgery. At the end of the observation period the eyes after surgery had a 2 to 8 times higher chance for a better function than those without treatment.

References

1. Ferris FL, Patz A (1984) Macular edema: a complication of diabetic retinopathy. Surv Ophthalmol 28[Suppl]:452–61
2. Klein R, Klein BE, Moss SE, et al (1984) The Wisconsin epidemiologic study of diabetic retinopathy: IV. Diabetic macular edema. Ophthalmology 91:1464–74
3. Nasrallah FP, Jalkh AE, VanCoppenrolle F, et al (1988) The role of the vitreous in diabetic macular edema. Ophthalmology 95:1335–9
4. Olk RJ (1986) Modified grid blue-green laser photocoagulation for diffuse diabetic macular edema. Ophthalmology 93:938–50
5. Lee Cm, Olk RJ (1991) Modified grid laser photocoagulation for diffuse diabetic macular edema: long-term visual results. Ophthalmology 98:1594–602
6. Ulbig MW, McHugh JDA, Hamilton AMP (1995) Focal diode laser treatment for diabetic macular edema. Br J Ophthalmol 79:318–21
7. Schepens CL, Avila MP, Jalkh AK, Tremple CL (1984) Role of the vitreous in cystoid in cystoid macular edema. Surv Ophthalmol 28:499–504
8. Lewis H, Abrams GW, Blumenkranz MS, Campo RV (1992) Vitrectomy for diabetic macular traction and edema associated with posterior hyaloid traction. Ophthalmology 99:753–9
9. Harbour JW, Smiddy WE, Flynn HW, Rubsamen PE (1996) Vitrectomy for diabetic macular edema associated with a thickened and taut posterior hyaloid membrane. Am J Ophthalmol 121:405–13
10. Tachi N, Ogino N (1996) Vitrectomy for diffuse macular edema in cases of diabetic retinopathy. Am J Ophthalmol 122:258–60
11. Pendergast SD (1998) Vitrectomy for diabetic macular edema associated with a taut premacular posterior hyaloid. Curr Opin Ophthalmol 9:71–5
12. Gandorfer A, Messmer EM, Ulbig MW, Kampik A (2000) Resolution of diabetic macular edema after surgical removal of the posterior hyloid and the inner limiting membrane. Retina 20:126–33
13. Otani T, Kishi S (2000) Tomographic assessment of vitreous surgery for diabetic macular edema. Am J Ophthalmol 129:487–94
14. Otani T, Kishi S (2002) A controlled study of vitrectomy for diabetic macular edema. Am J Ophthalmol 134:214–9

15. Hikichi T, Fujio N, Akiba Y, Takahashi M, Yoshida A (1997) Association between the short-term natural history of diabetic macular edema and the vitreomacular relationship in type II diabetes mellitus. Ophthalmology 104:473–8
16. Ladas ID, Theodossiadis GP (1993) Long-term effectiveness of modified grid laser photocoagulation for diffuse macular edema. Acta Ophthalmol 71:393–7
17. Otani T, Kishi S (2001) Tomographic findings of foveal hard exudates in diabetic macular edema. Am J Ophthalmol 131:50–4

Correspondence: Ulrike Stolba, Department of Ophthalmology, Rudolf Foundation Hospital, Ludwig Boltzmann Institute for Retinology and Biomicroscopical Laser Surgery, Juchgasse 25, A-1030 Vienna, Austria.

Vitrectomy for CME in retinal vein occlusions –
A new indication?

M. Velikay-Parel

University Eye Hospital, Vienna, Austria

Cystoid macular edema (CME) is the most common cause of visual impairment in vein occlusions. So far the "good clinical praxis in branch vein occlusions (BRVO)" and CME was a grid laser therapy [16, 18]. Vision improvement after grid laser occurs in 65% of the patients. If we look closer to what appears to be a remarkable advantage we find that the average vision improvement was just 1.3 lines, that 40% of the patients lost reading vision and patients with lower vision were less likely to achieve a good vision after grid laser. Furthermore, in patients with CME and capillary non perfusion laser failed to show any effect and in central retinal vein occlusions (CRVO) grid laser therapy also could not improve the visual prognosis.

As a consequence of these relatively poor treatment options we raised the following questions:

What can be done for those patients who do not respond to grid laser in BRVO?
Is there a better therapy for CME and BRVO?
Is there any help for patients with CRVO?

Reports on vision improvement after vitrectomy in diabetic patients with CME encouraged us to investigate vitrectomy as a therapy to improve function in those patients.

In a pilot study we performed vitrectomy on patients non responding to grid laser and found visual improvement. Looking up literature we found that within the last years in Japan several studies had been published on the same subject [8, 9, 11, 13, 17]. One study group operated on patients with attached posterior vitreous who did not achieve a good visual acuity after grid laser photocoagulation [17]. Other authors operated on patients with severe macula edema and BRVO and CRVO [8, 9]. Both reported improved visual recover in comparison to the patients of the branch vein occlusion study receiving standard grid laser therapy.

Our indications for vitrectomy were:
In acute CME the vision had to be 20/200 or less
In chronic CME a macular traction syndrom had to be proven with OCT.
All eyes had to have an attached posterior vitreous.
We operated on 15 patients with BRVO and 3 patients with CRVO.

Results

We found that in BRVO in acute CME 60% of the patients achieved a visual acuity of 0.7 or better. The drop out of perifoveal capillaries and avascular areas in the periphery were reperfused after surgery in 90% of the cases. In CRVO we observed a reduction of CME in all eyes, vision improved in two eyes.

We compared our results to those of others methods in eyes retinal vein occlusion:

One of the most well known methods within the last years is the sheathotomy first described by Osterloh et al. (1988). Opremcak et al. reported about a case series of 14 patients [14]. Mesters et al. [12] had the largest series of 43 patients and the control was performed on patients who refused operation (n = 25). 60% of his operated on patients improved 2 lines or more whereas his control group did not improve significantly. Unfortunately this study has several flaws: besides the fact that it is not randomized, Mesters does not differentiate between ischemic and non ischemic BRVO, which is important, since in ischemic BRVO visual prognosis is favorable in the natural course.

Secondly although the rationale to surgically remove the suggested reason of BRVO is striking, there is no prove whether the vitrectomy or the sheathotomy is the reason for the suggested anatomical improvement. Moreover the author himself states that although he completely separated adventitial tissue from artery to vene and therefore removed all obstacles additional internal limiting membrane peeling improved his results. This suggests that the effect of his therapy does not derive from sheathotomy. Since other authors were not able to have as good results with this method [11], Figureras compared the effect of vitrectomy with the effect of sheathotomy, where she found no significant diffference. (The paper is published in detail in the same book).

In all of the surgical BRVO studies the case selection was done regardless of the perfusion of the macula. This is surprising since Finkelstein [5] proved that 90% of the eyes with macula ischemia regain an visual acuity of 0.66 or better in natural course [1, 2]. It is therefore absolutely necessary to perform pilot studies only on eyes with perfused macula, which have a worse prognosis in BRVO.

Another treatment alternative in BRVO is triamcinolone acetonide intravitreale which already proved to be effective in other CME associated diseases [7]. So far it did not prove to be effective for BRVO or CRVO.

Intravitreal tissue plasminogen activator (TPA) injections failed to show any effect [6]. When applied as an retinal intravenous injection with high pressure patients with CRVO showed improved vision [19] when compared to the natural course of the CRVO study, but the method needs a special injection device and only 50% of the eyes (n = 30) had vision improvement of 3 lines or more at the last follow up.

The latest method in CRVO is the radial optic neurotomy by Opremcak [3, 15]. He reports on 11 patient, 73% of them showed visual improvement of five lines or more.

It seems that both methods bear an advantage for visual improvement for patients with CRVO when compared to the natural course.

Since this is a observational pilot study the clinical value is limited, but this applies to all studies on surgical treatments of CME in retinal vein occlusion at this point of time. Most of the studies do not differentiate ischemic from non ischemic BRVO or CRVO, control groups are missing and the number of eyes is very low. But in order to establish the evidence of treatment efficacy a randomized study on a large number of patients has to be performed. Since there are several treatment options indicating to be effective it is relevant to report on those in pilot studies and compare the results in order to choose the most promising method for an evidence based study.

At this point of time we can conclude that vitrectomy with posterior detachment of the vitreous is an effective alternative treatment in cases with severe CME. Secondly vision improvement is better when surgery was performed early. And patients with "old" vein occlusions and CME should be examined for vitreous traction with OCT and operated on when these are ascertained.

References

1. Battaglia-Parodi M, Saviano S, Bergamini L, Ravalico G (1999) Grid laser treatment of macular edema in macular branch retinal vein occlusion. Doc Ophthalmol 97(3–4):427–31
2. Battaglia-Parodi M, Saviano S, Ravalico G (1999) Grid laser treatment in macular branch retinal vein occlusion. Graefes Arch Clin Exp Ophthalmol 237(12):1024–7
3. Bynoe LA, Opremcak EM, Bruce RA, Lomeo MD, Ridenour CD, Letson AD, Rehmar AJ (2002) Radial optic neurotomy for central retinal vein obstruction. Retina 22(3):379–80; discussion 380–1
4. Elman MJ (1996) Thrombolytic therapy for central retinal vein occlusion: results of a pilot study. Trans Am Ophthalmol Soc 94:471–504
5. Finkelstein D (1992) Ischemic macular edema. Recognition and favorable natural history in branch vein occlusion. Arch Ophthalmol 110(10):1427–34
6. Glacet Bernard A, Kuhn D, Vine AK, Oubraham H, Coscas G, Soubrane G (2000) Treatment of recent onset central retinal vein occlusion with intravitreal tissue plasminogen activator: a pilot study. Br J Ophthalmol 84(6):609–13
7. Greenberg PB, Martidis A, Rogers AH, Duker JS, Reichel E (2002) Intravitreal triamcinolone acetonide for macular oedema due to central retinal vein occlusion. Br J Ophthalmol 86(2):247–8
8. Ishigooka, et al (2001) Indications and outcome of vitrectomy for macular edema secondary to branch vein occlusion. Jap J Ophthalmol 55(5):763–6
9. Iwaki, et al (2001) Outcome of vitreous surgery for macular edema secondary to vein occlusion. Jap J Ophthalmol 55(4):667–71
10. Le-Rouic JF, Bejjani RA, Rumen F, Caudron C, Bettembourg O, Renard G, Chauvaud D (2001) Adventitial sheathotomy for decompression of recent onset branch retinal vein occlusion. Graefes Arch Clin Exp Ophthalmol 239(10):747–51
11. Matawatari, et al (2000) Outcome of vitrectomy for macular edema in branch vein occlusion in its early stage. Jap J Ophthalmol 54(5):871–4
12. Mester U, Dillinger P (2002) Vitrectomy with arteriovenous decompression and internal limiting membrane dissection in branch retinal vein occlusion. Retina 22(6):740–6
13. Nakao, et al (2001) Changing patterns of retinal ischemia following vitrectomy for retinal branch vein occlusion. Jap J Ophthalmol 55(5):767–70
14. Opremcak EM, Bruce RA (1999) Surgical decompression of branch retinal vein occlusion via arteriovenous crossing sheathotomy: a prospective review of 15 cases. Retina 19(1):1–5
15. Opremcak EM, Bruce RA, Lomeo MD, Ridenour CD, Letson AD, Rehmar AJ (2001) Radial optic neurotomy for central retinal vein occlusion: a retrospective pilot study of 11 consecutive cases. Retina 21(5):408–15
16. Stefansson E (2001) The therapeutic effects of retinal laser treatment and vitrectomy. A theory based on oxygen and vascular physiology. Acta Ophthalmol Scand 79(5):435–40
17. Tachi, et al (1999) Vitrectomy for macular edema combined with retinal vein occlusion. Doc Ophthalmol 97:465–9
18. The Branch Vein Occlusion Study Group (1984) Argon laser photocoagulation for macular edema in branch vein occlusion. Am J Ophthalmol 98(3):271–82
19. Weiss JN (1998) Treatment of central retinal vein occlusion by injection of tissue plasminogen activator into a retinal vein. Am J Ophthalmol 126(1):142–4

Correspondence: Michaela Velikay-Parel, M.D., University Eye Hospital, Währinger Gürtel 18-20, A-1090 Vienna, Austria.

Comparative study of vitrectomy with and without vein decompression for branch retinal vein occlusion. A pilot study

M. S. Figueroa

Director of VitreoRetinal Department,
Hospital Oftalmológico Internacional,
Madrid, Spain

Abstract

Purpose: To prospectively compare results of vein decompression and vitrectomy with hyaloid removal for treating branch retinal vein occlusion (BRVO).

Methods: Thirty-five eyes with macular edema and visual acuity worse than 20/100 secondary to BRVO were included. Vitrectomy with posterior hyaloid removal and vein decompression at the arteriovenous crossing was performed on 15 patients (Group I); same technique without vein decompression was performed on 20 (Group II).

Results: Group I: After mean follow-up of 33 months, VA improved by two lines or more in 13/15 (87%), one line in 1/15 (6.5%) and remained unchanged in 1/15 (6.5%) eyes. Macular edema resolved in 14/15 (93%). No eyes developed new vessels.

Group II. After mean follow-up of 18 months, VA improved two lines or more in 16/20 (80%), remained unchanged in 2/20 (10%) and deteriorated in 2/20 (10%). Macular edema resolved in 16/20 (80%). No new vessels developed. No differences were found between groups in either age (p 0.566) or preoperative visual acuity (p 0.505). Despite a statistically significant difference in the duration of preoperative interval (p 0.004), no differences were found in post-operative visual results (p 0.147), resolution of macular edema (p 0.098) or prevention of neovascularization.

Conclusion: Results suggest that vitrectomy with posterior hyaloid removal without vein decompression can resolve macular edema, improve visual acuity and prevent development of new vessels in BRVO.

Introduction

Branch retinal vein occlusion (BRVO) is the second most common retinal vascular disease, affecting 1.6% of the population above the age of 40 [1]. Several studies have shown that the anterior location of the artery is one of the risk factors for BRVO [2–4]. Arteriosclerotic changes in the artery and the artery's anterior location to the vein cause an abrupt alteration of vein direction and a reduction of vein lumen. With increased compression, venous blood flow velocity at the crossing site gradually increases until local shear stress causes endothelial cell loss, thrombus formation and vein occlusion [5–7].

Several medical and surgical strategies have been employed to treat BRVO. The only therapy of documented value for BRVO is retinal argon laser photocoagulation. Laser photocoagulation has been shown to improve the visual prognosis in patients with secondary complications of BRVO, including persistent macular edema and retinal neovascularization. In the BRVO study, a comparison of the natural history of macular edema was performed, showing that laser treatment increases the probability of visual improvement, but the mean improvement in treated eyes was only 1.33 lines [8, 9]. Consequently, other surgical techniques are presently under investigation in an attempt to achieve better visual results. Among these are laser chorioretinal anastomosis and surgical vein decompression at the AV crossing.

In 1988 Osterloh and Charles gave the first description of surgical vein decompression at the arteriovenous (A/V) crossing in a patient with BRVO. During surgery, no changes in vein caliber or blood flow were detected, but 8 months later visual acuity improved from 20/200 to 20/25 [10]. Eleven years later, Opremcak and Bruce reported the first series of patients in whom vein decompression was performed. Following surgery, 67% of patients improved VA at a mean of 4 lines [11]. Shah et al. also found a substantial visual improvement in 4 of 5 eyes following vein decompression surgery [12]. In 2001, Mester et al. compared the results of surgical vein decompression in 40 patients with 22 controls, finding better VA in treated eyes [13]. In the same year, Dotrelova and coworkers reported three cases where VA improved 3.5 lines with the same surgical technique [14]. The only authors to have reported no visual improvement following surgery were Le Rouic et al. in a study performed on 3 eyes [15].

Moreover, other authors have reported improved VA following vitrectomy with posterior hyaloid removal without vein decompression [16, 17].

This paper reports the results of two prospective pilot studies on two consecutive series of patients surgically treated for BRVO. In one group the vitrectomy was followed by decompression of the vein at the A/V crossing, whereas in the other a vitrectomy with hyaloid removal was performed with no maneuvers at the crossing. The results of the two studies were retrospectively compared. To our knowledge, this is the first report to compare the results of these two surgical techniques in patients with BRVO.

Patients and methods

The study included 35 eyes of 35 patients with BRVO. All were operated on by the same surgeon (MSF). Between December 1998 and January 2000, vein decompression was performed in 15 patients (Group I). Between January 2000 and January 2001, vitrectomy with posterior hyaloid removal was performed in 20 patients (Group II). Primary outcome was visual acuity and secondary outcomes were resolution of macular edema and prevention of neovascularization. Informed consent was obtained from each patient.

Inclusion criteria were the same for both groups: BRVO cases presented for examination within one year of onset of symptoms, best-corrected Snellen VA equal to or worse than 20/100 and macular edema involving the fovea on slit-lamp examination. Any eyes presenting with posterior or anterior new vessels were excluded from the study. Patients with diabetic retinopathy or any other disease that could cause loss of vision were ineligible.

Best-corrected VA was checked prior to surgery and throughout the follow-up period. Using the Snellen chart, visual acuity was measured by masked observers who received no information on the procedures performed. Color fundus photographs were taken during all visits, and a flourescein angiography was performed before surgery, at 1, 3, 6, 9 and 12 months and then annually thereafter.

The results of the two prospective studies were retrospectively compared.

Surgical technique

In Group I, vitrectomy with posterior hyaloid removal and vein decompression at the AV crossing was performed. Decompression was done with a microvitreoretinal blade bent at the tip to separate the overlying arteriole from the venule, as previously described by Opremcak E.M. [11]. In cases where the tangential force required to separate the vessels was strong enough to endanger the integrity of the vein, horizontal or vertical scissors were used to complete decompression. Vitrectomy with posterior hyaloid removal was performed in the Group II. In this group, no maneuvers at the AV crossing were performed.

Statistical analysis

For data analysis, the Fisher exact test and the Mann-Whitney test were used. A finding was considered statistically significant at P < 0.05. The statistical package used was PRESTA PC, version 2.2.

Results

Group I. Surgical decompression

Fifteen eyes of 15 patients were included, 6 women and 9 men, with a mean age of 63 (51–80). The mean interval between the first symptoms and surgery was 28 days (7–75). The first step in surgery was to detach the posterior hyaloid, which was attached in 15/15 (100%) eyes. Decompression was successful in 11/15 (73%) patients (Fig. 1). In 4 cases where the integrity of the vein was endangered owing to strong attachment between the vessels at the crossing, decompression was not completed. During the procedure, no changes in vein caliber or blood flow were detected.

Despite successful decompression, 2 eyes developed venous collaterals 7 and 15 months after surgery, respectively (Fig. 2). Although successful decompression was performed in these two eyes 15 and 19 days after the occlusion, a severe vein stenosis persisted following surgery, making collaterals inevitable.

After a mean follow-up of 33 months (25–42 months) macular edema resolved in 14/15 (93%). Visual acuity improved 2 lines or more (2–8 lines) in 13/15 (87%), one line in one eye (6.5%) and remained the same in one patient (6.5%). Mean visual improvement was 4.5 lines in Snellen acuity, with a mean preoperative VA of 20/100 and a mean postoperative VA of 20/30. Mean time for VA improvement was 4.5 months (1.5–12 months). No relationship was found between the duration of the preoperative interval and visual results. Indeed, the patient with greatest VA improvement also had one of the longest preoperative intervals (45 days).

Six of fifteen eyes showed non-ischemic macular edema throughout the follow-up. Following surgery, the edema resolved in all of them and vision improved 4.5 lines (3–7 lines).

None of the eyes developed new vessels in either the anterior or posterior segments though 8/15 (53%) showed retinal ischemia larger than 5 disk diameters.

The following surgery-related complications were observed in this group during and after surgery: mild intraoperative retinal venous bleeding during the dissection in two eyes that resolved by increasing intraocular pressure; a macular hole 36 months after surgery in one eye despite macular edema resolution; and a nuclear cataract progression in most patients above the age of sixty.

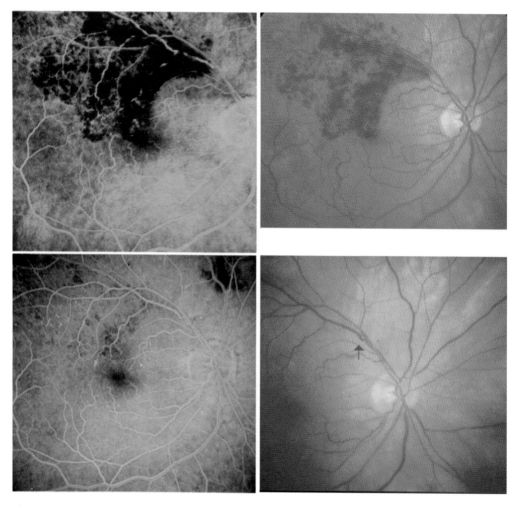

Fig. 1. Top left and right: Preoperative and color photographs. VA 20/100. Bottom left and right: Postoperative appearance 15 months after surgery. Following decompression, point of contact between the vessels is now visible (arrow). VA 20/20

Group II: Vitrectomy with posterior hyaloid removal

Twenty patients were included in this group (8 females and 12 males) with a mean age of 65 (56–71). The mean preoperative interval was 112 days (12 days–12 months). During surgery, the posterior hyaloid was detached in19/20 (95%), while one eye showed a pre-operative posterior hyaloid detachment.

After a mean follow-up of 18 months (14–25 months), macular edema resolved in 16/20 (80%) eyes. VA improved 2 lines or more (2–8 lines) in 16/20 (80%), remained the same in 2/20 (10%) and deteriorated one line in 2/20 (10%). Mean VA improvement was 3.5 lines, where the mean preoperative VA was 20/200 and the final postoperative VA was 20/40.

No eyes developed new vessels in either the posterior and anterior segments after a mean follow-up of 18 months.

During surgery, one case showed two peripheral retinal tears following posterior hyaloid detachment, which were treated with retinopexy and fluid/gas exchange. No other

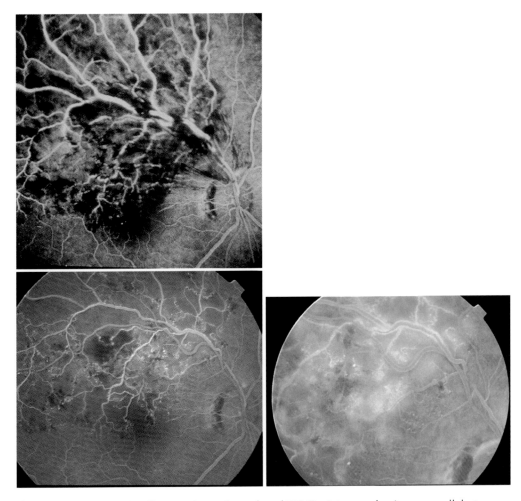

Fig. 2. Top: Preoperative fluorescein angiography of BRVO. Artery and vein are parallel at crossing. A thrombus is evident as a focal hyperfluorescence at the point of contact between the vessels. VA 20/100. Bottom left and right: Fluorescein angiography 28 months after surgery. Despite successful decompression 15 days after the occlusion, a severe vein stenosis persisted, making collaterals inevitable. VA 20/30

surgery-related complications were observed during or following surgery, except for the progression of nuclear cataracts.

Comparative study

No differences were found between the groups in terms of patients' age (P = 0.566; Mann-Whitney test). Nor were any differences found between the groups in terms of preoperative VA (P = 0.505; Mann-Whitney test). Nevertheless, there was a statistically significant difference in the preoperative interval, which was longer in the group where vitrectomy with posterior hyaloid removal was performed (P = 0.004; Fisher exact test). The mean preoperative interval was 28 days in Group I (7–75 days) and 3.5 months (12 days–12 months) in Group II. Despite this difference, no differences were found in final

Table 1. Comparative study

	Vitrectomy + decompression	Vitrectomy	P
Age	67 years	65 years	0.566
Mean preoperative VA	20/100	20/200	0.505
Mean preoperative interval	28 days	112 days	0.004
VA changes			
≥2 lines	13/15 (87%)	16/20 (80%)	
+1 line	1/15 (6.5%)	0/20	
no changes	1/15 (6.5%)	2/20 (10%)	0.147
−1 line	0/15	0/20	
≤2 lines	0/15	2/20 (10%)	
Macular edema resolution	14/15 (93%)	16/20 (80%)	0.365
New vessels (AS or PS) *	1/15	0/20	

*AC = anterior segment
PS = posterior segment

VA (P = 0.147; Mann-Whitney), resolution of macular edema (P = 0.365; Fisher exact test) or development of new vessels (0/15 in Group I and 0/20 in Group II) (Table 1).

Discussion

Branch retinal vein occlusion is the second most common cause of retinal vascular disease. This type of occlusion is most frequent in the superotemporal arcade because of the high density of A/V crossings. Two complications are most frequent: new vessels and macular edema. New vessels develop in approximately 20% of cases between 6 and 18 months after occlusion but the incidence of new vessels is determined by the size of the retinal ischemia. If the ischemia is smaller than 5 disk diameters, incidence will be near 11%; but if it is larger than 5 disk diameters, 36% of patients will develop retinal new vessels [9]. New vessels can also develop in either the disk or the anterior segment.

The second most common complication is macular edema, of which there are two types: ischemic and non-ischemic. An ischemic macular edema is characterized by an alteration of the foveal capillary net, which may or may not be associated with fluorescein leakage. In contrast, the non-ischemic macular edema is characterized by a normal foveal capillary net and leakage in the flourescein angiography. But the difference between these types of edema lies not only in their behavior during flourescein angiography but also in their natural evolution. The study by Finkelstein showed that the ischemic type tends to resolve spontaneously with an improvement in 90% of patients and mean final visual acuity of 20/30 without receiving any treatment. In his series, the non-ischemic form showed resolution of edema and improved visual acuity in 30% of cases; that is, 70% showed a persistence of edema with a final visual acuity of 20/100 with no treatment at all [18].

Thus, owing to the good natural evolution of the ischemic macular edema, most patients will not require any treatment. In eyes with the non-ischemic form, the results of the BRVO study indicate that grid laser treatment should be applied when visual acuity is worse than 20/40 three months after the occlusion. But the mean visual improvement in treated eyes was only 1.33 lines in the BRVO study [8]. Consequently, other surgical techniques are at present under investigation in an attempt to achieve better visual results. Among these are laser-induced chorioretinal anastomosis and surgical vein decompression at the AV crossing.

But laser-induced chorioretinal anastomosis was reported to be successful in only 3 of 6 eyes with BRVO, where visual acuity improved in 66% [19]. Moreover, severe complications including choroidal neovascularization, segmental retinal ischemia, choroidovitreal neovascularization, preretinal fibrosis with or without associated retinal traction and vision-limiting hemorrhages [20–23].

The second technique under investigation is surgical vein decompression, with good visual results reported by several authors. In December 1998 we began a prospective pilot study to determine whether BRVO was reversible by A/V decompression and what effect surgery had on the secondary complications of the disease. But to analyze the effectiveness of decompression, the procedure must be performed very early in the course of the disease, because experimental histological studies have shown irreversible capillary closure four days after the occlusion [24]. However, the state of the foveal capillary net cannot be determined by a fluorescein angiography so early in the course of the disease. Thus, we performed surgery on patients with macular edema and vision of 20/100 or worse as soon as possible, regardless of the type of edema.

In our series, complete decompression could not be performed in four eyes. Strong adherence between the vessels at the A/V crossing posed a serious risk of vein damage. The results of these four patients were included in Group I because maneuvers at the crossing were performed even though decompression was not completed.

In spite of the success of vein decompression in 11 of 15 operated eyes, two developed retinal venous collaterals. Although successful decompression was performed in these two eyes 15 and 19 days after the occlusion, a severe vein stenosis persisted following surgery, making collaterals inevitable.

Nevertheless, macular edema resolved in 14 of 15 eyes, that is, 93%, after a mean follow-up of 33 months. It is worth noting that no relationship was found between the duration of the preoperative interval and the incidence of resolution of macular edema. Edema resolved both in eyes that were operated on as soon as 7 days after the occlusion and in eyes operated as late as 75 days after the occlusion. Therefore, this finding would not appear to support the idea that decompression is the cause of edema resolution.

Disappearance of macular edema in our study was associated with visual improvement of one line or more in 93% of eyes with a mean improvement of 4.5 lines. But this significant visual improvement could be due to the high proportion of patients with ischemic macular edema. Although we were unable to determine the state of the foveal capillary net preoperatively owing to intraretinal hemorrhages, 9 eyes showed ischemic macular edema during the follow-up. So what happened in patients with the non-ischemic form of the disease, which is believed to have a worse prognosis? Of the 15 eyes operated on, 6 showed the non-ischemic form and vision improved in all at a mean of 4.5 lines (3–7 lines). This improvement was truly significant compared to that described in the BRVO study, where the mean improvement in treated eyes was 1.3 lines [8].

Neither our study nor any previous ones have found a relationship between the duration of the preoperative interval and visual results, which is surprising if the mechanism of improvement is understood to be vein decompression. Indeed, the patient with the best visual acuity after surgery also had one of the longest pre-operative intervals, that is, 45 days.

Surgery did not only improve visual acuity, but also prevented the development of new vessels in both groups, the second most common complication following BRVO.

All the above factors led us to pose the question of whether the absence of new vessels and the resolution of macular edema could be the result of the detachment of the posterior hyaloid and the removal of vitreous gel rather than of vein decompression. Thus, in January 2000 we undertook a new study to determine whether vitrectomy with posterior hyaloid removal with no vein decompression could achieve resolution of macular edema, visual improvement and prevention of the development of new vessels. To obtain valid results, inclusion criteria had to be the same as in the previous study: that is, eyes with macular edema secondary to BRVO and best-corrected VA of 20/100 or worse. Surgery was also performed as soon as possible following the diagnosis.

Retrospective comparison of results between the Group I and Group II revealed no differences in either patients' age or preoperative visual acuity. But there was a statistically significant difference in the duration of the preoperative interval, which was longer in Group II. Despite this difference, no differences were found in final visual acuity, resolution of macular edema or prevention of neovascularization.

Therefore, our findings would suggest that posterior hyaloid detachment and vitreous removal might be sufficient to resolve macular edema, improve visual acuity and prevent the development of new vessels in patients with BRVO, making maneuvers at the crossing unnecessary. Recent reports by Tachi and Saika would support our findings on vitrectomy with hyaloid removal. Tachi and co-workers reported 27 patients where macular edema resolved and VA improved following phacoemulsification and pars plana vitrectomy with posterior hyaloid detachment [16]. They found that VA improvement was better in those eyes that had higher visual acuity before surgery. Saika et al. combined this technique with a gas/air tamponade and found that VA improved substantially when surgery was performed no later than 11 months after the occlusion [17].

But what might be the mechanism for macular edema resolution and visual improvement following a vitrectomy with hyaloid removal?

It should be emphasized that nearly all the eyes in this study showed an attached posterior hyaloid during surgery. Detachment of the posterior hyaloid and removal of the vitreous gel may improve the oxygen supply to ischemic inner retina by way of fluid currents in the vitreous cavity, as Stefansson et al. reported in 1990 [25]. The improvement in the preretinal oxygen tension levels may cause vessel constriction and lower intravascular pressure, reducing edema formation according to Starling's law [26]. This may cause the resolution of macular edema in BRVO, in a manner similar to the resolution of diabetic macular edema following vitrectomy, and it also may explain the inhibitory effect that vitrectomy has on retinal neovascularization.

But it is also possible that the removal of vitreous gel causes resolution of macular edema because intravitreal cytokines are eliminated. Vascular endothelial growth factor (VEGF) is a cytokine produced by hypoxic retina in central retinal vein occlusion and diabetic retinopathy, inducing capillary permeability and angiogenesis [27, 28]. It has recently been reported that VEGF leads to endothelial cell hypertrophy and capillary luminal narrowing, causing more ischemia and more VEGF production [29]. Vitreous removal, by eliminating this cytokine and perhaps other cytokines as well, may alter this vicious circle, inducing the resolution of macular edema and the improvement of visual acuity found in our study. Nevertheless, these are only hypotheses that must be tested by future studies.

Although there are numerous potential complications associated with these surgical techniques, including retinal tears or detachment, vitreous hemorrhage, retinal gliosis at the incision site or nerve fiber layer defects, in our series they were very uncommon. Only one eye showed retinal tears during surgery, which were successfully treated with retinopexy and fluid/gas exchange. Our most common complication was the acceleration of nuclear sclerotic cataract formation, which is inherent to vitrectomy.

In summary, our study would suggest that vitrectomy with posterior hyaloid removal might resolve macular edema, improve visual acuity and prevent development of new vessels in patients with BRVO, making maneuvers at the crossing unnecessary. Nevertheless, this is only a pilot study: a larger number of patients would be necessary to confirm our findings. Moreover, only randomization with a control group could determine the effectiveness of these surgical techniques.

References

1. Mitchell P, Smith W, Chang A (1996) Prevalence and association of retinal vein occlusion in Australia. The Blue Mountains Eye Study. Arch Ophthalmol 114:1243–7
2. Fryczkowski AW, Sato SE (1987) Scanning electron microscopy evaluation of arteriovenous crossing phenomenon. Contemp Ophthalmic Forum 5:184–92
3. Duker JS, Brown GC (1989) Anterior location of the crossing artery in branch retinal vein occlusion. Arch Ophthalmol 107:998–1000
4. Weinberg D, Dodwell DG, Fern SA (1990) Anatomy of arteriovenous crossing in branch retinal vein occlusion. Am J Ophthalmol 109:298–302
5. Rabinowicz IM, Litman S, Michaelson IC (1969) Branch venous thrombosis – a pathological report. Trans Ophthalmol Soc UK 88:191–210
6. Staurenghi G, Lonati Ch, Aschero M, Orzalesi N (1994) Arteriovenous crossing as a risk factor in branch retinal vein occlusion. Am J Ophthalmol 117:211–13
7. Kumar B, Yu D, Morgan WH, et al (1998) The distribution of the angioarchitectural changes within the vicinity of arteriovenous crossing in branch retinal vein occlusion. Ophthalmology 105: 424–7
8. Argon laser photocoagulation for macular edema in branch vein occlusion. The Branch Vein Occlusion Study Group (1984). Am J Ophthalmol 98:271–82
9. Argon laser scatter photocoagulation for prevention of neovascularization and vitreous hemorrhage in branch vein occlusion. A randomised clinical trial. The Branch Vein Occlusion Study Group (1986) 104:34–41
10. Osterloh MD, Charles S (1988) Surgical decompression of branch retinal vein occlusion. Arch Ophthalmol 106:1469–71
11. Opremcak EM, Bruce RA (1999) Surgical decompression of branch retinal vein occlusion via arteriovenous crossing sheathotomy. Retina 19:1–5
12. Shah GK, Sharma S, Fineman MS, et al (2000) Arteriovenous adventitial sheathotomy for the treatment of macular edema associated with branch retinal vein occlusion. Am J Ophthalmol 129:104–6
13. Mester U, Dillinger P (2001) Treatment of retinal vein occlusion. Vitrectomy with arteriovenous decompression and dissection of the internal limiting membrane. Opthalmologe 98:1104–9
14. Dotrelova D, Dubska Z, Kuthan P, Stepankova J (2001) Initial experience with surgical decompression of the vein in branch retinal vein occlusion. Cesk Slov Oftalmol 57:359–66
15. Le Rouic JF, Bejjani RA, Rumen F, et al (2001) Adventitial sheathotomy for decompression of recent onset branch retinal vein occlusion. Graefes Arch Clin Exp Ophthalmol 239:747–51
16. Tachi N, Hashimoto Y, Ogino N (1999) Vitrectomy for macular edema combined with retinal occlusion. Documenta Ophthalmologica 97:465–9
17. Saika S, Tanaka T, Miyamoto T, Ohnishi Y (2001) Surgical posterior vitreous detachment combined with gas/air tamponade for treating macular edema associated with retinal vein occlusion: retinal tomography and visual outcome. Graefes Arch Clin Exp Ophthalmol 239:729–32
18. Finkelstein D (1992) Ischemic macular edema. Recognition and favorable natural history in branch vein occlusion. Arch Ophthalmol 110:1427–34
19. Fekrat S, Goldberg M, Finkelstein D (1998) Laser-induced chorioretinal venous anastomosis for nonischemic central or branch vein occlusion. Arch Ophthalmol 116:43–52
20. Eccarius SG, Moran MJ, Slingsby JG (1996) Choroidal neovascular membrane after laser-induced chorioretinal anastomosis. Am J Ophthalmol 122:590–1
21. Yarng S-S, Hsieh C-L (1996) Chorioretinal neovascularization following laser-induced chorioretinal venous anastomosis. Ophthalmology 103:136
22. Browning DJ, Rotberg MH (1996) Vitreous hemorrhage complicating laser-induced chorioretinal anastomosis for central retinal vein occlusion. Am J Ophthalmol 122:588–9
23. Luttrull JK (1997) Epiretinal membrane and traction retinal detachment complicating laser-induced chorioretinal venous anastomosis. Am J Ophthalmol 123:698–9
24. Minamikawa M, Yamamoto K, Okuma H (1993) Experimental retinal branch vein occlusion. 4. Pathological changes in the middle and late stage. Nippon Ganka Gakkai Zasshi 97:920–7

25. Stefánsson E, Novack RL, Hatchell DL (1990) Vitrectomy prevents retinal hypoxia in branch retinal vein occlusion. Invest Ophthalmol Vis Sci 31:284–9
26. Arnarsson A, Stefánsson E (2000) Laser treatment and the mechanism of edema reduction in branch retinal vein occlusion. Invest Ophthalmol Vis Sci 41:877–9
27. Pe'er J, Folberg R, Itin A, et al (1998) Vascular endothelial growth factor up regulation in human central retinal vein occlusion. Ophthalmology 105:412–16.
28. Amin RH, Frank RN, Kennedy A, et al (1997) Vascular endothelial growth factor is present in the glial cells of the retina and optic nerve of human subjects with nonproliferative diabetic retinopathy. Invest Ophthalmol Vis Sci 38:36–47
29. Funatsu H, Yamashita H, Ikeda T, et al (2002) Angiotensin II and vascular endothelial growth factor in the vitreous fluid of patients with diabetic macular edema and other retinal disorders. Am J Ophthalmol 133:537–43

Correspondence: Marta S. Figueroa, M.D., PhD., Director of VitreoRetinal Department, Hospital Oftalmológico Internacional, Santa Hortensia 58, E-28002 Madrid, Spain, E-mail: figueroa@lander.es

Radial optic neurotomy for central retinal vein occlusion-first results

S. Binder, S. Brunner, and A. Abri

Department of Ophthalmology, The Ludwig Boltzmann Institute for Retinology and
Biomicroscopic Laser Surgery, Rudolf Foundation Clinic, Vienna, Austria

Introduction

Central vein occlusion (CVO) is a common retinal vascular disorder with potentially blinding complications. The two mayor complications associated with CVO are reduced vision resulting from macular involvement, which might be present as macular edema, macular haemorrhage or macular nonperfusion and neovascular glaucoma secondary to iris neovascularisation, which might result in pain and blindness [1].

Under the many different terminologies used for the different types of CVO related to the findings on fluoresceinangiography the most appropriate is possibly the term perfused and non perfused [2]. Although the exact area of non perfusion is not always clear, it was proposed by Margalal et al. that the existence of 10 disc areas of retinal nonperfusion is necessary to define ischemia [3].

There is a strong association with hypertension, cardiovascular disease and diabetes mellitus in 50–70% of the affected patients, and most of them are over 50 years of age [4].

Treatment so far has been directed to prevention of complications with panretinal laser coagulation or grid pattern treatment for macula edema. Results of the Central Vein Occlusion Study (88–92) [5] have shown, that patients with low visual acuity at onset (less than 20/200) had only a 20% chance for improvement at outcome, perfused or not perfused. Out of 728 eyes 547(74.4%) were considered as perfused at the study onset, after 4 months additional 15% converted into nonperfused and during the next 32 months additional 19% became non perfused, a total of 34%. As far as prophylactic panretinal photocoagulation for nonperfused CVO was concerned the study demonstrated, that this does not totally prevent the development of iris neovascularisation and prompt regression of NV is more likely to occur in eyes following treatment when those eyes have not been previously treated.

Grid pattern photocoagulation for macular edema showed no visual benefit in this disease when the CVOS macular edema eligibility crtierias were met [5, 6].

Histopathologic studies by Green et al. of 29 eyes with CVO have shown a thrombosis of the central retinal vein in the area of the lamina cribrosa as a constant finding [7].

Left with little effective treatment for CVO, Opremcak et al. [8] developed a surgical technique which is supposed to decompress the CVO via a radial optic neurotomy (RON), performed after vitrectomy from a transvitreal approach. Improvements in 73% (8/11) were reported with this technique, the surgery was evaluated as being safe.

In this article we describe our first experiences with RON in a consecutive series of patients with CVO which was supplemented by the removal of the inner limiting membrane (ILM) in eyes with cystoid macular edema to allow further improvement of the macular function.

Patients and methods

Patients were selected on a non randomized case by case basis. They were eligible for the surgery if detoriation of vision over 3 months or non-perfused CVO was present and the visual acuity was 20/200 or lower. Reported onset of the disease should not exceed 12 months.

The natural course of the disease and the possible treatment alternatives were explained to each patient, as well as the fact that this was a new surgical intervention. Patients were included if they were able and willing to come for follow up every three months for at least one year. An informed consent was signed in each case.

Examinations performed included best corrected visual acuity, biomicroscopy of the anterior and the posterior segment, fundus colour photography, fluorescein angiography (Heidelberger Engineering, HRA) multifocal ERG examination (multiSCAN, Munich) and optical coherence tomography (OCT, Zeiss) pre – and post operatively, after one month and every 3 months thereafter.

The surgery was performed by one surgeon (S.B) after surgical training on cadaver eyes – which had their corneas removed for corneal transplantation and were donated from the Institute of Pathology – to determine the route of the knife and its depth. Preoperatively the site of incision was carefully selected according to the fluorescein angiogram to avoid cutting of larger vessels.

In general the technique described by Opremcak and his knife* was used. except that in addition to the p.p. Vitrectomy the ILM was carefully removed after indocyanine staining before the RON was performed.

Results

Between December 2001 and March 2003, 12 eyes of 12 patients could be included in the study. The medium follow-up was 6.8 months(3–18 months). All surgeries were performed in general anesthesia. No combined procedures were performed in this series, because we felt that the intraoperative pressure raise necessary during and after the radial incision to avoid haemorrhage might cause dislocation of the posterior chamber implant.

The medium age of the patients was 77.7 years (50–91), 5 were female, 7 were male.

Preoperative data

Associated cardiovascular risk factors were present in 9/12 (75%), 4 patients had a medically controlled wide angle glaucoma, one patient was pseudophakic.

An ischemic CVO was present in 8 cases before surgery, in 2 eyes a perfused CVO was diagnosed, but visual detoriation progressive due to a large macular edema and under 20/200.

One patient had anterior ischemic optic neuropathy with already considerable optic damage, and in one patients a Leber's Congenital Opticoneuropathy was present.

In 40% (5/12) of the patients the other eye had marked reduced vision. In 2 patients the other eye had also a non perfused CVO, in 2 patients a terminal age-related macular degeneration was present and in one patient a Leber's Congenital Optico–Neuropathy.

The *surgery* was uneventful in all cases.

As *postoperative complications* a mild intravitreal hemmorrharge was observed in 2 eyes and a haemorrhage around the incision observed in 3 eyes, both absorbed at the latest within 21 days (Table 1).

Table 1. Complications (n = 12)

Intraoperative	0
Postoperative	
• mild vitr. hemorrh.	2
• Hemorrh. around incision	3
• (resorbed after max. 21 days)	
• Persistent	
• Macular edema	2
• Rubeosis and sec. Glaucoma after 12 weeks	1

Visual outcome

The best corrected visual acuity at the last visit was taken for evaluation.

The preoperative visual acuities ranged between 0.05 and light perception, no useful reading acuity was recorded in this group.

Postoperatively visual acuity ranged between HM and 0.2, a reading acuity of Jg 5 was present in one case.

Mild visual improvement between one and 3 lines was reported in 75% (9/12) at the last control follow-up.

Fluorescein angiography

More than 10 disc diameters of non perfusion was present in 8 cases, in 2 the retinas were perfused preoperatively.

A massive macular edema was present in 10 of 12 eyes.

Improved perfusion – defined by rapid absorption of hemorrharges and loss of venous congestion – developed in 80% (8/10) during the first 1–3 months (Fig. 1).

An arterio-venous anastomosis on the incision site was observed in one eye.

Progression of ischemia was observed in one eye 2 months after surgery, which resulted in the development of severe rubeosis iridis with secondary glaucoma (Table 1). This diabetic patient, was pseudophakic, had a compensated glaucoma preoperatively and laser treatment for massive ischemia preoperatively as well (Fig. 2).

Macular edema slowly reduced in 8/10 patients, but some residual hyper fluorescence could be seen at last visit in 4 of them. In 2 eyes the macular edema remained unchanged to the preoperative status (Table 1).

Optical coherence tomography (OCT)

Measurements were taken at 3 different sites preoperatively and compared with the values obtained at the same locations postoperatively.

Parallel with the reduction of hyperfluorescence on fluorescein angiography a decrease of the medium value from 598.3 (364–672 µm) to 441.4 (154–604) was documented in 80% (8/10) (Fig. 3).

Again, 2 eyes had unchanged values.

Multifocal electroretinography (mERG)

The medium potential measured was 66.0 nVol preoperatively and 65.9 nVol postoperatively. It remained unchanged during the observation period (Fig. 4).

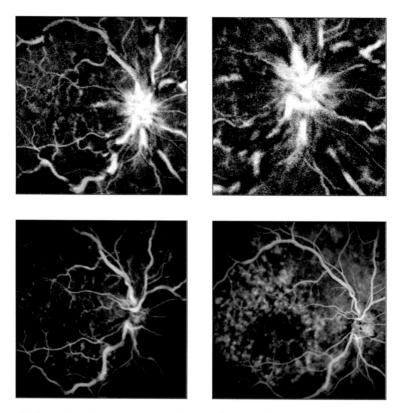

Fig. 1. Case Nr 2, male, 63y: pre (superior line) and 6 months postoperative (inferior line) early and late phase fluoresceinangiogramm VA preop:0.05 NRA postop 0.15, Jg 14

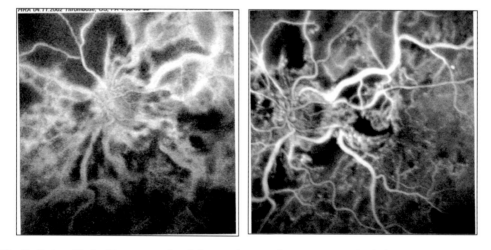

Fig. 2. Patient Nr 6., 82 years, male, diabetes, chronic glaucoma, pseudophakia, scatter laser treatment before surgery Pre-(left) and postoperative (right) fluorescence angiography after 3 months shows unchanged ischemia

Discussion

Prognosis for non perfused CVO in general is unfavourable and 60% of all cases with CVO develop finally a n.p. CVO. In addition a vision of 20/200 and lower is a predictor for further vision loss even in perfused eyes [1].

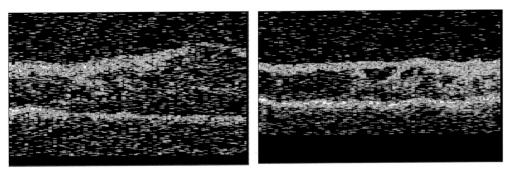

Fig. 3. Case Nr 2, pre(left) – and 6 months postoperative (right) OCT shows a reduction of the macular edema, but not a complete absorption

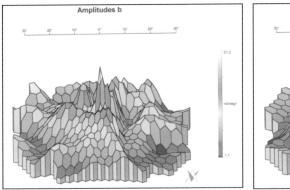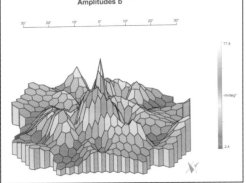

Fig. 4. Case Nr 2: Multifocal ERG (Retiscan) pre (left) – and postoperatively (right) after 6 months shows almost unchanged values

The current treatment options are very limited and medical treatment so far has failed in the cure of this disease [9]. Grid laser-treatment has shown no visual improvement in eyes with macular edema and panretinal laser does not prevent the development of rubeosis iridis in all cases [5].

A chorioretinal anastomosis is difficult to perform with laser treatment and was achieved in the clinical situation in only 30%. Complications related to this treatment have been observed [10].

Recently favourable results have been reported with high-dose Triamcinolone-Acetonite [11] along with a large percentage of secondary glaucoma and the disadvantage of an transient effect. Opremcak's surgical technique seems to be safe and the effect was also shown experimentally by Lit et al. [12]. This is in contrast to earlier reports from Vasco–Pasada and Arcieniegas [13, 14] who tried to open the lamina cribrosa from an external approach.

No intraoperative complication were observed in our first series and our clinical results are comparable to those published by Opremcak [9]. However the visual improvements we observed were only moderate, and no useful reading vision was achieved. This could be explained by the rather long history of our cases and most likely an earlier intervention might improve this condition. In addition most of our cases had non perfused CVO.

Interestingly, the macular oedema decreased but was not completely absorbed during our observation period. Whether the removal of the ILM helps in further absorption is questionable and needs further examination. Clearly in all these cases the ILM was very taught and strongly adherent and could not be removed safely and completely without a dye.

Almost no change of the potential values was observed with mERG. A possible explanation for this might be, that a considerable damage of the retinal layers has already occurred.

Although some additional information was gained with this study, it has its weakness in is small case number and the lack of a control group.

Conclusion

Radial optic neurotomy is a technically feasible and promising surgical procedure with the potential to restore some vision in eyes with CVO. A prospective trial is needed to explore its value further.

References

1. Clarkson JG (2001) Central retinal vein occlusion. In: Stephen JR, Andrew P (eds) Schachat; Retina, Vol 2, 3rd ed. Mosby 75:1368–75
2. Hayreh SS (1983) Classification of central retinal vein occlusion. Ophthalmology 90:458–74
3. Margalal LE, Donooso LA, Sanborn GE (1982) Retinal ischaemia and risk of neovascularisation following central retinal vein obstruction. Opthalmology 89:1241–5
4. Gutman FA (1983) Evaluation of a patient with central retinal vein occlusion. Ophthalmology 90:481–3
5. The Central Vein Occlusion Study Group (1997) Natural history and clinical management of central retinal vein occlusion. Arch Ophthalmol 115:486–91
6. Klein ML, Finkelstein D (1987) Laser photocoagulation of macular edema in central retinal vein occlusion. Symposium on Central Vein Occlusion, 10th Macula Society Meeting, Cannes, France
7. Green WR, Chan CC, Hutchins GM, et al (1981) Central retinal vein occlusion: a prospective histopathologic study of 29 eyes in 28 cases. Retina 1:27–55
8. Opremcak EM, Bruce RA, Lomeo MD, Ridenour CD, Letson AD, Rehmar AJ (2001) Radial optic neurotomy for central retinal vein occlusion: a retrospective pilot study of 11 consecutive cases. Retina 21(5):408–15
9. Aggermann T, Brunner S, Binder S (2003) The challenge of retinal vein occlasions. Br J Ophthalmol (Submitted)
10. McAllister IL, Douglas JP, Constable IJ, Yu DY (1998) Laser-induced chorioretinal venous anastomosis for nonischemic central retinal vein occlusion: evaluation of the complications and their risk factors. Am J Ophthalmol 126(2):219–29
11. Jonas JB, Kreissig I, Degenring RF (2002) Intravitreal triamcinolone acetonide as treatment of macular edema in central retinal vein occlusion. Graefes Arch Clin Exp Ophthalmol 240(9):782–3
12. Lit E, Tsilimbaris M, Gotzaridis E, D'Amico DJ (2002) Lamina puncture: pars plana optic disc surgery for central retinal vein occlusion. Arch Ophthalmol 120(4):495–9
13. Vasco–Pasada J (1972) Modification of the circulation in the posterior pole of the eye. Ann Ophthalmol 4:48–59
14. Arciniegas A (1984) Treatment of the occlusion of the central retinal vein by section of the posterior ring. Ann Ophthalmol 16:1081–6

Correspondence: Susanne Binder, M. D., Professor and Chairman, Department of Ophthalmology, The Ludwig Boltzmann Institute for Retinology and Biomicroscopic Laser Surgery, Rudolf Foundation Clinic, Juchgasse 25, A-1030 Vienna, Austria, E-mail: susanne.binder@kar.magwien.gv.at

Structural changes following photodynamic therapy evaluated by Optical Coherence Tomography (OCT)

I. Krebs, S. Binder, and U. Stolba

Department of Ophthalmology,
The Ludwig Boltzmann Institute of Retinology and Biomicroscopic Laser Surgery,
Rudolf Foundation Hospital, Vienna, Austria
(Chairman: Prof. Dr. Susanne Binder)

Optical Coherence Tomography (OCT) is a non invasive and non-contact imaging modality producing cross sectional images of retinal tissues [1]. The OCT is analogous to B-mode ultrasound except that light is used rather than sound waves. This provides a higher resolution of 10–20 microns.

There is a false colour scheme employed to differentiate the structures of the cross-sectional images. Highly reflective structures like the nerve fiber layer and the pigmentepithelium are coloured with bright colours (white or red). The area of decreased reflectivity between these highly reflective layers is coloured yellow or green and corresponds to the neurosensory retina. Spaces filled with fluid, like a detachment of the neurosensory retina or the vitreus gel, show extremely low reflection and are coloured blue to black. Neovascular membranes are highly reflective and coloured red. Computer controlled manually placed cursers are used to measure the distance between the highly reflective surface of the retina and the retinal pigmentepithelium corresponding to the retinal thickness. The retinal thickness is increased in cases of retinal edema. Besides measuring the retinal nerve fiber thickness in glaucoma cases the OCT was previously used for preoperative evaluation of macular holes [2, 3] or epiretinal membranes [4, 5]. Measurement of the retinal thickness was helpful in evaluating the changes of diabetic macular edema after photocoagulation or pars plana vitrectomy [6, 7]. OCT was used to compare the changes of the retinal structures in age related macular degeneration (AMD) with biomicroscopic findings [8, 9].

Photodynamic Therapy (PDT) is a new therapy option in cases of choroidal neovascularisation due to AMD, pathologic myopia and other cases. The beneficial effect in comparison to the natural course has been proven in randomised clinical studies (TAP [10] and VIP [11] study). The eligibility for this therapy and the indications for retreatment base on fluoresceinangiographic (FA) findings. We compared the structural changes found in the OCT images following PDT with the fluorescein angiograms. Measurements of the retinal thickness were performed to quantify the decrease of retinal edema and the effect of the PDT.

Patients and methods

Optical coherence tomography and fluorescein angiography of a series of patients treated with PDT were examined. We included only eyes with classic subfoveal choroidal neovascularisation without any occult parts in the FA [12]. Classic membranes are well defined, measurements of the greatest diameter of the membrane are easily done in FA and OCT. We wanted to compare the OCT images of a group with similar angiographic findings. Eyes with subfoveal choroidal neovascularisations due to age related macular

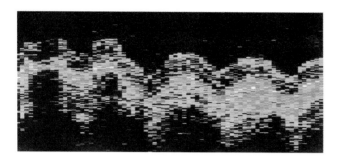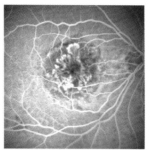

Fig. 1. The limits of OCT are demonstrated. The OCT of this patient suffering from Morbus Parkinson can not be interpreted although the FA is of sufficient qualitiy

degeneration (AMD), pathologic myopia and multifocal choroiditis were included. The patients had to fulfil the general criteria for PDT and PDT was performed according to the TAP guidelines.

Retreatment was performed when we noted any leakage in the late phase angiograms at the three months check-ups.

OCT, FA and distance acuity were performed at baseline examination, after 6 weeks, 3 months and afterwards every 3 months.

The best corrected distance acuity was tested with ETDRS Charts in 4 m distance [13].

The fluorescein angiography and the measurement of the lesion size was performed with the Heidelberg Retina Angiograph. 6–8 pictures were taken in the early phase after injection, then every 15 seconds, after 1 minute, 2 minutes and finally late pictures after 5 and 10 minutes. Optical Coherence Tomography (OCT) was performed with enlarged pupils with the Optical Coherence Tomography-Scanner (Zeiss). Six horizontal scans through the centre of the lesion with a length of 2.83 mm were performed. The retinal thickness was measured in front of the membrane and immediately near the membrane.

Results

Insufficient central fixation in patients with poor visual acuity in both the eyes prevented scans of sufficient quality through the centre of the lesion in four eyes. These patients could not be included. One patient with Morbus Parkinson (the scan and FA picture is shown in Fig. 1), and one patient with posterior staphyloma could not be included either. Finally 43 eyes met the criteria of inclusion.

29 patients (30 eyes) were female and 13 (13 eyes) male. The mean age was 70 years ranging from 26 to 92. 23 eyes suffered from choroidal neovascularisations due to AMD, 18 eyes due to pathologic myopia and 2 eyes due to multifocal chorioiditis.

At baseline examination the classic neovascular membrane was visible as a hyper-reflective band anterior to the pigment epithelium, sometimes separated from the pigmentepithelium by a zone of lower reflectivity as is shown in Fig. 2. The boundaries of the membrane are well defined, the measurement of the diameter of the lesion in the OCT is possible. The results of the measurements in OCT and FA are almost the same. Some of the membranes showed only a bumplike thickening of the high reflective zone corresponding to the pigmentepithelium and the neovascular membrane. In spite of the absence of a separation zone the area of the membrane could be identified and the diameter of the lesion could be measured. The mean values of the greatest horizontal diameter measured with OCT and FA were almost the same (1666 µm in the OCT and

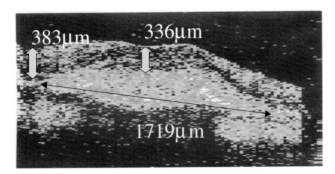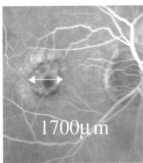

Fig. 2. The measurement of the diameter of the lesion is marked with black arrows in the OCT and the corresponding diameter in the FA with a white arrow. The grey Arrows show the locations of the measurements of the retinal thickness in front of the membrane and immediately beside the membrane. The highly reflective (red) zone anterior to the retinal pigmentepithelium (RPE)-choriocapillaris complex represents the choroidal neovascularisation

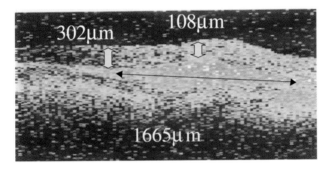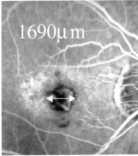

Fig. 3. OCT and FA of the eye presented in Fig. 2 two years after the first treatment: There is a remarkable decrease of retinal thickness, the thickness of the membrane-RPE complex is reduced, the area of low reflectivity posterior to the RPE is smaller but still present

1659 μm in the FA). The difference between the measurements was not more than 0.4 mm in any case and in 80% of the eyes under 0.1 mm.

After 6 weeks we found a decrease of the mean values of the retinal thickness compared with baseline examination. In 58% there was an increase of the retinal thickness after 3 months compared with the values of the week 6 examination and these eyes were retreated. 11% of the eyes were retreated although there was a decrease of retinal thickness. After 6 months 11% of the eyes needing retreatment showed an increase of retinal thickness and 19% a decrease of retinal thickness compared to the values of the month 3 examination. Significant leakage in the FA and an increase of retinal thickness in the OCT are signs of activity of the membrane and these eyes need retreatment. One of these cases with detachment of the neurosensory retina is shown in Fig. 4. After 18 months in 81% of the eyes no significant leakage had occurred in the FA and the retinal thickness did not increase compared with the month 15 examination. Figure 3 shows one of these eyes with decreased retinal thickness after two PDT treatments. The thickness of the membrane-pigmentepithelium complex is also reduced. The hyporeflective area behind the membrane due to absorption of the light is smaller than in the images before treatment, but still present. In 11% a retinal atrophy occurred. The retinal thickness was subnormal (under 150 μm), the area behind the pigmentepithelium is hyperreflectve because of the increased penetration of the light through the fibrotic scar. In the FA late staining is present (one of these cases is presented in Fig. 5).

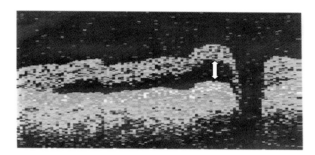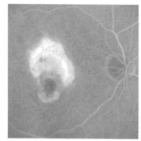

Fig. 4. There is a large amount of fluid in the retina, the neurosensory retina is detached (the area of low reflectivity marked with a white arrow), these are signs of an active membrane needing retreatment

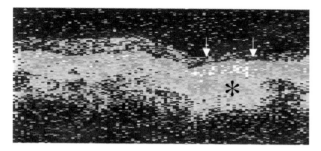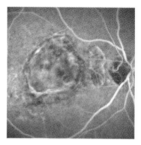

Fig. 5. In this case retinal atrophy occurred after PDT: The retinal thickness is subnormal (marked with arrows), there is an increase of penetration of the light, the decreased area of hyperreflectivity is marked with an asterix

In most of the eyes it was possible to achieve inactivity of the CNV after multiple treatment with late staining in the FA and minimal retinal fluid in the OCT. But there were cases responding not well after PDT. Retinal hemorrhages [14], sometimes extensive, have been described before. Another complication fortunately not so often seen occurred in one of our patients. After the first retreatment a contraction of the neovascular membrane occurred with starfolds of the retina in the red free images. Furthermore there was a huge detachment of the neurosensory retina. In the OCT the retinal thickness increased, a large minimal reflective area, separated by a hyperreflective septum is seen in front of the hyperreflective band of the CNV due to cystoid macular edema. Subretinal surgery was offered to the patient but he refused to further treatment (Fig. 6 shows images of this case).

Discussion and conclusion

Measurement of the retinal thickness appeared to be very useful in objectively monitoring changes in macular edema in diabetic cases or eyes with branch vein occlusion [16]. The reproducibility of OCT examinations has been proven before [17, 18]. We used measurements of the retinal thickness for objectively evaluating the effect of PDT in eyes with classic subfoveal CNV. A significant decrease of macular edema after 6 weeks up to 18 months was observed. The amount of leakage in the FA correlated well with the retinal thickness measured with the OCT and the documentation was more precisely with the help of OCT.

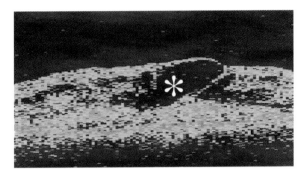 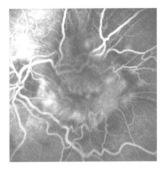

Fig. 6. Patient WK, male, 68 years. 1 month after the second PDT a contraction of the neovascular membrane occurred (star folds in the FLA) and the amount of intraretinal fluid increased very much. Cystoid macular edema is present (the very low reflective spaces are marked with an asterix)

In addition OCT provides a structural assessment of the macular region. A classification system of the changes of retina following PDT in AMD was developed by Adam H Rogers et al. based on FA and OCT findings [19]. Our own experiences correlate well with the findings of this recently published article. We also found similar structural changes in cases of pathologic myopia and multifocal choroiditis. OCT can provide further information of the amount of fluid in the retina and the activity of the choroidal neovascularisation. To summarize, OCT can probably not replace FA and ICG but provides significant further information in the monitoring of the arrest or progression of choroidal neovascularisations.

References

1. Hee MR, Izatt JA, Swanson EA, Huang D, Schuman JS, Lin CP, Puliafito CA, Fujimoto JG (1995) Optical coherence tomography of the human retina. Arch Ophthalmol 113(3):325–32
2. Ullrich S, Haritoglou C, Gass C, Schaumberger M, Ulbig MW, Kampik A (2002) Macular hole size as a prognostic factor in macular hole surgery. Br J Ophthalmol 86(4):390–3
3. Gobel W, Schrader WF, Schrenker M, Klink T (2000) Findings of optical coherence tomography (OPT) before and after macular hole surgery. Ophthalmologe 97(4):251–6 (German)
4. Abri A, Stolba U, Krebs I, Mihalics Ch, Brunner S, Binder S (2000) Retrospektive Studie von 57 Fällen mit Macular pucker. Retrospective study of 57 cases with Macular pucker. Spektrum Augenheilkd 14/5:259–61
5. Azzolini C, Patelli F, Codenotti M, Pierro L, Brancato R (1999) Optical coherence tomography in idiopathic epiretinal macular membrane surgery. Eur J Ophthalmol 9(3):206–11
6. Martidis A, Duker JS, Greenberg PB, Rogers AH, Puliafito CA, Reichel E, Baumal C (2002) Intravitreal triamcinolone for refractory diabetic macular edema. Ophthalmology 109(5):920–7
7. Massin P, Duguid G, Erginay A, Haouchine B, Gaudric A (2003) Optical coherence tomography for evaluating diabetic macular edema before and after vitrectomy. Am J Ophthalmol 135(2):169–77
8. Puliafito CA, Hee MR, Lin CP, Reichel E, Schuman JS, Duker JS, Izatt JA, Swanson EA, Fujimoto JG (1995) Imaging of macular diseases with optical coherence tomography. Ophthalmology 102(2):217–29
9. Hee MR, Baumal CR, Puliafito CA, Duker JS, Reichel E, Wilkins JR, Coker JG, Schuman JS, Swanson EA, Fujimoto JG (1996) Optical coherence tomography of age-related macular degeneration and choroidal neovascularization. Ophthalmology 103(8):1260–70
10. Treatment of Age-Related Macular Degeneration with Photodynamic Therapy (TAP) Study Group (1999) Photodynamic therapy of subfoveal choroidal neovascularization in age-related macular degeneration with verteporfin: one-year results of 2 randomized clinical trials – TAP report. Arch Ophthalmol 117(10):1329–45

11. Verteporfin in Photodynamic Therapy (VIP) Study Group (2001) Photodynamic therapy of sub-foveal choroidal neovascularization in pathologic myopia with verteporfin. 1-year results of a randomized clinical trial – VIP report no. 1. Ophthalmology 108(5):841–52

12. Macular Photocoagulation Study Group (1991) Subfoveal neovascular lesions in age-related macular degeneration. Guidelines for evaluation and treatment in the macular photocoagulation study. Arch Ophthalmol 109(9):1242–57

13. Ferris Fld, Kassoff A, Bresnick Gh, et al (1982) New visual acuity charts for clinical research. Am J Ophthalmol 94:91–6

14. Theodossiadis GP, Panagiotidis D, Georgalas IG, Moschos M, Theodossiadis PG (2003) Retinal hemorrhage after photodynamic therapy in patients with subfoveal choroidal neovascularization caused by age-related macular degeneration. Graefes Arch Clin Exp Ophthalmol 241(1):13–8 (Epub 2002 Dec 05)

15. Imasawa M, Iijima H, Morimoto T (2001) Perimetric sensitivity and retinal thickness in eyes with macular edema resulting from branch retinal vein occlusion. Am J Ophthalmol 131(1):55–60

16. Hee MR, Puliafito CA, Wong C, Duker JS, Reichel E, Rutledge B, Schuman JS, Swanson EA, Fujimoto JG (1995) Quantitative assessment of macular edema with optical coherence tomography. Arch Ophthalmol 113(8):1019–29

17. Massin P, Vicaut E, Haouchine B, Erginay A, Paques M, Gaudric A (2001) Reproducibility of retinal mapping using optical coherence tomography. Arch Ophthalmol 119(8):1135–42

18. Koozekanani D, Roberts C, Katz SE, Herderick EE (2000) Intersession repeatability of macular thickness measurements with the Humphrey 2000 OCT. Invest Ophthalmol Vis Sci 41(6): 1486–91

19. Rogers AH, Martidis A, Greenberg PB, Puliafito CA (2002) Optical coherence tomography findings following photodynamic therapy of choroidal neovascularization. Am J Ophthalmol 134(4):566–76

Correspondence: Ilse Krebs, M.D., The Ludwig Boltzmann Institute of Retinology and Biomicro-scopic Laser Surgery, Department of Ophthalmology, Rudolf Foundation Hospital, Juchgasse 25, 1030 Vienna, Austria.

Optical coherence tomography (OCT) for idiopathic macular holes and macular pucker

G. Ripandelli,[1,2] C. Scassa,[1] A. Coppè[1], and M. Sciamanna[1]

[1] Fondazione G.B. Bietti per lo Studio e la Ricerca in Oftalmologia, Rome, Italy
[2] Policlinico Universitario "Campus Bio-Medico" di Roma, Rome, Italy

Abstract

Purpose: The authors report their experience, starting from 1997 up to today, in the utilization of Optical Coherence Tomography (OCT) technique for the diagnosis and the morphological evaluation of macular pucker (MP) and idiopathic full-thickness macular holes (MH).

Materials and Methods: Different cases and studies based on OCT examination for the clinical diagnosis of idiopathic MP and MH are briefly reported.

Results: Optical coherence tomography examination may visualize the different morphological aspects of MP and MH and may detect their changements with time.

Conclusions: Optical coherence tomography is a high resolution, non–invasive diagnostic technique that permits a detailed evaluation of various macular pathologies. This examination frequently helps to select the cases that are more likely to benefit from surgery.

Introduction

Optical coherence tomography (OCT) is a non-invasive, no-contact diagnostic technique for high resolution, cross-sectional imaging of the retina that measures the optical reflectivity of the tissue by means of low-coherence or white light interferometry principle [1–4]. The OCT two-dimensional scans acquired during the examination are processed by a computer and represented in a false-color scale: bright colors (from red to white) correspond to regions of high relative optical reflectivity or backscattering and dark colors (from blue to black) represent areas of minimal or no relative reflectivity. The axial resolution of the scans in the first and the second OCT version was evaluated to be about 10–12 microns and the field of view of approximately 35° with a dilated pupil. In the latest version, the OCT III Stratus, the axial resolution of the scans reaches a value of about 8–10 microns.

Retinal thickness and retinal reflectivity are the two main keys to interpret an OCT scan. The mean standard deviation (SD) of the retinal and central foveal thickness in normal human eyes has been calculated to be respectively 230 ± 15 microns and 152 ± 21 microns [1, 5]. The inner limiting membrane of the normal retina is well defined due to the non-reflectivity of the vitreous and the backscattering of the retina; the posterior boundary of the neurosensory retina is defined by a highly reflective red layer which corresponds to the retinal pigment epithelium (RPE) and choriocapillaris depicted together. The photoreceptor layer (PRL) appears as weakly backscattering, while an intermediate reflectivity (from yellow to green) is observed for the remaining layers of the retina.

Thanks to the great resolution of its scans, the OCT examination allows an objective assessment of the morphology of the retina and, in cases of macular holes (MH) and macular pucker (MP), may give quantitative information as the MH diameter, the retinal thickness and the evaluation of intraretinal fluid accumulation. Dense corneal, lens, vitreous opacities may limit the performance and the interpretation of the scans.

OCT for macular pucker

Idiopathic epiretinal proliferations can be responsible for different macular pathologies with a serious decrease of the visual acuity (VA). The resolution of vitreoretinal proliferations may be accomplished by pars plana vitrectomy and membrane peeling. However, the preoperative predictive factors for wich cases are more likely to benefit from surgery are controversials. Various prognostic factors that may influence the postoperative outcomes, as the preoperative VA, the duration of symptoms, the presence and the amount of a cystoid macular edema, the thickness of the epiretinal membrane, have been evaluated by different authors with conflicting results [6–11].

Since its creation, the great usefulness and reliability of the informations that OCT scans provide on the macular morphology and macular diseases has been more and more confirmed and reported in various studies [12–16]. Cases of MP show at OCT a retinal thickening with a variable reduction of the intraretinal reflectivity, consistent with fluid accumulation. Epiretinal membranes may appear as intravitreal, high-reflective bands connected to the inner retinal surface or as highly backscattering plaques tightly adherent to the inner retinal surface (Figs. 1, 2).

Wilkins and Puliafito [12] observed that " . . . quantitative measurements and the assessment of membrane adherence with OCT may be useful in characterizing the surgical prognosis of eyes with an epiretinal membrane." In an oral presentation, Azzolini reported " . . . better postoperative VA outcomes in eyes with partially adherent epiretinal membranes compared to eyes with totally adherent epiretinal membranes" (Vail Vitrectomy Meeting, March 12–15, 2000, Vail, Colorado).

In cases of MP, our experience is consistent to what reported by other authors: OCT gives precise anatomical details that may result as prognostic factors for the postoperative outcomes.

We employed OCT, among other diagnostic exams, in a prospective study carried out between February 1997 and January 1999 including 84 eyes of 84 patients (52 F, 32 M, mean age 56.3 ± 12.4 yrs.; VA ranging from 20/200 to 20/40) with a diagnosis of MP.

In 75 on 84 eyes (89.2% of cases) the OCT scans of the macular region revealed the presence into the vitreous cavity of highly backscattering bands that were partially adherent to the inner retinal surface (PAM), whereas in 9 on 84 eyes (10.8% of cases) OCT scans showed an increased reflectivity of the inner retinal surface, consistent with the presence of a tightly adherent epiretinal membrane (TAM).

In PAM eyes (89.2% of the eyes) that underwent surgery, a postoperative improvement of the VA was observed. The TAM eyes (10.8% of the eyes) that underwent surgery had no postoperative improvement of the VA, and a decrease of the VA was observed in some cases. Some eyes with the same preoperative VA showed different preoperative values of foveal thickness and different postoperative VA outcomes. On the other hand, some eyes with same VA and same preoperative foveal thickness had different postoperative VA outcomes.

After 1 year of follow-up the mean macular thickness values were similar in both groups.

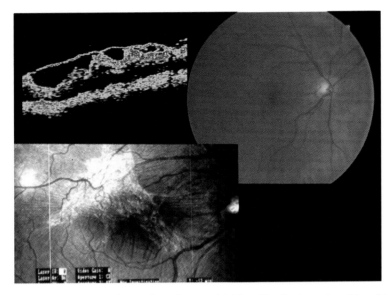

Fig. 1. Vitreomacular traction and macular edema. A highly reflective intravitreal band is connected to the macula determining foveal thickening and presence of non-reflective, cystic spaces beneath the fovea

These observations could confer to the morphology of the epiretinal membranes and its evaluation by means of OCT, an important role in the decision for surgery and for the prediction of postoperative functional recovery.

In TAM cases is possible to suppose a iatrogenic, intraoperative damage caused by the attempt to remove the membrane, or might be supposed a preoperative damage of the nerve fiber layer and/or of the inner retinal layers caused by the strong adherence of the membrane itself.

Functional informations of the macular region obtained with microperimetry and focal ERG could support the morphological evaluation obtained with OCT and may help to detect risk cases for a postoperative decrease of the VA.

OCT for macular holes

Macular pseudoholes (MPH) partial-thickness and full-thickness MH may be detected and followed in their morphological changes. In these cases, OCT gives quantitative informations as the diameter of the lesion and the amount of the retinal edema, helps in monitoring the evolution of both partial-thickness and full-thickness MH and in the decision for surgery [14].

In the surgical decision for MH repair, our experience suggests that not only the estimation of the time of onset of MH but also their morphological evaluation could play a role as predictive factor for postoperative results [17, 18].

In highly myopic eyes the presence of vitreous opacities and of dystrophic processes along the posterior pole may lead to a difficult fundus examination. In these cases OCT scans permit a better evaluation of the vitreoretinal relationships on the macular area and may reveal anatomical details not detected with other diagnostic exams.

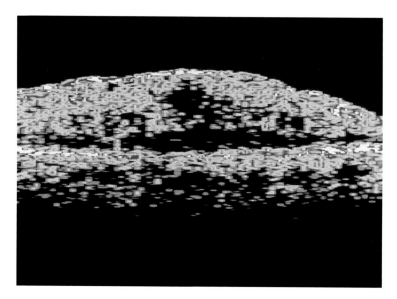

Fig. 2. Epiretinal membrane tightly adherent to the inner retinal surface. OCT scans show an increased foveal thickness with loss of the normal foveal contour

In a group of 24 consecutive high myopic patients (myopia over 14 negative diopters) that were examined in our clinic, OCT showed that 6 eyes had an asymptomatic MH and in 4 of these 6 eyes the MH was bilateral. In no one of the 6 eyes the MH was detected before at slit-lamp fundus examination and with indirect ophthalmoscopy. This was probably due to the small diameter of the MH (330 microns on average) and to the weak contrast between the neuroretinal layers and the retinal pigment epithelium (RPE). In all the 6 eyes the MH was located paracentral to the fovea; the visual acuity of the 6 eyes ranged from 20/100 to 20/40. In 2 of these 6, MH was associated with a shallow, inferior retinal detachment.

Conclusions

Thanks to the accuracy and great resolution of the scans, we believe that OCT is a determinant examination for a precise assessment of the vitreoretinal relationship on the posterior pole. In our clinical practice, OCT is a fundamental tool for the diagnosis, the clinical and the surgical approach of macular diseases.

References

1. Hee MR, Izatt JA, Swanson EA, et al (1995) Optical coherence tomography of the human retina. Arch Ophthalmol 113:325–32
2. Huang D, Swanson EA, Lin CP, Schuman JS, Stinson WG, Chang W, Hee MR, Flotte T, Gregory K, Puliafito CA, Fujimoto JG (1991) Optical coherence tomography. Science 254:1178–81
3. Swanson EA, Izatt JA, Hee MR, Huang D, Lin CP, Schuman JS, Puliafito CA, Fujimoto JG (1993) In vivo retinal imaging by optical coherence tomography. Op Lett 18:1864–6
4. Puliafito CA, Hee MR, Schuman JS, Fujimoto JG (1996) Principles of operation and technology. In: John H. Bond publisher. Optical coherence tomography of ocular diseases. Thorofare, NJ- USA: Slack Inc., 1996 chap. 1:3–15
5. Hee MR, Puliafito CA, Wong MS, Duker JS, Reichel E, Rutledge B, Schuman JS, Swanson EA, Fujimoto JG (1995) Quantitative assessment of macular edema with optical coherence tomography. Arch Ophthalmol 113:1019–29

6. Margherio RR, Cox MS, Trese MT, et al (1985) Removal of epimacular membranes. Ophthalmology 92:1075–83
7. Trese MT, Chandler DB, Machemer R (1983) Macular pucker. I. Prognostic criteria. Graefes Arch Clin Exp Ophthalmol 221:12–5
8. Rice TA, De Bustros S, Michels RG, et al (1986) Prognostic factors in vitrectomy for epiretinal membranes of the macula. Ophthalmology 93:602–10
9. Mc Donald HR, Verre WP, Aaberg TM (1986) Surgical management of idiopathic epiretinal membranes. Ophthalmology 93:978–83
10. Pesin SR, Olk RJ, Grand MG, et al (1991) Vitrectomy for premacular fibroplasia. Prognostic factors, long-term follow-up and time course of visual improvement. Ophthalmology 98:1109–14
11. Michels RG (1981) Vitreous surgery for macular pucker. Am J Ophthalmol 92:628–39
12. Puliafito CA, Hee MR, Lin CP, Reichel E, Schuman JS, Duker JS, Izatt JA, Swanson EA, Fujimoto JG (1995) Imaging of macular diseases with optical coherence tomography. Ophthalmology 102:217–29
13. Wilkins JR, Puliafito CA, Hee MR, Duker JS, Reichel E, Coker JG, Schuman JS, Swanson EA, Fujimoto JG (1996) Characterizaton of epiretinal membranes using optical coherence tomography. Ophthalmology 103:2142–51
14. Hee MR, Puliafito CA, Wong C, Duker JS, Reichel E, Schuman JS, Swanson EA, Fujimoto JG (1995) Optical coherence tomography of macular holes. Ophthalmology 102:748–56
15. Hee MR, Puliafito CA, Wong C, Reichel E, Duker JS, Schman JS, Swanson EA, Fujimoto JG (1995) Optical coherence tomography of central serous chorioretinopathy. Am J Ophthalmol 120:65–74
16. Hee MR, Puliafito CA, Duker JS, Reichel E, Coker JG, Wilkins JR, Schuman JS, Swanson EA, Fujimoto JG (1998) Topography of diabetic macular edema with optical coherence tomography. Ophthalmology 105:360–70
17. Ripandelli G, Coppè AM, Bonini S, Giannini R, Curci S, Costi E, Stirpe M (1999) Morphological evaluation of full-thickness idiopathic macular holes by optical coherence tomography. Eur J Ophthalmol 9:212–6
18. Kelly NE, Wendel RT (1991) Vitreous surgery for idiopathic macular holes: results of a pilot study. Arch Ophthalmol 109:654–9

Correspondence: Guido Ripandelli, Fondazione "G.B. Bietti" per lo Studio e la Ricerca in Oftalmologia, Piazza Sasseri 5, I-00161 Rome, Italy.

Fundus autofluorescence mapping using a confocal scanning laser ophthalmoscope

A. Bindewald, S. Schmitz-Valckenberg, and F. G. Holz

Department of Ophthalmology, University of Bonn, Germany

Visualization of the retinal pigment epithelium (RPE) in vivo has proven difficult in the past for various reasons, including the optical properties of the eye and the small size of the cellular elements, forming a single layer between the neurosensory retina and Bruch's membrane. With the advent of scanning laser ophthalmoscopy it is now possible to image topographic distribution and intensity of fundus autofluorescence (AF) derived from accumulations of lipofuscin (LF) in the lysosomal compartment of RPE cells. Excessive lipofuscin storage in the RPE cytoplasm occurs not only in association with age but also with many hereditary and degenerative retinal diseases including age-related macular degeneration (AMD), Stargardt disease, Best disease, and pattern dystrophies. It represents a common pathogenetic downstream pathway for various heterogenous etiologies.

LF in the RPE mainly derives from incomplete degradation of phagocytosed distal segments of photoreceptor outer segments, and is composed of various biomolecules including lipids, protein, and retinoids. Some of its constituents such as A2-E have recently been shown to possess toxic properties and seem to play a pathophysiological role in diseases including age-related macular degeneration.

Visualizing lipofuscin in vivo may help to better understand the significance of these metabolic alterations in the pathogenesis of retinal disorders. In addition, fundus AF imaging can be useful in the preclinical diagnosis of hereditary retinal disease. Dynamic alterations of intrinsic RPE fluorescence change may be applicable for monitoring effects at the level of the RPE of novel therapeutic modalities. Furthermore, identification of high-risk characteristics in patients with age-related macular degeneration with this technique may be helpful in evaluating future therapies and designing studies.

Recording AF images with the Heidelberg Retina Angiograph (HRA)

The spatial distribution and intensity of fundus AF is recorded with the HRA using the argon laser excitation wavelength of 488 nm. Emission is detected with a barrier filter above 500 nm. The quality of AF images is largely dependent on the quality of the media. Lens opacities represent the most common reason for poor image quality. Especially yellowish cataracts absorb light in the wavelength range used for AF imaging. In the FAM-Study we use the following *standard operating procedure* to achieve optimal and comparable AF images with the HRA:

- Argon laser calibration
- Sensitivity adjustment
- Focussing in reflection and redfree mode
- Aquisition: 15 single 30° images 512 × 512 pixel in series mode
- 9 images for automated alignment
- Calculation of mean image

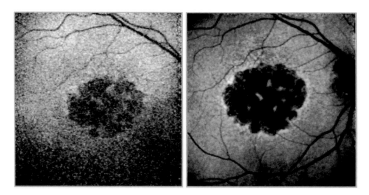

Fig. 1. The effect of lens opacities on the quality of AF images: in presence of cataract (left) and after cataract extraction with intraocular lens implantation (right)

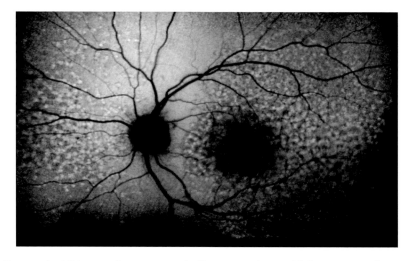

Fig. 2. Panoramic AF image after automated alignment using Heidelberg Eye Explorer Software

In interpreting AF images it should be considered that there are *other fluorophores than RPE-LF* that show up in the wavelength for excitation and emission used here. These are usually of much lower intensity. However, especially in diseases associated with exudation, additional fluorophores may occur which make differentiation from RPE-LF difficult.

FAM-Study

Together with other ophthalmic centers throughout Germany a multicenter, prospective *FAM-Study* (*F*undus *A*utofluroescence in Age-related *M*acular Degeneration-Study) has been initiated within the Priority Research Program AMD of the German Research Council (Deutsche Forschungsgemeinschaft). Study aims include detection of AF variation in eyes with AMD, classification of abnormal autofluorescence (AF)-patterns in the junctional zone of geographic atrophy (GA) and their impact on spread of atrophy and visual loss, the effect of elevated AF on the function of apposing photoreceptors as well as modification of the cSLO-device for *in vitro* mapping of RPE-LF.

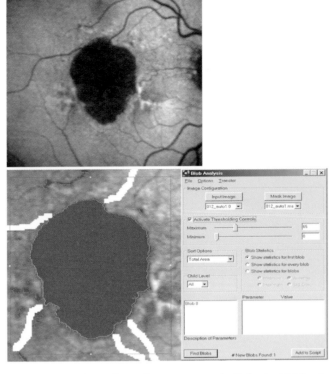

Fig. 3. Automated delineation of atrophy at the posterior pole (Schmitz-Valckenberg et al., Graefe's Archive 2001)

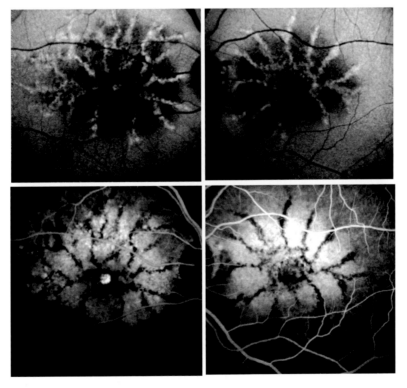

Fig. 4. Fundus AF image (top) and fluorescein angiogram (bottom) in a patient with autosomal dominant pattern dystrophy and a macular hole (right eye)

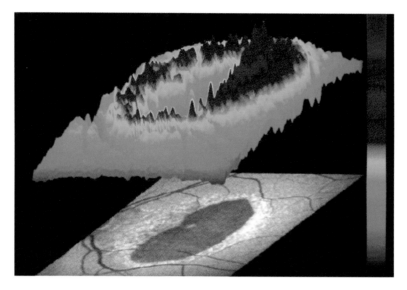

Fig. 5. Color-coded intensities of AF signals. There is an increased AF in the junctional zone of a kidney-shaped patch of geographic atrophy associated with age-related macular degeneration

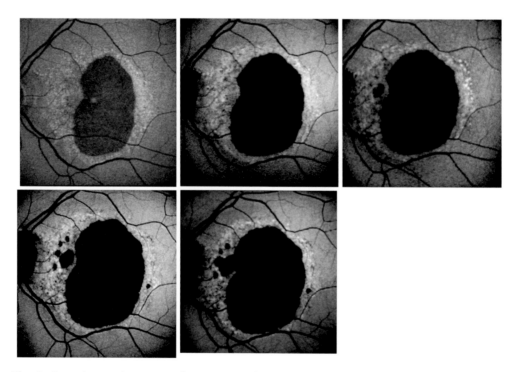

Fig. 6. Over time, enlargement of existing atrophy or occurrence of new atrophic patches in this elderly patient with advanced AMD occurred only in areas with abnormally high AF at baseline, reflecting the pathophysiological role of excessive lipofuscin accumulation in RPE-cells (Holz et al. IOVS 2001)

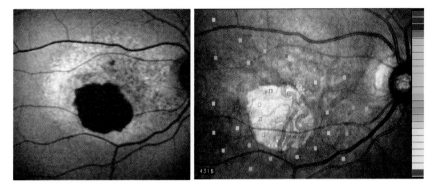

Fig. 7. Retinal function in areas with abnormal AF was assessed with static fundus automated full-threshold static fundus perimetry and mean deviation values were compared with age-corrected normal values. There were variable degrees of functional impairment in areas with increased AF signals indicating interference of excessive LF accumulations in the RPE with photoreceptor function (Bultmann et al. submitted)

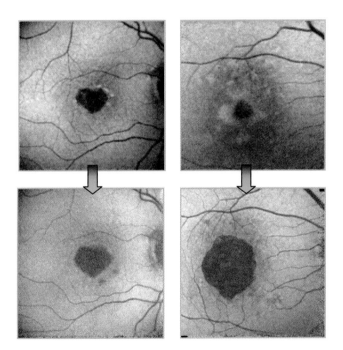

Fig. 8. Spread of atrophy over one year's time. While the pattern of focal increased AF in the junctional zone of GA shows only little enlargement (left), marked spread occurs in presence of larger areas of elevated AF at the margin of the atrophic patch (right)

Autofluorescence findings in retinal disease

AF images in eyes with geographic atrophy in late stage AMD show variable patterns of abnormal AF in the junctional zone. Phenotypic subtypes include focal, band, patchy and diffuse pattern of abnormal AF, whereby the latter type can be classified into reticular, fine-granular branching and fine granular with peripheral punctate. Areas of increased AF obviously indicate incipient atrophy as they precede the development and enlargement of outer retinal atrophy, which may reflect the pathophysiological role of excessive LF accumulations in the RPE and allows for identification of prognostic determinants. Patterns of abnormal AF showed a high degree of symmetry between eyes. Also in eyes with soft drusen, focal elevated AF may evolve into atrophy over time.

In other diseases abnormal variation in fundus AF can also be identified. Cone dystrophies may be associated with a distinct ring of increased AF surrounding the macula without corresponding funduscopic or angiographic changes. In Acute zonal occult outer retinopathy (AZOOR) we have seen areas with elevated AF correspond with the visual field loss whereas other examination techniques fail to detect abnormalities in these areas. In Stargardt disease focal flecks typically fluoresce brightly and may fade as atrophy develops. There is phenotypic variability with regard to diffuse AF change in Stargardt disease. While some patients demonstrate an increase in AF over normally appearing retina, the level is within the normal range in others. Changes in atrophic areas are best followed with AF imaging over time.

When *retinal sensitivity* was tested using macular perimetry with another SLO, elevated AF was associated with variable degrees of functional impairment of apposing photoreceptors.

Besides imaging LF content in the RPE cell layer HRA-AF imaging is a very accurate method for *recording atrophy of the outer retina*. As in those areas the RPE and, therefore, LF fluorophores, are absent, these areas appear dark with very low or absent AF signal. Thus, atrophic patches are more readily defined than on funduscopy, and their detection would not require injection of fluorescein to demonstrate corresponding window defects. For longitudinal analyses and *automated quantitation* of atrophic areas we have customized an image analysis software as recently published (Schmitz-Valckenberg et al. 2002). Automated computerized image analysis of the digital images allows for accurate detection and measurement of the size of atrophic areas, and will be useful in longitudinal natural history studies of retinal diseases associated with atrophy and for monitoring effects of future therapeutic interventions to slow down disease progression.

Summary

In summary, fundus AF imaging provides information over and above conventional fundus photographs or fluorescence angiography. This method gives clues for better understanding of pathogenetic mechanisms in various retinal diseases and is useful for monitoring the course of diseases as well as the effect of current and future therapeutic interventions.

References

1. Bellmann C, Holz FG, Schapp O, Volcker HE, Otto TP (1992) Topography of fundus autofluorescence with a new confocal scanning laser ophthalmoscope. Ophthalmologe 94:385–91
2. Bellmann C, Jorzik J, Spital G, Unnebrink K, Pauleikhoff D, Holz FG (2002) Symmetry of bilateral lesions in geographic atrophy in patients with age-related macular degeneration. Arch Ophthalmol 120:579–84
3. Bellmann C, Spital G, Unnebrink K, Schütt F, Pauleikhoff D, Holz FG (2002) Bilaterality of geographic atrophy of the retinal pigment epithelium associated with age-related macular degeneration. Archiv Ophthalmol 120:569–84
4. Bültmann S, Schmitz-Valckenberg S, Bindewald A, Holz FG, Rohrschneider K (2003) Fundus perimetry and fundus autofluorescence in the junctional zone of geographic atrophy in patients with age-related macular degeneration. (submitted)

5. Holz FG, Bellmann C, Schütt F, Völcker HE (1999) Patterns of increased in vivo fundus auto-fluorescence in the junctional zone of geographic atrophy of the retinal pigment epithelium associated with age-related macular degeneration. Graefe Arch Clin Exp Ophthalmol 237: 145–52

6. Holz FG, Schütt F, Kotpiz J, Kruse FE, Cantz M, Völcker HE (1999) Inhibition of lysosomal degradative functions in RPE cells by a retinoid component of lipofuscin. Invest Ophthalmol Vis Sci 40:737–43

7. Holz FG, Staudt S, Bellmann C, Völcker HE (2001) Fundus autofluorescence and development of geographic atrophy in age-related macular degeneration. Invest Ophthalmol Vis Sci 42: 1051–6

8. Holz FG (2001) Autofluoreszenz-Imaging der Makula. Ophthalmologe 98:10–18

9. Lois N, Halfyard AS, Bird AC, Fitzke FW (2000) Quantitative evaluation of fundus autofluores-cence imaged "in vivo" in eyes with retinal disease. Br J Ophthalmol 84:741–5

10. Lois N, Owens SL, Coco R, Hopkins J, Fitzke FW, Bird AC (2002) Fundus autofluorescence in patients with age-related macular degeneration and high risk of visual loss. Am J Ophthalmol 133:341–9

11. Bergmann M, Schütt F, Holz FG, Kopitz J (2001) Does A2-E, a retinoid component of lipofus-cin and inhibitor of lysosomal degradative functions, directly affect the activity of lysosomal hydrolases? Exp Eye Res 72:191–5

12. Schmitz-Valckenberg S, Jorzik J, Unnebrink K, Holz FG (2002) Analysis of digital scanning laser ophthalmoscopy fundus autofluorescence images of geographic atrophy in advanced age-related macular degeneration. Graefe Arch Clin Exp Ophthalmol 240:73–8

13. Schutt F, Bergmann M, Holz FG, Kopitz J (2002) Isolation of intact lysosomes from human RPE cells and effects of A2-E on the integrity of the lysosomal and other cellular membranes. Graefes Arch Clin Exp Ophthalmol 240:983–8

14. Schutt F, Ueberle B, Schnolzer M, Holz FG, Kopitz J (2002) Proteome analysis of lipofuscin in human retinal pigment epithelial cells. FEBS Lett 25(528):217–21

15. von Ruckmann A, Fitzke FW, Bird AC (1995) Distribution of fundus autofluorescence with a scanning laser ophthalmoscope. Br J Ophthalmol 79:407–12

16. von Ruckmann A, Schmidt KG, Fitzke FW, Bird AC, Jacobi KW (1998) Fundus autofluorescence in patients with hereditary macular dystrophies, malattia leventinese, familial dominant and aged-related drusen. Klin Monatsbl Augenheilkd 213:81–6

Correspondence: Dr. Almut Bindewald, Department of Ophthalmology, University of Bonn, Sigmund-Freud-Strasse 25, D-53105 Bonn, Germany.

Multifocal electroretinography (mfERG) in macular disorders

A. Abri, S. Binder, A. Assadoullina, S. Brunner, E. Harrer,
and E. Golestani

Department of Ophthalmology, Rudolf Foundation Hospital, Vienna, Austria

Introduction

Multifocal electroretinography (mfERG) is a new technique that allows an objective analysis of the local functions in patients with different retinal diseases.

The basic work was done by Marmarelis and co-workers in 1979 which was clinically applied by Sutter and Tran [2].

Two mfERG systems are widely used: VERIS™ System Technology and RETIscan contributed by LKC and Roland Consult Instruments, respectively.

Method

The guidelines for the performance of the mfERG have recently been established by the International Society for Clinical Electrophysiology of Vision (www.iscev.org)

The technique of the mfERG procedure in Rudolf Foundation

The multifocal ERG was recorded using Retiscan (version 3.1, Roland Consult, Wiesbaden, Germany). The stimulus array consisted of 103 hexagonal elements, were presented on a high resolution cathode-ray tube monitor (60 Hz). The eye-monitor distance was 33 cm. The central 30° of the retina was simulated by flickering hexagons independently between black and white according to a pseudorandomized binary m-sequence (mean luminance 180 cd/m^2). Hexagon size war scaled with eccentricity to evoke focal responses of approximately the same amplitude in the response arrays. Each record was collected in 5–6 segments each 45 seconds. Every active m-sequence lasted 16.6 ms and war followed by a rest interval of 66.4 ms before the next active m-sequence was started.

Pupils were fully dilated with cyclopentolat 1%. Lens of +3.0 diopter were added to the lens holder in front of the eye, which was refracted for best visual acuity for far distance. A diagonal cross was the fixation target and the fellow eye was occluded. DTL conjuctival electrode was used for the recording. The reference electrode was attached to the lateral margin of the same eye. Ground electrode is placed on the forehead after cleaning and use of conductive paste (Fig. 1).

The typical mfERG record is a biphasic wave with a negative deflection (a-wave) followed by positive one (b-wave).

The recording signals were amplified (50000×) and band pass filtered (10–300 Hz).

The quality of the records was controlled by real-time monitoring. The presence of "blind spot" was an indication for good quality of recording.

The noisy records were discarded and rerecorded.

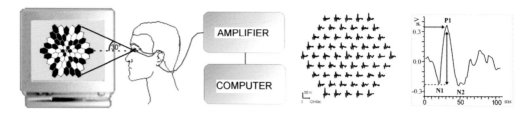

Fig. 1. Scheme of mfERG system with typical trace array in a normal eye (reprinted from M.W. Seeliger et al. [3] with the permission of the publisher)

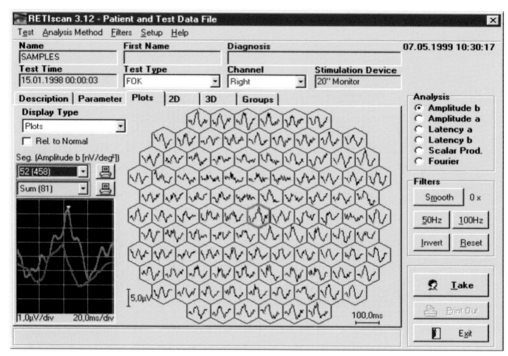

Fig. 2a–d. Types of mfERG representations: **a** plots, **b** 3D picture, **c** rings, **d** quadrants

Display features

Different functional features like plots (Fig. 2a), 2D, 3D (Fig. 2b), Rings (Fig. 2c) and Quadrants (Fig. 2d) can be used. We use the plots for evaluation of the records and 3Ds only for demonstration (waveform information is lost and noise artifacts could be amplified).

The following clinical cases should highlight the importance of mfERG for functional follow-up after therapy or for evaluation of natural history.

Case 1 shows follow-up in angiographic and mfERG patterns of patient after CNV membrane excision with autologous retinal pigment epithelium transplantation (Fig. 3), case 2 shows it after photodynamic therapy (Fig. 4). After therapy the maximal potential value for b-wave is increased and potential configuration becomes narrower.

Case 3 demonstrates also an increase of potential values of central retina after successful macular hole surgery (Fig. 5); in case 4 (Fig. 6) of retinitis pigmentosa we consider a decrease of potentials in the periphery in early cases with progression towards center with diminishing of potentials in the late cases.

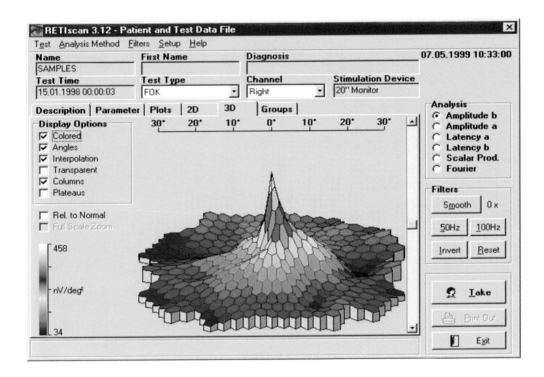

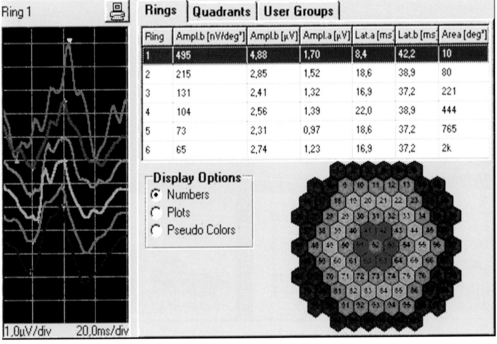

Fig. 2a–d. *Continued*

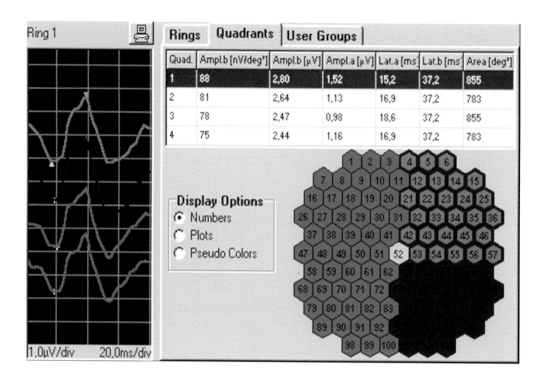

Quad.	Ampl.b [nV/deg³]	Ampl.b [μV]	Ampl.a [μV]	Lat.a [ms]	Lat.b [ms]	Area [deg²]
1	88	2,80	1,52	15,2	37,2	855
2	81	2,64	1,13	16,9	37,2	783
3	78	2,47	0,98	18,6	37,2	855
4	75	2,44	1,16	16,9	37,2	783

Fig. 2a–d. *Continued*

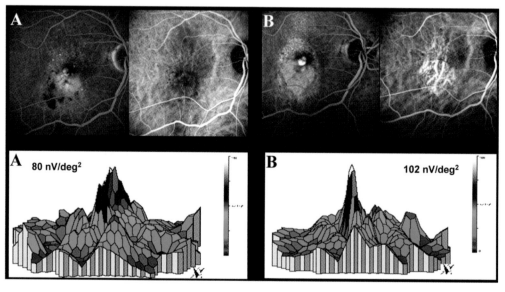

Fig. 3. FLA-, ICG- and mfERG-findings preoperative and after membranectomy and autologous RPE transplantation. **A** Preoperative (visual acuity 0.05; no reading acuity), **B** postoperative (visual acuity 0.16; reading acuity Jg 16)

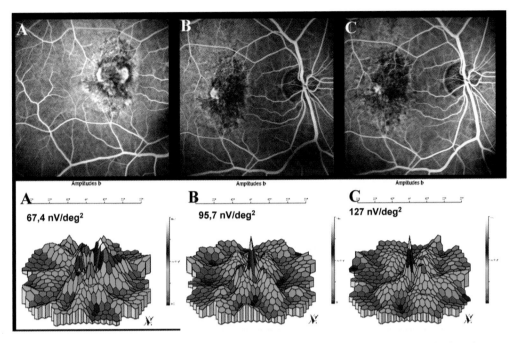

Fig. 4. FLA- and mfERG-findings before therapy and after 1. and 2. PDT treatment **A** before therapy (visual acuity 0.1; reading acuity Jg 16), **B** after 1. PDT (visual acuity 0.52; reading acuity Jg 5), **C** after 2. PDT (visual acuity 0.74; reading acuity Jg 3)

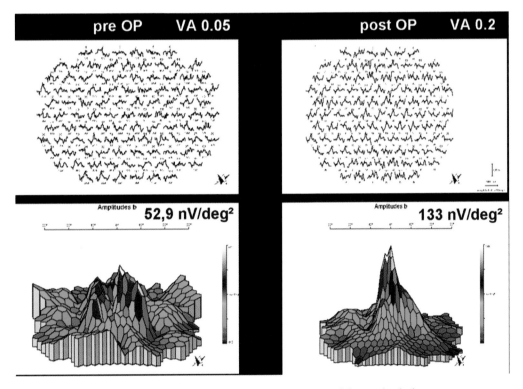

Fig. 5. mfERG-findings preoperative and after successful macular hole surgery

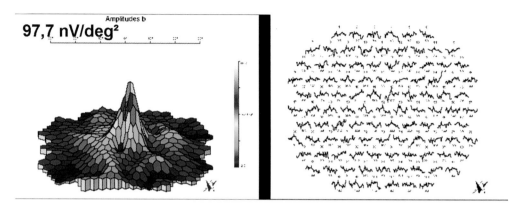

Fig. 6. mfERG-findings in case of Retinitis Pigmentosa

References

1. Marmarelis PZ, Marmarelis VZ (1978) The white noise method in system identification. In: Marmarelis PZ, Marmarelis VZ (eds) Analysis of physiological systems. New York: Plenum, pp 134–9
2. Sutter EE, Tran D (1992) The field topography of ERG components in man – I. The photopic luminance response. Vision Res 32:433–46
3. Seeliger MW, Jurklies B, Kellner U, Palmowski A, Bach M, Kretschmann U (2001) Multifokale Elektroretinographie (mfERG). Ophthalmologe 98:1112–29

Correspondence: Dr. Ali Abri, Department of Ophthalmology, Rudolf Foundation Hospital, Juchgasse 25, A-1030 Vienna, Austria, E-mail: ali.abri@kar.magwien.gv.at

Standards of reading performance and visual acuity measurements in maculopathy-reliability and validity analyses of vision tests

W. Radner, E. Stifter, S. Richter-Mueksch, Ch. Kiss, and M. Velikay-Parel

Department of Ophthalmology and Optometry, University of Vienna, Austria

Determination of visual performance is one of the most important clinical examinations in ophthalmology. Thus, the results of vision tests have to be accurate, reproducible, and comparable. To achieve this, the testing parameters of the various measurement procedures have to be uniformly standardized [12, 14, 15, 18, 33, 45] for both distance acuity and reading performance.

Required standards for visual acuity tests

The definition of visual acuity (VA) is based on the visual angle, considering the testing distance and optotype size. In Europe, the EN ISO 8596 defines an official international standard, evaluating VA with the logarithmically graded "Landolt optotypes" [4, 12, 14, 15]. In accordance with the recommendations of the Committee on Vision of the National Academy of Sciences-National Research Council (NAS-NRC) [33], the design principles of the Bailey-Lovie charts [5] have been applied to the development of the ETDRS charts [18, 19], which have become the standard method for measuring VA (LogMAR) in large clinical studies [20, 29, 30, 32, 40, 41, 46, 47]. For these charts, five of the ten Sloan letters [42] are used per line. These optotypes are of approximately equal legibility and, as a group they are equivalent to the Landolt rings [42, 43]. The separation of the letters within and between the lines is uniform, so that the contour interaction is controlled [5, 18, 27, 33, 45]. This design provides constant geometric proportions for all testing distances [5, 45]. The only stimulus variable is the optotypes' size, which is graduated in 0.1-log unit steps (ratio: 1.26:1) equivalent to the logarithmical scaling defined by the EN ISO 8596 [12, 14, 15]. Thus, these standards provide internationally comparable measures of the distance VA, although the procedures, the design of the test items, and the notations vary [4, 7, 33].

Since reading performance is an important clinical parameter of macular function [16, 17, 22, 34, 36, 39], the above standards have to be also applied to reading tests [33]. The print sizes of the test paragraphs are required to be logarithmically scaled, and in addition the reading test items should be as comparable as possible [6, 37, 38] to allow accurate and standardized measurements of reading acuity and/or reading speed at every viewing distance.

Standardized reading tests

Some of these required principles of the above outlined standardization for vision tests [4, 12, 14, 15, 33] have already been used for the design of new reading charts [6, 31, 37]. Bailey and Lovie [6] used unrelated words of similar legibility to simultaneously determine reading acuity and speed, a method that has also been applied to the MNRead Acuity Chart [31] and to our German "Radner Reading Charts" (RR Charts) [37]. However, differences in the philosophy of sentence standardization exist between the later two chart systems that use single sentences: The sentences of the MNRead Acuity Chart have 3 lines and 60 characters, including spaces, but their number (10–14 words), length, and position of words vary considerably [31]. For calculating reading speed, it is assumed that these represent 10 words of a supposed average English word length of 6 characters. In contrast, our goal for the "Radner Reading Charts", which were developed for clinical use in all ophthalmologic patients, was to create "sentence optotypes" in order to minimize variations between the test items and to keep the geometric proportions as constant as possible at all distances. Thus, in cooperation with psychologists, linguists, and schools, we developed a series of test sentences that are highly comparable in terms of the number of words (14 words), word length, position of words, lexical difficulty, and syntactical complexity, by establishing over 30 definition rules [37]. The 24 most similar of these 32 sentences were selected statistically [37, 38] by evaluating their reliability and validity for measuring reading speed [38] and were then used for the Radner Reading Charts. Thus, our concept of "sentence optotypes" for reading charts should be capable to provide standardized clinical measurements of reading acuity and speed [37, 38].

Vision tests: test-retest reliability and validity

For distance visual acuity measurements, reliability and validity have been evaluated for various procedures [3, 11, 27, 45] by assessing the test-retest reliability by calculating the correlations between repeated measurements [2, 3, 11, 27]. Lovie-Kitchin [27] compared the distance VA measurements obtained with the Snellen, Bailey-Lovie, Illiterate E, and Flom S-charts and found a high test-retest reliability for all of these four charts (r = 0.94 – 0.99). In addition, the high correlations among these charts (r = 0.91 – 0.96) indicated that, with all of them, valid measures of distance VA could be made [27]. Similarly, Camparini and coworkers [11] have reported a good reproducibility for the ETDRS standard procedure and for their "ETDRS Fast Procedure". Using a computerized testing system to reduce the variability of VA measurements, Arditi and Cagenello [3] ascertained in a test-retest setting for the ETDRS charts that the upper limits for test-retest reliability of VA measurements can best be measured within ±0.1 log units [3].

To our opinion, such statistical evaluations and standardization i.e. validity, test-retest reliability, interchart reliability as well as variance component analyses should be performed for every clinical method, and particularly for function-based vision tests such as reading tests.

However, for reading parameters similar investigations (validity, test-retest reliability, interchart reliability as well as variance component analyses) have only been analysed for the "Radner Reading Charts" whereas, until that statistical analyses have only been applied of reading speed measurements [25, 1, 2, 16, 36, 38]: For the Minnesota Low-vision Reading Test [25], it has been shown that single sentences can provide valid and reproducible reading speed measurements in low-vision patients when these sentences are presented one-by-one on single printed cards or in the form of a computerized test [1, 2] and Elliott et al. have evaluated the validity and reliability of a reading speed test for potential vision measurements in patients with normal vision, cataract, central and peripheral vision loss [16, 36]. For our "sentence optotypes," the validity of reading speed measurements has been shown for students and blue-collar apprentices [38].

To assess the statistical reliability of our standardized Radner Reading Chart system for clinical diagnosis and follow-up, we analyzed the test-retest and inter-chart reproducibility and performed a "variance component analysis" to determine the sources of variability under clinical conditions and the test-retest and the inter-chart reproducibility of the available reading parameters. We have found that this system has a high test-retest and inter-chart reliability for individuals with a range of VA levels, with most of the variance being attributed to inter-individual variability.

Why variance component analyses

Statistical evaluations of test-retest and inter-chart reliability can only establish whether a particular source of variation (e.g. different charts, two test days, different patients) has a significant influence on the variability of the testing procedure; in contrast, the variance component analyses used in the present study make it possible to quantify the contributions of these sources to the total variability. For our "Radner Reading Chart" system we have identified the sources of variability for all measured variables and for the three groups of individuals with different VA and found that the individuals were predominantly responsible for the variability in the results, whereas test replication and reading charts had only a minor influence on the whole variance. The influence of the patients increased with visual impairment, indicating that the functional disability affects the variables. This, particularly, held true for the maximum reading speed, a finding that is in accordance with previous studies that have identified reading speed as a performance-based parameter sensitive to functional visual loss [1, 2, 10, 16, 22, 24, 26, 28, 44]. On the other hand the CPS showed a different proportion of the "variance component estimates" than did the other reading parameters. As much as 67% of the whole variance came from unidentified sources. One explanation for this difference might be that the CPS is not a measurement like reading acuity or speed, since it is set by the examiner at the smallest print size the patient can read with optimal reading speed [13, 16, 31]. Therefore, the examiner's subjective decision is one of the most likely unidentified sources of variability and may have contributed significantly to the variability we observed.

Definitions of reading parameters

In several clinical studies we have developed and used several parameters to define reading performance in patients.

1) **Reading acuity:** To avoid confusion and to be psychophysically more accurate with definitions we suggest to express logarithmically scaled reading acuity in terms of LogRAD (=Log-Reading-Acuity-Determination) which is the reading equivalent of LogMAR (=Log-Minimal-Angle-of-Resolution) since reading acuity does not express the minimal angle of resolution.

2) **LogRAD-score:** Reading errors can be included into the measured reading acuity in terms of a reading score [radner, MN-read) i.e. for our reading charts the LogRAD-Score which is calculated as follows: LogRAD-Score = Reading acuity (LogRAD) plus 0.005 times the number of syllables of the incorrectly read words (LogRAD-Score = LogRAD + 0.005 × # of syllables of incorrectly read words).

3) **Reading speed:** Reading speed is determined in words per minute. Clinically reading speed can be differentiated into two parameters i.e. (a) the mean reading speed and (b) the maximum reading speed. Another relevant parameter is to show reading performance of single patients or patient groups by graphically represent reading speed based upon reading acuity. Such representations can show the decline of reading speed with smaller print sizes and also indicate the reading speed at different LogRAD measures (Fig. 1).

Reading Speed

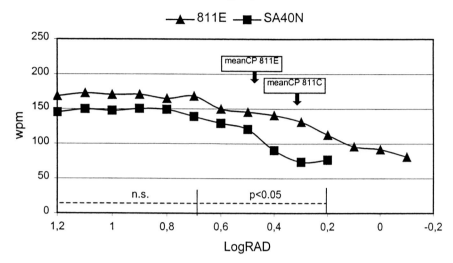

Fig. 1. Reading speed based upon reading acuity: Graph represents the different reading perform-ances of patients who received a diffractive multifocal IOL (811E) and a refractive multifocal IOL (AR 40)

4) **Critical Print Size (CPS):** Another method to define a limit of reading performance is the critical print size (CPS), which is defined as the smallest print size a patient can read with maximum reading speed [13, 16, 31].

5) **LogMAR/LogRAD-ratio:** A clinically relevant parameter seems to be the LogMAR/LogRAD ratio which compares distance and reading acuity by calculating the ratio of the achieved reading acuity in percentage of the distance acuity. In several clinical studies the LogRAD/LogMAR ratio showed considerable differences between distance acuity and reading acuity in several macular diseases indicating that dis-tance acuity alone is not capable to measure the real functional impairment in several ophthalmologic diseases.

Why not Jaeger charts

As early as 1854 Professor Jaeger was the first postulating that macular function can be best measured by real life performance tests and recommended to do this by measuring reading acuity. His Jaeger charts have become an international standard. However, even in the original versions which were distributed in the mid-19th century in German, French and English these Jaeger charts differed significantly in text, print size and fonts. The English versions changed over time and so did their scaling of the print sizes and for the current German version it is not even possible to elucidate its origin. The later is not comparable anymore to one of the original versions of Professor Jaeger from 1854 to 1896 and is not even comparable to the modified version of Professor Fuchs from 1902. In addition, this current German version also is not at all comparable to the English ver-sions. Its smallest print size is equivalent to a visual acuity measure of about 0.8 (visus) and, in addition, the English, French and German versions differs significantly in scaling. Further, the scaling of the German version is by far not logarithmically (Fig. 2). The dif-ferences between the smaller print sizes are too big whereas with greater print sizes (between Jaeger 8 to 16) these differences decreased below half of a logarithmical step.

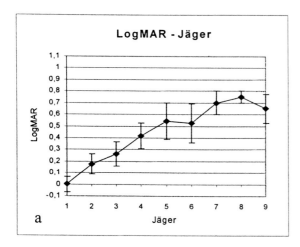

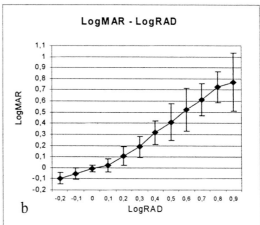

Fig. 2. Reading acuity compared to distance acuity (LogMAR; n = 300 patients). (**a**) The scaling of the German Jaeger charts is not logarithmically and clinically appropriately scaled. Note the plateau between Jaeger 5 and Jaeger 6. In a clinical study we have uncovered that Jaeger 5 and 6 of the current available version of the Jaeger charts are of equal print size! Together with the non-logarithmical, clinically inappropriate scaling these and several other qualitative deficiencies of this version should not be used for clinical diagnosis anymore. In addition, it cannot be used for statistical analyses and is therefore obsolete for scientific studies. (**b**) The logarithmical scaling of the Radner Reading charts results in reading acuity measures which are comparable with that achieved with the LogMAR charts

It has to be noted at this point that Jaeger 5 and Jaeger 6 have been uncovered being of the same print size in a clinical study which has finally led us to microscopically measure the letter height of the print sizes.

The current versions of the Jaeger charts do by far not meet the requirements of the current standards for visual acuity measurements and are not comparable between different languages anymore. These charts have never been standardized and it is not possible to measure other clinically relevant reading parameters such as the reading speed, the CPS or a distance acuity/reading acuity ratio.

In contrast, standardized reading charts have been designed following the modern optometric requirements for visual acuity tests and have been psychophysically standardized in volunteers. Additionally, with the new standardized test systems several reading parameters can be evaluated and used for more accurate diagnoses as has been shown in several clinical studies.

Clinical relevance of standardized reading charts

In several studies we have investigated whether our German Radner Reading Charts, which were designed to conform to current international standards and the psychophysical requirements for controlling optical item interactions, can provide reliable and reproducible results, as has already been demonstrated for distance acuity charts [3, 11, 27, 45]. Recently, the "Radner Reading Charts" have successfully been used to evaluate differences in reading performance between patients with different multifocal intraocular lens systems [39]. In addition, another study with these charts revealed a significantly altered reading performance in patients with anisometropic amblyopia [34], indicating that the real functional impairment is clearly underestimated when only distance VA is measured in this disease [34]. Furthermore, in patients with subfoveal occult choroidal neovascularization in age-related macular degeneration, reading acuity and speed measured with the Radner Charts were shown to correlate significantly with the size of the absolute scotomata but not to that of the relative scotomas [17]. In another study we compared the reading performance of patients with drusen maculopathy to that of patients with subfoveal CNV scares showing a considerably difference in reading performance between these two diagnoses despite comparable distance visual acuity. This again indicated that distance visual acuity alone is an insufficient measure for macular functional impairment (Richter-Mueksch S et al. ARVO 2003; Paper).

Summary

New standardized reading charts have been developed according to the requirements for international standards of visual acuity tests. In addition, for our German version we have analysed the reliability and the validity of the measured parameters. With such test systems it is possible to simultaneously measure several reading parameters and improve the diagnosis of the patients. For clinical routine it makes even a difference for diagnosis when listening to the patients reading performance without any stop watch measurements. With our standardized Radner Reading Charts we have shown a considerable difference between reading acuity and distance acuity for different macular and other ophthalmologic diseases indicating that with distance acuity alone it is not possible clinically show the full functional impairment.

References

1. Ahn S, Legge G, Luebker A (1995) Printed cards for measuring low-vision reading speed. Vision Res 35:1939–44
2. Ahn S, Legge G (1995) Psychophysics of reading-XIII. Predictors of magnifier aided reading speed in low vision. Vision Res 35:1931–8
3. Arditi A, Cagenello R (1993) On the statistical reliability of letter-chart visual acuity measurement. Invest Ophthalmol Vis Sci 34:120–9
4. Bach M, Kommerell G (1998) Sehschärfenbestimmung nach Europäischer Norm: wissenschaftliche Grundlagen und Möglichkeiten der automatischen Messung. Klin Monatsbl Augenheilkd 212:190–5
5. Bailey IL, Lovie JE (1976) New design principles for visual acuity letter charts. Am J Optom Physiol Opt 53:745–53
6. Bailey IL, Lovie JE (1980) The design and use of a new near-vision chart. Am J Optom Physiol Opt 57:378–87
7. Bailey IL, Bullimore MA, Raasch TW, Taylor HR (1991) Clinical grading and the effects of scaling. Invest Ophthalmol Vis Sci 32:422–32
8. Bland JM, Altmann DG (1986) Statistical methods for assessing agreement between two methods of clinical measurement. Lancet 1:307–10
9. Brown B, Yap MKH (1995) Differences in visual acuity between the eyes: determination of normal limits in a clinical population. Ophthal Physiol Opt 15:163–9
10. Bullimore MA, Bailey IL (1995) Reading and eye movements in age-related maculopathy. Optom Vis Sci 72(2):125–38
11. Camparini M, Cassinari P, Ferrigno L, Macaluso C (2001) ETDRS-Fast: Implementing psychophysical adaptive methods to standardized visual acuity measurement with ETDRS-Charts. Invest Ophthalmol Vis Sci 42:1226–31
12. CEN (European Committee of Norms) (1996) Europäische Norm Sehschärfenprüfung EN ISO 8596. Berlin: Beuth-Verlag
13. Chung STL, Mansfield JS, Legge GE (1998) Psychophysics of reading. XVIII. The effect of print size on reading speed in normal peripheral vision. Vision Research 38:2949–62
14. Colenbrander A (1988) Consilium Ophthalmologicum Universale Visual Functions Committee, Visual Acuity Measurement Standard. Ital J Ophthalmol 11:5–19

15. DIN 58220 "Sehschärfenbestimmung" Teil 3, 5 and 6 (1997) Beuth Verlag, Berlin

16. Elliott D, Patel B, Whitaker D (2001) Development of a reading speed test for potential-vision measurements. Invest Ophthalmol Vis Sci 42:1945–9

17. Ergun E, Maar N, Radner W, Barbazetto I, Schmidt-Erfurth U, Stur M (2003) Scotoma Size and reading speed in patients with subfoveal occult choroidal neovascularization in age related macular degeneration. Ophthalmology 110:65–9

18. Ferris F, Kassoff A, Bresnick G, Bailey I (1982) New visual acuity charts for clinical research. Am J Ophthalmol 94:91–6

19. Ferris F, Sperduto R (1982) Standardized illumination for visual acuity testing in clinical research. Am J Ophthalmol 94:97–8

20. Friedmann S, Munoz B, Rubin G, West S, Bandeen-Roche K, Fried L (1999) Characteristics of discrepancies between self-reported visual function and measuring reading speed. Salisbury Eye Evaluation Project Team. Invest Ophthalmol Vis Sci 40:858–64

21. Geer I, Westall CA (1996) A comparison of tests to determine acuity deficits in children with amblyopia. Ophthal Physiol Opt 16:367–74

22. Hazel CA, Petre KL, Armstrong RA, Benson MT, Frost NA (2000) Visual function and subjective quality of life compare in subjects with acquired macular disease. Invest Ophthalmol Vis Sci 41:1309–15

23. John PWM (1971) Statistical design and analysis of experiments. New York: The Macmillan Company

24. Legge GE, Rubin GS, Pelli DG, Schleske MM (1985) Psychophysics of reading – II. Low vision. Vision Res 25:253–66

25. Legge GE, Ross JA, Luebker A, LaMay JM (1989) Psychophysics of reading VIII. The Minnesota Low-Vision Reading Test. Optom Vis Sci 66:843–53

26. Legge G, Ross J, Isenberg L, LaMay J (1992) Psychophysics of reading – XII: Clinical Predictors of low vision reading speed. Invest Ophthalmol Vis Sci 33:667–72

27. Lovie-Kitchin JE (1988) Validity and reliability of visual acuity measurements. Ophthal Physiol Opt 8:363–70

28. Mackensen G (1962) Die Untersuchung der Lesefähigkeit als klinische Funktionsprüfung. Fortschr Augenheilkd 12:344–79

29. Macular Photocoagulation Study Group (1982) Argon laser photocoagulation for senile macular degeneration: Results of a randomized clinical trial. Arch Ophthalmol 100:912–18

30. Macular Photocoagulation Study Group (1986) Argon laser photocoagulation for neovascular maculopathy: Three year results from randomized clinical trials. Arch Ophthalmol 104:694–701

31. Mansfield J, Ahn S, Legge G, Luebker A (1993) A new reading-acuity chart for normal and low vision. Opt Soc Am Techn Digest 3:232–5

32. Munoz B, West SK, Rubin GS, Schein OD, Quigley HA, Bressler SB, Bandeen-Roche K, and the SEE Study Team (2000) Causes of blindness and visual impairment in a population of older Americans. Arch Ophthalmol 118:819–25

33. NAS-NRC Committee on Vision (1980) Recommended standard procedures for the clinical measurement and specification of visual acuity. Adv Ophthalmol 41:103–48

34. Osarovsky-Sasin E, Richter-Mueksch S, Pfleger T, Stifter E, Velikay-Parel M, Radner W (2002) Reduced Reading ability of eyes with anisometropic amblyopia. Invest Ophthalmol Vis Sci 43: Abstract 4691. ARVO 2002

35. Patel B, Elliott DB, Whitaker D (2001) Optimal reading speed in simulated cataract: development of a potential vision test. Ophthal Physiol Opt 21:272–6

36. Pesudovs K, Patel B, Bradbury JA, Elliott DB (2002) Reading speed test for potential central vision measurement. Clin Experiment Ophthalmol 30:183–6

37. Radner W, Obermayer W, Richter-Mueksch S, Willinger U, Velikay-Parel M, Eisenwort B (2002) The validity and reliability of short German sentences for measuring reading speed. Graefe's Arch Clin Exp Ophthalmol 240:461–7

38. Radner W, Willinger U, Obermayer W, Mudrich C, Velikay-Parel M, Eisenwort B (1998) [A new German Reading Chart for the simultaneous evaluation of reading acuity and speed] [Article in German] Klin Monatsbl Augenheilkd 213:174–81

39. Richter-Mueksch S, Weghaupt H, Skorpik C, Velikay-Parel M, Radner W (2002) Reading performance with a refractive multifocal and a diffractive bifocal intraocular lens. J Cataract Refract Surg 28:1957–63

260   W. Radner et al.: Standards of reading performance and visual acuity measurements

40. Rubin G, West S, Munoz B, Bandeen-Roche K, Zeger S, Schein O, Fried L (1997) A comprehensive assessment of visual impairment in a population of older Americans. The SEE Eye Evaluation Project. Invest Ophthalmol Vis Sci 38:557–68
41. Rubin GS, Munoz B, Bandeen-Roche K, West S (2000) Monocular versus binocular visual acuity as measures of vision impairment and predictors of visual disability. The SEE Project Team. Invest Ophthalmol Vis Sci 41:3327–34
42. Sloan L, Rowland WM, Altmann A (1952) Comparison of three types of test target for the measurement of visual acuity. Q Rev Ophthalmol 8:4–16
43. Sloan LL (1959) New test charts for the measurement of visual acuity at far and near distances. Am J Ophthalmol 48:807
44. Stangler-Zuschrott E (1990) [Decreased reading speed and rapid fatigue as signs of disordered visual function] [Article in German] Klin Monatsbl Augenheilkd 196:150–7
45. Wesemann W (2000) [Visual acuity measured via the Freiburg Visual Acuity Test (FVT), Bailey Lovie Chart and Landolt Ring Chart] [Article in German] Klin Monatsbl Augenheilkd 219:660–7
46. West S, Munoz B, Rubin G, Schein O, Bandeen-Roche K, Zeger S, German S, Fried L (1997) Function and visual impairment in a population-based study of older adults. The SEE Eye Evaluation Project. Invest Ophthalmol Vis Sci 38:72–82
47. West SK, Rubin GS, Broman AT, Munoz B, Bandeen-Roche K, Turano K (2002) How does visual impairment affect performance on tasks of everyday life. Arch Ophthalmol 120:774–80

Correspondence: W. Radner, Department of Ophthalmology and Optometry, University of Vienna, Währinger Gürtel 18-20, A-1090 Vienna, Austria.

Recent trends in ocular drug delivery

J.-M. Parel[1], P. J. Milne[2], and R. K. Parrish[3]

[1] Henri and Flore Lesieur Chair in Ophthalmology and Director, Ophthalmic Biophysics Center, Bascom Palmer Eye Institute, University of Miami School of Medicine, Miami, Florida, USA; Professeur Associé Emeritus Universités de Paris Hôtel-Dieu Hospital, Paris, France; Professeur Visiteur, University of Liège, Department of Ophthalmology, Centre Hospitalier Universitaire Sart-Tilman, Liège, Belgium
[2] Associate Professor, Ophthalmic Biophysics Center, Bascom Palmer Eye Institute, University of Miami School of Medicine, Miami Florida USA and Department of Atmospheric Chemistry, University of Miami Rosenstiel School of Marine and Atmospheric Science, Key Biscayne, Florida, USA
[3] Associate Dean for Graduate Medical Education and Professor of Ophthalmology, Bascom Palmer Eye Institute, University of Miami School of Medicine, Miami Florida USA

I. Introduction

Modern discovery techniques are leading to an ever increasing numbers of drugs and drug candidates. Together with the deeper understanding of ocular physiological processes and the molecular pathogenesis of disease states, this stimulates potential interest in drug modalities for treatment and control of several ocular conditions. Because of the potency and specificity of newer therapeutic agents, increasing attention must be paid to the delivery schemes clinicians use for the targeting of drugs and pro-drugs to their specific sites of action. An instance of the challenges of this are to be seen in the consideration of peptide and oligonucleotide sequences newly developed from molecular biological fields such as proteomics and gene therapy which may require highly controlled delivery of non-traditional drugs, biomolecules and agents to intended targets at the cell layer and specific cell type level [21] to be both effective and safe for treatment.

A. General considerations for drug delivery

1. Delivery systems for target drugs and treatment conditions

Treatment of the outermost ocular surfaces is familiarly sought for conditions such as conjunctivitis, blepharitis and keratitis, and is thus consistent with the conventional dosage delivery forms exemplified by eye-drops of suitable solutions and formulations. Conventional dosage as eye-drops accounts for the majority of currently available commercialized formulations. Because of patient familiarity, safety, efficacy and cost-advantages of such a delivery path, it is not surprising that attempts at intraocular treatment applied through the cornea with topical application of solutions have also been sought for a range of pathologies such as glaucoma, uveitis, wound healing, and herpes simplex and even for immune response modulation. The efficacy of topical therapy ultimately depends upon the physiological consideration that drainage from the eye is typically significantly greater than achievable drug uptake rates.

After instillation of a traditionally formulated ophthalmic drug solution as eye-drops (1 drop ~ 40–50 μL), the drug-lacrimal fluid mix may only experience tissue contact times of a few minutes due to either normal (0.5–2.2 μl/min; average 1.2 uL/min) or stimulated

(3–400 µl/min) lacrimal fluid production. Drainage of tears through the upper and lower canaliculi into the lacrimal sac is promoted by blinking. Transnasal absorption after drainage to the nasolacrimal duct not only removes the drug from the target ocular tissues but may, via absorption and systemic circulation, result in unintended delivery to non-target tissues (e.g. Meseguer et al., 1994 [56]).

2. Physiological considerations

As well as containing distinct tissue structures of several specific physiological functions in a intricately compartmentalized volume, the eye has a variety of protective mechanisms to ensure proper vision through the active cleaning and filtration of interior and exterior visual surfaces. These include tissue drainage, tear film renewal and the tear response, aqueous humor flow, absorption and drainage via the vascularization of the conjunctiva, in addition to the impermeability of blood-eye barrier. Intrinsic ocular absorption is also limited by structural features unique to the relatively impermeable corneal barrier.

Structurally, the cornea contains three lamellar sorptive barriers, the epithelial membrane, the endothelium and the inner stroma. The outermost epithelial layer is approximately five to seven cell layers in thickness. Constantly irrigated by tear film serving to dilute and disperse topically applied medication, the epithelium has a lipophilic character which acts as a barrier to the penetration of charged or polar drug molecules. Epithelial cell tight junctions, composed of the band of specialized proteins that form apical boundaries of epithelial cell layers, further preserve the integrity of epithelial layers by serving as a barrier to paracellular transport. Transcellular permeability in the corneal epithelial layer is physiologically regulated, serving as it does for maintenance of corneal hydration. Even for drugs of moderate lipophilicity (e.g. dexamethasone, sodium phosphate timolol maleate) up to half of the permeability resistance is provided by the epithelial layer. For more hydrophilic drugs (e.g. pilocarpine HCl, epinephrine) corneal resistance is even higher. The stroma, composing some 85% of the corneal thickness beneath the corneal epithelium, is composed of fibrillar bundles of collagen. The highly hydrophilic corneal stroma is significantly resistant to the passage of lipophilic substances and low molecular weight drugs. The corneal endothelium is a single-cell layer and is not normally a barrier to drug penetration.

As the sclera has a total surface area greater than 16 cm², it represents a favorably large candidate entry path for ocular drug delivery. Scleral composition is a hypocellular fiber matrix consisting of heterogeneous bundled structures of collagen fibrils embedded in a glycosaminoglycan ground matrix [3, 41, 80, 82]. The predominant scleral collagen is of Type I [38], but types III, IV, V, VI, VII and XIII are also present [19, 40].

Measurements of the permeability of scleral tissues has been the subject of several studies [2, 55, 75, 84]. These investigations reveal that scleral permeability declines exponentially with molecular weight of the permeant, but that molecular size (hydrodynamic radius) is an even better predictor of penetration. Compounds of moderately high MW (>50 kD) are to some extent transferable across the sclera. Chemical selectivity between compounds such as proteins (e.g. bovine serum albumin and immunoglobulin) and carbohydrates (e.g. dextrans) of comparable molecular weight have been demonstrated. Other predictable aspects of scleral permeability include:

  i) increased permeability with surgical thinning of the sclera
 ii) increased permeability with increasing tissue hydration [18]
iii) increased permeability with increasing temperature [84]
 iv) increased permeability with reduced intraocular pressure [72]

These observations are all consistent with paracellular transport through a collagen fiber matrix rather than through active transcellular pathways. At least one fiber matrix model of the permeability of sclera and cornea has been presented [28]. In vivo permeability studies of the sclera have also been carried out [15, 16] which indicate greater permeability to hydrophilic over lipophilic molecules [23, 27].

3. Pharmacokinetic considerations

Relevant physicochemical properties of drugs and drug formulations intended for ocular instillation include aqueous solubility, lipophilicity, molecular size and shape, degree of ionization, and ionic and electrophoretic charge.

II. Clinical needs and approaches

A. Anterior segment

Despite evident accessibility, delivery of drugs to the anterior segment of the eye (cornea, conjunctiva, anterior chamber, iris and lens) is challenging in view of the inherent protective mechanisms which function to shield the visual pathway from external biological agents, particulates, and chemicals.

1. Topical delivery

A primary limitation to the topical application of ophthalmic therapeutic agents is their rapid and efficient drainage associated with high tear fluid turn over from the eye's outer surface. Less than 5% of drugs applied as aqueous solutions typically actually penetrate the cornea to reach underlying tissues [48]. Much of the instilled dosage may also be removed by incidental systemic uptake through either conjunctival microvasculature or via the nasolacrimal duct. To ameliorate such essentially wasteful drug losses through these paths, modern drug delivery strategies are directed towards increasing drug bioavailability through retentive strategies, aimed at deliberately prolonging the contact time of the therapeutic agent with one or more ocular surface components. To enhance drug-tear film residence on the ocular surface and cul de sac, punctual occlusion is often used.

Drug delivery formulations designed to improve ocular bioavailability by modifying the drug delivery vehicle to impart increased retention or contact time may employ approaches such as adhesion or gelation to reduce drainage or flushing rates. In this manner, ointments have been used to increase ocular contact times. However, if the ointment vehicle significantly blurs patient vision or leads to other discomfort it maybe of lesser treatment value due to poor compliance. Suitable oil or hydrophobic bases may enable higher effective concentrations of lipophilic compounds, such as corticosteroids, to be applied to the eye than can be provided in the form of aqueous suspensions of the same drug. Modification of drug vehicle viscosity by incorporation of water soluble and otherwise inert polymers is also commonly employed in ocular formulations. Typical polymer systems for such applications include polyvinyl alcohol, polyvinyl pyrrolidone, polyacrylates, methyl cellulose etc [86].

2. Gel and colloidal systems

Polymeric gel delivery systems, applied either as preformed vehicles or as formulations which undergo gelation in situ following their topical application, are designed to extend ocular residence time via enhanced viscosity or favorable mucoadhesive properties to the mucin components of ocular surfaces. Gel forming systems are typically liquids whose structural aggregation changes via enhanced physical cross-linkages brought about altered physiological conditions. Thus the existing pH, temperature or electrolyte composition of tear fluids may serve to trigger transition from a more or less easy flowing liquid phase to a gel state at the eye surface [33, 58, 70]. The sought for phase transitions are often reversible.

Bioadhesion is promoted though the formation of moderately strong, non-covalent interactions between polymer hydrophillic functional groups and the mucin coatings of the conjunctiva, cornea and sclera. Desired polymer characteristics include the ability to form hydrogen bonds, ionizable anionic charge groups, moderate to high molecular weight, but retaining sufficient chain flexibility and surface energies to enable spreading over ocular mucin layers. Polymers having these bioadhesive properties include poly-acrylic acid, carbophil, hyarulonic acid, pullulan, carboxymethyl cellulose and chitosan [68, 73].

3. Colloidal dispersion systems for lipophilic drugs

Emulsions and microemulsions (liposomes) are colloidal dispersions of immiscible liquids that are thermodynamically stabilized typically by the preferential adsorption of amphi-philic surfactants at their interfaces. In microemulsions, surfactant concentrations may be 10% or more by weight, compared to 0.1% or less in typical emulsions. The stability and other physicochemical properties of the system may additionally be modified by the presence of co-surfactants, often in the form of low MW alcohols. This results in a greatly increased interfacial area between the dispersed oily and the carrier aqueous phases, together with smaller "droplet" sizes (~10 to 100nm). Formulations of these basic components can be tailored to tolerance by the eye [85]. From the standpoint of drug deliv-ery, a key advantage of microemulsions as delivery vehicles is markedly increased solubilization of drugs. This is especially so for lipophilic drugs, whose instillation into the polar aqueous environment of ocular surfaces would otherwise be problematic. Addi-tional possibilities, such as tailoring the surface charge of nanodroplets to favor their binding to negatively charged corneal surfaces and thus enhance ocular residence times [14], or modifying the kinetics of the drug delivery to better match desired pharmacoki-netic profiles remain to be shown for these systems.

Assuming that the drug retains its chemical stability and efficacy in the microemul-sive environment, its subsequent rate of clearance will be determined largely by the size and composition properties of the carrier system.

B. Posterior segment

1. Subconjunctival injection

Subconjunctival injection, despite its possible lower convenience, is often a clinically pre-ferred means of attaining elevated intraocular drug concentration for both the anterior and posterior segments of the eye, although there is evidence that subconjunctival injec-tion also leaks out into the tear film layer and drug gets absorbed also through the cornea. Both antimicrobial and antimetabolite drugs may be delivered in this manner [69, 79]. Studies have demonstrated that this more direct route provides higher therapeutic pene-tration to the aqueous humor and the vitreous than anteriorally applied devices and strate-gies such as topical drops, scleral shields, presoaked contact lenses, peribulbar injections [29, 57, 91] or systemic administration. The pathways of drug transport and distribution following subconjunctival administration are known to be dependent upon the specific

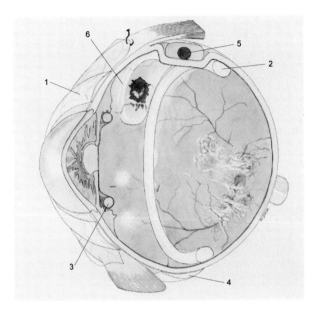

Fig. 1. Intraocular controlled drug release inserts potential locations: 1) subconjunctival, 2) intra-vitreal, 3) endocapsular, 4) suprascleral, 5) in a buckle groove – 6) over a melanoma. (Courtesy of G. Simon, MD, PhD)

physicochemical characteristics of the drug [54, 62], but the details of the exact routes appear to be limited and confounded by injection site, injection volume, and even the animal model being studied [5, 25, 50].

2. Implants and bioerodible inserts

Another approach to achieving either site specific delivery or more favorable retention time in the eye seeks to employ either spatial or temporal control over the release of a given therapeutic agent by use of controlled drug delivery technologies (Fig. 1). Such delivery systems are typically based on manufacture of a synthetic polymer carrier device for the target drug, and are designed for greater efficacy, patient compliance and or convenience. Controlled release strategies may also reduce incidences of toxicity or side effects. Controlled release over time, either for an extended period (days to months) or at a specifiable time during the course of a treatment allows for improved control of rapidly metabolized or eliminated drugs. Extended duration delivery of a drug from a well tolerated implant device obviates repeated drug administration, advantageous in situations where specialized delivery (e.g. by repeated injections) is impractical.

Repeated application of drugs results in sub-optimal drug concentrations associated with bolus injections, a factor to be considered with medications that have specified therapeutic concentration windows (Fig. 2a). Peak concentrations associated with an injection may lead to either widely varying concentrations over the treatment cycle, attaining both sub-therapeutic concentrations at the treatment site and at levels prone to producing unwanted side effects systemically. Rapidly metabolized drugs in particular benefit from having their dosage rate matched to their elimination kinetics, for instance in the case of pain treatment. If many drugs, such as 5-FU (5-fluorouracil), clear the vitreous cavity in a 4 to 8 hours, a few, like triamcilonone acetonide as Machemer's team has shown [1], have an inherently slower release kinetics (Fig. 2b) and, given the same effec-

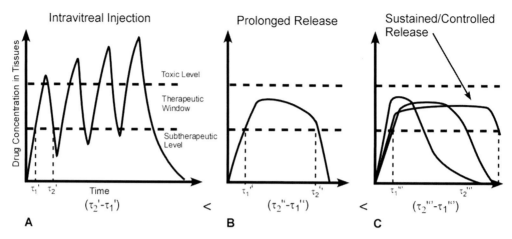

Fig. 2. Schema of intraocular pharmacokinetics with T_2–T_1 representing therapeutic time window. **A** A single injection produce a short lasting (~4 hrs) burst effect while with multiple injections, drug accumulation in tissues may reach toxic levels. **B** Prolonged release systems (e.g. Kenalog) give greater T_2–T_1 but rarely more than 2 weeks. **C** General pharmacokinetics of drug release implants. Controlled drug release device produce a square pattern where T_2–T_1 may reach over 12 months

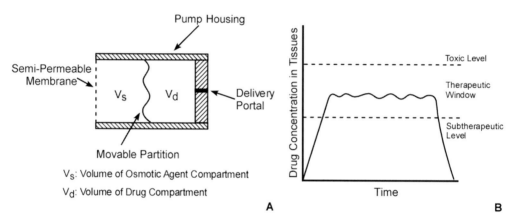

Fig. 3. Osmotic pump concept. **A** Schema of one of the devices that can be re-loaded in situ using a 30 ga needle. **B** Typical pharmacokinetics pattern. In most devices, the semi-permeable membrane is made of polyvinyl alcohol (PVA) which has the propensity to elicit fibrotic encapsulation which can slow the release with time

tiveness, are better suited to slow release implants. For ophthalmic applications, a major concern is the sensitivity of the retina to drugs currently in development such as those developing from proteomics and biotechnological are expected to heighten the need for optimal drug delivery both in time and to specific sites [66].

A diversity of polymer structures and systems have and continue to be developed for controlled drug release [26, 83], with different polymer backbones allowing for versatility in meeting requirements of either the drug or the treatment site, and even for the principle of the release mechanism (Fig. 2c). An important primary design consideration is the subsequent fate of the polymer system after the drug release. Non degradable, yet biocompatible, polymer systems such as patches or inserts can usually be removed (Fig. 3). Polymers that are broken down by either biodegradation or erosion and then

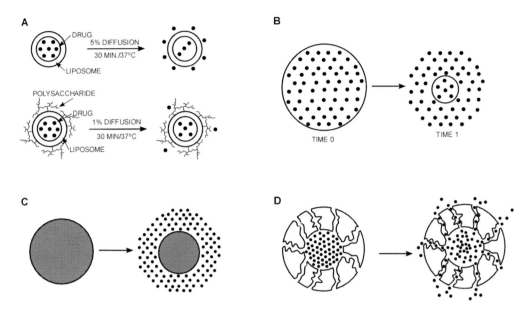

Fig. 4. Biodegradable drug delivery systems (**A**) liposomes, (**B**) bioerodible surface erosion (e.g. co-drugs, (**C**) polymer-drug matrix, (**D**) matrix coated with a semi-permeable biodegradable membrane

safely excreted from the body are advantageous in that a recovery step is not needed. Degradation of a polymeric system in the body refers to chemical bond cleavage to smaller sub-units, whereas erosion of a polymeric system is the physical dissolution and diffusion leading to depletion. In practice, both mechanism will occur to variable extent depending on the polymeric system.

Polymeric controlled drug release systems may delay the rate at which drug molecules are exposed to aqueous solution by having the polymer matrix, dissolving at a slow rate, act as a barrier to the immediate aqueous environment (Fig. 4). Alternately, polymer coating may act as a diffusional barrier. In porous polymer systems the diffusional velocity of the drug molecule to the external cellular environment may simply be reduced sufficiently to result in slow release. Hydrogels based on poly(HEMA), a normally insoluble polymer well tolerated as contact lens material, have been suggested for this purpose [53].

The homo- and heteropolymers of lactic and glycolic acids (PLGA) show good biocompatability, as demonstrated by their long standing use as resorbable surgical sutures. In the eye, these poly(ester) systems degrade at predictable and reproducible rates into the parent acids, which may be further metabolized to the hydroxy acids in the eye or else removed by the blood stream or filtration. Poly(esters), such as those based on either poly(lactic acid), poly(glycolic acid) or their copolymers (PLGA) are easily synthesized to yield desired mechanical, thermal and biological properties, and form solid solutions with a range of target drugs. Implantable, biodegradable PLGA devices, plugs and inserts have been shown to be well tolerated in animal models [39, 59]. Facile control over dissolution rates of PLA, PGA and PLGA has been demonstrated [88], potentially allowing for sustained drug release periods between 1 week and 1 month.

Using PLGA is advantageous as varying the ratio of polylactic to polyglycolic moeities modifies both the polymer's physical characteristics and drug release kinetics. Develop-

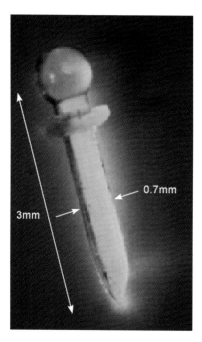

Fig. 5. Biopin. The biodegradable device was made of PLGA 90/10, a biomaterial that has the potential for drug loading using the matrix concept. It was shown to be safe when implanted in the rabbit retina-choroid-sclera layers

mental work performed in a rabbit model shows low lactide/glycolide ratios to biodegrade very rapidly. Only very small fragment of a 10/90 PLGA biopin implant [63] could be found 3 weeks after subconjunctival implantation although a 90/10 implant was still visible at 3 months. Biodegradation was found to be function of the implant location; a 90/10 implant inserted in the retina-choroid-scleral tissue was still visible at 9 months (Fig. 5). The drug loading also modified biodegradation characteristics, the higher the drug fraction, the more fragile the implant became and the more quickly it dissolved. In ophthalmology, each specific medical application imparts restrictions on the size and shape of the implant which must be miniaturized for easy insertion and minimal trauma to adjacent tissues. Optimizing the implant requires maximizing drug loading.

For the "C-ring", an implant primarily developed in our laboratories to prevent recurrent proliferative vitreoretinopathy (PVR), we used a 50/50 PLGA and maximized the drug concentration to 30% (Fig. 6). Experimental in vitro testing showed the implant drug release to be non-linear; with a rapid burst followed by a logarithmic decay. As each drug has a site-specific toxic to therapeutic threshold, a burst release could easily endanger intraocular tissues in the immediate postoperative period. To prevent burst release and optimize delivery, the "C-ring" implant was externally coated with a drug-free polymer which, while dissolving, produced a semi-permeable barrier over the 5FU-PLGA matrix and slowed biodegradation time. As the coating was only several micrometers in thickness, a delivery system was designed to avoid punctures that could be made during insertion with a tying forceps. The coated implant was shown to be safe when inserted in the vitreous cavity of rabbits and found to dissolve in 60 days when inserted under the anterior conjunctiva and in 3 to 4 months when inserted in the vitreous cavity [36]. In an experimental animal model of PVR, Rubsamen et al. [71] demonstrated the implant to be efficacious at preventing retinal detachment compared to a control implant without

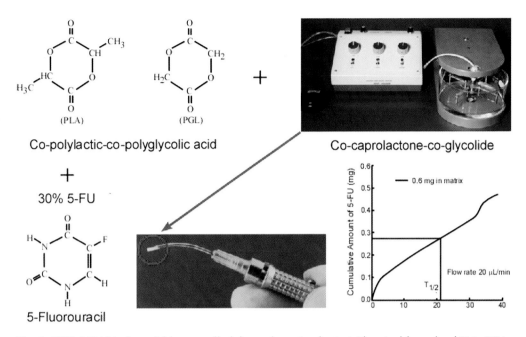

Fig. 6. BPEI 5-FU biodegradable controlled drug release implant. **a**) Chemical formula of PLA, PGA, and 5-FU, **b**) implant coating apparatus, **c**) implant in delivery inserter, **d**) implant's pharmacokinetics measured in vitro

drug. In an ongoing European Phase I clinical study led by Professor Christophe Baudouin and performed on 150 patients, the EC approved implant (Corneal SA, Paris) was shown at 1 year follow-up to be safe as an antiproliferative adjunct to trabeculectomy (Fig. 7). Efficacy studies of the "C-ring" in patients will require several additional years of follow-up.

3. Transcorneal and transscleral iontophoresis

As a drug delivery modality, iontophoresis refers to the application of an electric field and associated current to enhance transport of ionized drug molecules across otherwise impermeable tissue barriers and boundaries. Ocular (transcorneal) uses of this approach date back to von Sallman [90] with earlier accounts at the turn of the century by Wirtz. While reasonably well understood for increased permeability through the skin (stratum corneum), clinical development and ophthalmic use of the technique has been hampered by a lack of systematic scientific study of the mechanism for drug penetration through ocular tissues. It is also true that many of the scientific investigations of underlying mechanisms have been conducted on ex- vivo explant skin tissue, and in arrangements of very different or lesser relevance to ophthalmic therapeutic situations. Similar consideration applies to the exact experimental definition of passive diffusion of target drugs that an iontophoretric approach may be compared to. However, interest in iontophoresis has been demonstrated in animal model studies for range of medicines including antibiotics [6, 7], steroids [10, 46], antifungals [32], antivirals [47, 74] as well as fluorescein tracers [53a].

Significant methodological variables include the intensity and duration of the applied current, which may be both AC and DC, as well as both continuous and pulsed, in addi-

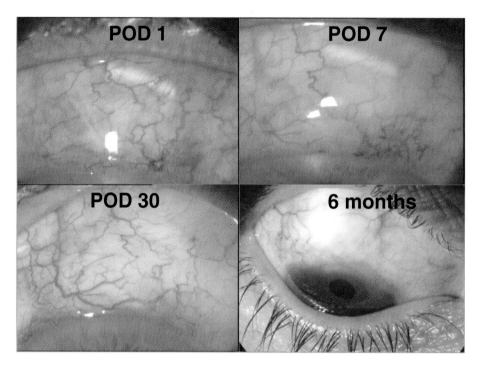

Fig. 7. Clinical appearance of the 5-FU CDR implant (courtesy of Christophe Baudouin, MD, PhD, Centre Hospitalier Universitaire XV–XX, Paris)

tion to the geometric configuration and placement of electrodes on ocular surfaces. Physicochemical characteristics of the drug molecules, such as their degree of ionization, molecular weight, size and shape at physiological pH, and ionic strength, and solvent composition are relevant. In general, negatively charged molecules are expected to penetrate scleral and corneal surfaces better than positively charged ones [24, 93]. It is usually beneficial to adapt the electric field protocol to the ionization state (charge) of the target molecule. However, increased permeability of zwitterionic or even neutral molecules appears to be facilitated by iontophoresis.

Proposed mechanisms underlying enhanced permeant flux across tissue barriers that have been suggested include:

i) passive diffusion, notably as enhanced through skin or tissue pathways such as follicles, capillaries, imperfections and intercellular gaps, ii) electrical repulsion, especially of charged species, iii) electrosmosis of solvent molecules and their entrained solutes and even iv) electrical potential alteration of lipid-bilayer structures allowing formation of voltage-dependent pores.

A concern over the use of iontophoresis for a general, or even a specialized, drug delivery mechanism is the degree of variability reported in some studies (e.g. Barza et al. [7]) and thus the general possibility of reduced effectiveness during repeated therapeutic application. Systemized studies of iontophoretic delivery using well optimized protocols including artifact-free sampling of attained therapeutic concentrations of delivered drugs are lacking. A second area of concern is patient safety. Historically, there exist reports of several difficulties including corneal scarring and tissue damage [35, 37]. Even a cursory examination of some of these early reports reveals that sub-optimal electrode geometries and excessive current densities were sometimes employed in order to "demonstrate" the desired effects, enhanced permeant concentrations. Better understanding of the pharma-

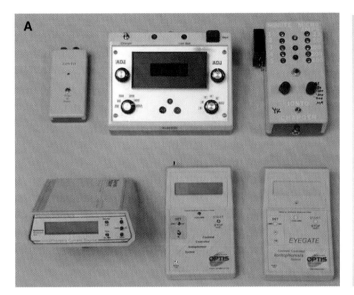
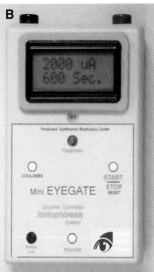

Fig. 8. CCI power unit. **A** Evolution 1980 to 2001. **B** The mini-CCI apparatus (2002) is processor controlled for treatment flexibility and 9 Volts DC battery operated for patient safety, the device monitors current delivery, calculate total charge, and alerts the physician if inadequate fluidic contact occurs

cokinetics of sought for treatment regimes on both healthy and diseased eyes are needed for refinement of the iontophoretic delivery approach.

A variant of the basic iontophoretic technique, Controlled Coulomb Iontophoresis, designed to maximize drug transfer while preventing tissue burns has been proposed [77, 61] and tested in several animal studies [9, 10, 12, 89]. These studies demonstrated transepithelial electrical fields less than 2 Volts were sufficient for optimal drug transfer and that most of the field-loss occurred at the return electrode interface over bare skin. The studies also showed current densities greater than $50\,mA/cm^2$ thermally affected tissues, especially the conjunctival epithelium where burns occurred at 100 to $140\,mA/cm^2$. These preliminary studies showed how to optimize the CCI instrument for clinical use. The instrument consists of a portable 9-Volt battery powered microprocessor system that controls electrical field, current and application time as well as warning the physician when treatment is completed and when the applicator is not appropriately connected or positioned. The device automatically calculates and indicates total charge delivered (A/s) which facilitates medical record keeping (Fig. 8). For transcorneal applications, the applicator has a central $0.5\,cm^2$ circular 5 mm deep cavity filled with the drug solution surrounded by a soft skirt to seal the ocular surface and minimize damage to the epithelium (Fig. 9). For transscleral applications, the $0.5\,cm^2$ contact area is shaped to conform to the ocular globe and consists of a fluidic annulus that is positioned on the limbus and anterior sclera. A central opening permits visualization of the cornea, anterior and posterior segment during treatment with the slit-lamp or operation microscope (Fig. 10). The treatment current level can be varied over a wide range, but for safety reasons is limited to 2.5 mA. The CCI provides a >5 hrs total treatment time at maximum current level. Rabbit studies performed at a current density of $5\,mA/cm^2$ demonstrated treatment time greater than 10 min did not substantially increase retinal drug concentrations (Chapon et al. 1999). An experimental trial with the antiviral ganciclovir showed a 10 min transscleral application produced a higher retinal concentration at 5 days than a single intravitreal

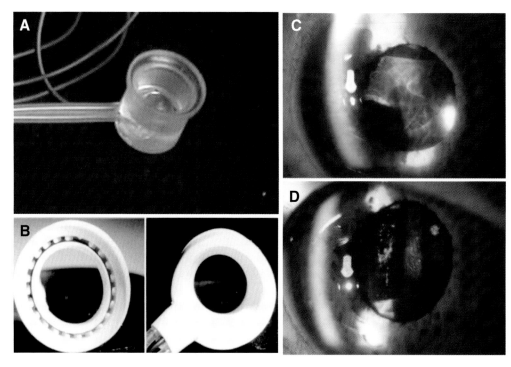

Fig. 9. CCI transcorneal (**A**) and transscleral (**B**) applicators. The skirt of the devices made of medical grade silicone rubber fits the scleral contour, both have cavities containing the drug solution which is infused and aspirated via 2 parallel fluidic lines. The annular platinum electrode is deeply recessed to prevent tissue contact. Patient with intraocular inflammation before (**C**) and 24 hrs after (**D**) a single CCI application of solumedrol (courtesy Francine Behar-Cohen MD, PhD, Rothschild Foundation, Paris)

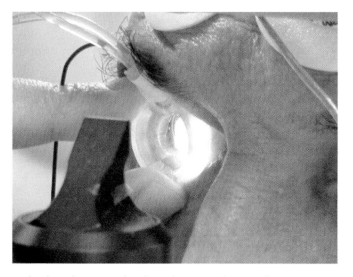

Fig. 10. CCI transscleral applicator in the clinical setting. The visual axis remains free for slit-lamp examination during treatment. The EKG-type return electrode can be seen on the patient forehead. The two fluidic lines and the lead to the internally located platinum electrode are at 12 O'clock

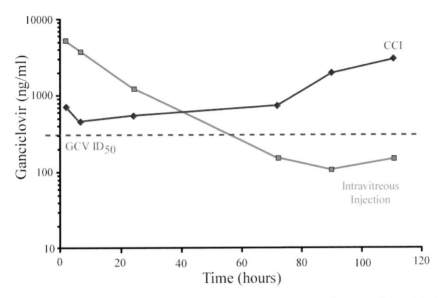

Fig. 11. Typical retinal pharmacokinetics after one CCI treatment with antiviral ganciclovir. The retinal drug levels remain above ID^{50} and tend to increase with time whereas with a single intravitreal injection, it decreases below therapeutic threshold at 60 hrs

injection (Fig. 11). The study found very elevated concentration of the drug in both corneal and scleral tissues that tapered with time. We surmised the large amount of drug stored in these tissues was slowly released intraocularly, therefore increasing the retinal drug concentration over time.

Kinetic studies have shown drug concentration at 4 min to be over 65% the concentration at 10 mins. In a phase I clinical study, Behar-Cohen and team sought to use lower currents (~400 µA) and shorter durations (~4 min) leading to a controlled surface charge as low as 0.4 Coulombs/cm^2. Using this protocol, successful treatment of uveitis via localized delivery of solumedrol in patients was demonstrated [22, 34] as well as treatment of corneal edema and intraocular inflammation [65] and infectious keratitis [92].

The logarithmic relation between tissue drug concentration and application time in the direct current (DC) regime is probably related to a saturation field effect. The tissue response slowly increases its ohmic resistance at longer treatment times. Alternative iontophoresis is surmised to solve this problem by rapidly de-phasing cellular polarity but this phenomenon has not been scientifically proven. To investigate this effect, an alternating current (AC) iontophoretic system based on the principles of Coulomb has recently been designed (Fig. 12) for comparative studies in the rabbit. The programmable system allows modulation of the bias signal as well as current rise time, pulse shape and frequency. This system could be used to improve the non-invasive transfer of drugs and large molecular weight moeities such as plasmids and oligonucleotides for gene therapy [11, 78] and antiVEGF factors in the retina to avoid the repeated intravitreal injections currently performed for age related macular degeneration (AMD).

C. Vitreoretinal compartment

The vitreous is a highly diluted aqueous gel (~1% solids) composed of hyaluronic acids held in a very loose collagen matrix. Although some drugs have been shown to freely diffuse within the vitreous, both the position of injection and the volume injected may

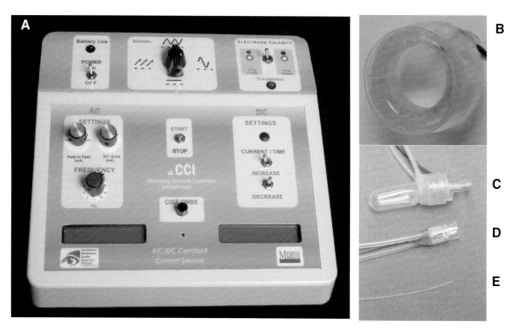

Fig. 12. The alternative CCI instrument (**A**) as the same safety features but produces different waveforms with adjustable bias level and signal frequency. It automatically calculates and continuously indicates the cumulative treatment charge. Ongoing testing makes use of a drug-gel loaded corneoscleral applicator (**B**) fitting rabbits as well as applicators for rats (**C**), mice (**D**) and an endo-ocular electrode (**E**)

markedly affect drug distribution and clearance rates. Predominant clearance pathways include diffusion into the posterior chamber, egress from the anterior chamber as well as elimination through the blood-retinal barrier. Aqueous soluble drugs are expected to equilibrate quickly, with typical clearance rates yielding drug half-lives of the order of 5 to 20 hours [30, 51].

1. Systemic drug delivery

Drug delivery to the posterior segment of the eye via systemic administration generally offers reduced facility as a treatment option, and will in any event be limited to drugs that are tolerated systemically. A consideration of the circulation of the posterior segment [60], reveals that the retina and the choroid are supplied by relatively few vessels, namely the retinal artery and a few, short posterior arteries. Additionally, the outer third of the retinal layer and region of the macula are essentially avascular and are supplied with needed nutrients from the choroid circulation. On the other hand the fine capillary network of the chorio capillaries underlying the retinal pigment epithelium has been demonstrated [17] to exhibit high permeability to substances of molecular weight (MW) of up to that of albumin (67 kDa), consistent with the physiological need to maintain retinal glucose and key transport proteins [81]. The above is consistent with a view of the vitreoretinal compartment being essentially a privileged space, with the tight junctions of the blood-retinal barrier serving to restrict paracellular access of many low MW drugs into this part of the eye. A possibly important therapeutic consideration is that the integrity of the blood retinal barrier maybe reduced or wholly compromised in conditions that are likely to require drug administration to the posterior segment in the first place. This may be true for instances of inflammation and tumors. Since epithelia with barrier-function typically express transporter systems for the selective transport and molecular exchange, treatment strategies with pro-drugs targeted to such transporters or the co-application of drugs with certain barrier permeability mediators that are taken up by the cells [31].

2. Direct intravitreal injection

Drug injection into the vitreoretinal compartment through the pars plana has long been used as a means of delivering desired therapeutic concentration of given drugs to the posterior segment. Traditionally reserved for ocular conditions that pose greatest chance of visual loss (e.g. tumors, PVR, bacterial endophthalmitis, severe inflammatory conditions), the procedure does involve some risk, often stemming from the extrinsic need to scrupulously ensure sterility of injected drugs. Injected volumes are appropriately small (typically 0.5 mL to 1.0 mL) although even then, anterior chamber paracentesis may be needed to remove aqueous humor, minimizing ocular pressure elevation. Repeated intravitreal injection may, however, have an attendant risk of complications such as cataract formation, retinal disturbance or detachment, and in immunocompromised patients, endophthalmitis. Direct intravitreal antibiotic injection remains the recommended drug delivery option for endophthalmitis [8], and is usually associated with a sampling of ocular fluids for purposes of culture or identification of the infectious agent.

3. Intravitreal implants

Apart from the osmotic pump developed by Ashton [67] for release of antiviral ganciclovir (Vitrasert, Alcon. TX), no other FDA approved controlled drug release system are commercially available. Recently, Ashton and Jaffe experimentally tested an osmotic pump loaded with with co-drug 5FU-triamcilonone [94] and several teams have experimentally investigated biodegradable implants based on uncoated PLGA matrices [52, 95, 97].

Intravitreal silicone oil that has been used to maintain the retina attached after vitrectomy [96], can also be used as a reservoir for slow drug release. As Refojo and his colleagues have shown, the lighter than water 1000 and 5000 cts silicon oils in clinical use today, both trimethyl terminated polydimethylsiloxanes [64], readily adsorb lipophilic compounds such as the anti-proliferative agents caramustine (BCNU) [4], retinoic acid [87], and alpha tocopherol (vitamin E) [49]. When silicone oil is mixed with a hydrophilic drug, the drug moiety remains in suspension and, after implantation, slowly diffuses outward along the concentration gradient at the oil bubble-retina interface. The drug is absorbed by retinal and choroidal tissues, and in patients having had a total lensectomy-vitrectomy, by the ciliary body and iris. Using non-steroidal anti-inflammatory drugs (NSAID), such as acetylsalicylic acid (aspirin), [44, 45], have recently shown this method to be safe and efficacious in the rabbit model (Fig. 13). Other low molecular weight medications could be released in this fashion, including corticosteroids, such as dexamethasone and Anacortave. It is to be determined if very high molecular weight moieties, such as oligonucleotides, peptides and anti-VEGF (e.g. RhuFabV2), can be released from the drug-oil suspension.

III. Conclusions and future directions

The choices of available therapeutic agents and drug delivery approaches continue to expand rapidly. Widespread acceptance of many of these newer technologies into mainstream ophthalmology remains a challenge on several fronts. Controlled clinical trials are required to establish both the safety and long term efficacy of novel drug delivery

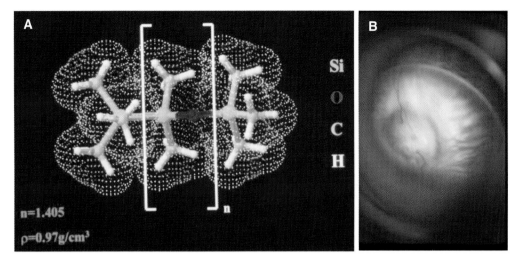

Fig. 13. Tri-dimensional representation of silicone oil trimethyl terminated polydimethylsiloxane (**A**) and fundus appearance (**B**) at postoperative day 56 of a rabbit implanted with a 1.67 mg/ml acetylsalicylic acid loaded-silicone oil

approaches and the formulations. These expensive and lengthy investigations remain a barrier to commercialization and clinical adoption over more conventional treatments. The promise of proteomic and molecular biologically based therapeutic agents which require focused pharmacological delivery and targeting of new drugs is particularly challenging. Neuroprotective agents or vectors for gene transfer which may hold great promise for conditions, such as glaucoma and other degenerative diseases of the choroid and retina, are developing faster than our clinical facility of delivering their desired therapeutic features at appropriate sites of action. Ultimately an ideal drug design goal will be the incorporation of all the desired pharmacological features – stability, solubility, ability to transfer across membranes and tissue barriers, cellular and subcellular targeting – directly into the drug itself. Indeed, recent efforts in this direction have raised promising new approaches for some drugs [76]. However newer drug delivery approaches are often complex in their operating principles, and they are likely to continue to further challenge our understanding of ocular physiology.

IV. Acknowledgements

The authors gratefully acknowledge the scientific leadership and moral support of EWD Norton MD who first promoted these studies over 21 years ago.

The treatment concepts were developed with clinical input from Karl Olsen, MD, Yoshiko Takesue, MD, PhD, Francine Behar-Cohen, MD, PhD, Janet L Davis, MD, Scott Cousins, MD, Sonia Yoo MD, Gerhard Kieselbach, MD, Martina Kralinger, MD and Christophe Baudoin, MD, who also provided scientific support in the analysis of the results from the experimental animal research as well as clinical data from patient treated with the devices described herein.

The drug release systems were developed in collaboration with polymer chemists Franck Villain, PhD, Valerie Jallet, PhD, Sandrine Gautier, PhD, Pascal Chapon, PhD, and Fotios Andreopoulos, PhD. The chemists also directed pharmacokinetic analysis.

The instrumentation shown herein was developed at the BPEI's Ophthalmic Biophysics Center with the collaboration of Izuru Nose, BSEE, William Lee, David Denham MSME and Lidet Abiy BS. Noel Ziebarth BS, helped with drawings and figures.

Animal experiments were performed in accordance with the Association for Research in Vision and Ophthalmology Statements for Use of Animals in Ophthalmic Vision and Research under ACUC protocols written with the collaboration of Bobby Collins, DVM. Animal care was provided by Eleut Hernandez LAT and his staff at the McKnight Vision Research Center, University of Miami School of Medicine. Histology was read by ocular pathologists Robert Rosa, MD and Sander Dubovy, MD.

The authors gratefully acknowledge support from the departments of: Professor Kenji Oshima of the University of Fukuoka, Japan; Professor Yves Pouliquen of the University of Paris, France; Professor Michel Vert of the University of Montpellier, France; and Professor Gerhard Kieselbach of the University of Innsbruck, Austria.

The authors have no financial interest in the technology described herein. Intellectual property belongs to the University of Miami. The studies were supported in part by the Henri and Flore Lesieur Foundation, Corneal SA, the Florida Lions Eye Bank, Research to Prevent Blindness and the Veterans Hospital Administration.

V. References

1. Antoszyk AN, Gottleib JL, Machemer R, Hatchell DL (1993) The effects of intravitreal triamcinolone acetonide on experimental preretinal neovascularization. Graefes Arch Clin Exp Ophthalmol 231:34–40
2. Ambati J, Gragoudas ES, Miller JW, You TT, Miayamoto K, Delori FC, Adamis AP (2000) Transscleral delivery of bioactive protein to the choroid and retina. Invest Ophthalmol Vis Sci 41:1186–91
3. Ambati J, Adamis AP (2002) Transscleral drug delivery to the retina and choriod. Prog Retin Eye Res 21:145–51
4. Arroyo MH, Refojo MF, Araiz JJ, Tolentino FL, Cajita VN, Elner VM (1993) Silicone oil as a delivery vehicle for BCNU in rabbit proliferative vitreoretinopathy. Retina 13:245–50
5. Barza M, Kane A, Baum JL (1981) The difficulty of determining the route of intraocular penetration of gentamicin after subcojunctival injection in the rabbit. Invest Ophthalmol Vis Sci 20:509–14
6. Barza M, Peckman C, Baum J (1986) Transscleral iontophoresis of cefazolin, tiarcillin and gentamycin in the rabbit. Ophthalmology 93:133–8
7. Barza M, Peckman C, Baum J (1987) Transscleral iontophoresis of gentamycin in monkeys. Invest Ophthalmol Vis Sci 29:1033–7
8. Baum J, Peyman GA, Barza M (1982) Intravitreal administration of antibiotic in the treatment of bacterial endophthalmitis III, Consensus. Surv Ophthalmol 26:204–6
9. Behar-Cohen FF, Parel JM, Pouliquen Y, Thillaye-Goldenberg B, Goureau O, Heydolph S, Courtois Y, De Kozak Y (1997) Iontophoresis of dexamethasone in the treatment of endotoxin induced uveitis in rats. Exp Eye Res 65:533–45
10. Behar-Cohen FF, Salvodelli M, Parel JM, Goureau O, Thillaye-Goldenburg B, Courtois Y, de Kozak Y (1998) Reduction of corneal edema in endotoxin-induced uveitis after application of L-NAME as nitric oxide inhibitor in rats by iontophoresis. Invest Ophthalmol Vis Sci 39:897–904
11. Behar-Cohen F, DeKozak Y, Voigt M, Parel J-M, Goureau O, Chauvaud D (1999) Ocular Coulomb Controlled Iontophoresis (CCI) of NOS II Antisens oligonucleotides in endotoxin-induced-uveitis in rats. ARVO Invest Ophthalmol Vis Sci 40:s869
12. Behar-Cohen F, El Aouni A, Le Rouic JF, Parel J-M, Renard G, Chauvaud D (2001) Iontophorèse: revue de la littérature et perspectives. J Fr Ophtalmol 24(3):319–27

13. Behar-Cohen FF, Gautier S, El Aouni A, Chapon P, Parel J-M, Renard G, Chauvaud D (2001) Methylprednisolone concentrations in the vitreous and the serum after pulse therapy. Retina 21:48–53

14. Benita S, Levy MJ (1993) Submicron emulsions as colloidal drug carriers for intravenous administration: comprehensive physico-chemical characterization. J Pharm Sci 82:1069

15. Bill A (1964) The drainage of albumin from the uvea. Exp Eye Res 3:179–87

16. Bill A (1965) Movement of albumin and dextran through the sclera. Arch Ophthalmol 74:248–52

17. Bill A (1968) Capillary permeability to an extravascular dynamics of myoglobin, albumin and gammaglobulin in the uvea. Acta Physiol Scan 73:204–19

18. Boubriak OA, Urban JP, Akhtar S, Meek KM, Bron AJ (2000) The effect of hydration and matrix composition on solute diffusion in rabbit sclera. Exp Eye Res 71:503–14

19. Chapman SA, Ayad S, O'Donoghue E, Bonshek RE (1998) Glycoproteins of trabecular meshwork, cornea and sclera. Eye 12:440–8

20. Chapon P, Voigt M, Gautier S, Behar-Cohen F, O'Grady G, Parel J-M (1999) Intraocular tissues pharmacokinetics of ganciclovir transscleral coulomb controlled iontophoresis in rabbits. ARVO Invest Ophthalmol Vis Sci 40:S189

21. Chaum E, Hatton MP (2002) Gene therapy for genetic and acquired retinal diseases. Surv Ophthalmol 47(5):449–69

22. Chauvaud D, Behar-Cohen FF, Parel J-M, Renard G (2000) Transscleral iontophoresis of corticosteroids: Phase II Clinical trial. ARVO Invest Ophthalmol Vis Sci 41(4):S79

23. Chein DS, Homsy JJ, Gluchowski C, Tang-Liu DD (1990) Corneal and conjunctival/scleral penetration of p-aminoclonidine, AGN 190342, and clonidine in rabbit eyes. Curr Eye Res 9:1051–9

24. Church AI, Bara M, Baum J (1992) An improved apparatus for transcleral iontophoresis of gentamicin. Invest Ophthalmol Vis Sci 33:3543–5

25. Conrad JM, Robinson JR (1980) Mechanisms of anterior segment absorption of pilocarpine following subconjunctival injection in albino rabbits. J Pharm Sci 69:875–84

26. Deshpande AA, Heller J, Gurny R (1998) Bioerodible polymers for ocular drug delivery. Crit Rev Ther Drug Carrier Syst 15:381–420

27. Edelhauser HF, Maren TH (1988) Permeability of human cornea and sclera to sulfonamide carbonic anhydrase inhibitors. Arch Ophthalmol 106:1110–15

28. Edwards A, Prausnitz MR (1998) Fiber matrix model of sclera and corneal stroma for drug delivery to the eye. AIChE J 44:214–25

29. Erkin Ef, Gunenc, Oner FH, Gelal A, Erkin Y, Guven H (2001) Penetration of amikacin into aqueous humor of rabbits. Ophthalmologica 215:299–302

30. Friedrich S, Cheng YL, Saville B (1997) Drug distribution in the vitreous humour of the human eye: the effects of intravitreal injection position and volume. Curr Eye Res 16:663–9

31. Frohlich E (2002) Structure and function of blood-tissue barriers. Dtsch Med Wochenschr 127:2629–34

32. Grossman R, Lee DA (1998) Transscleral and transcorneal iontophoresis of ketoconazole in the rabbit eye. Ophthalmology 96:724–9

33. Gurny R (1981) Preliminary study of prolonged acting drug delivery systems for the treatment of glaucoma. Pharm Acta Helvetica 56:130–2

34. Halhal M, Renard G, Bejjani RA, Behar-Cohen F (2003) Corneal graft rejection and corticoid iontophoresis: 3 case reports. J Fr Ophtalmol 26(4):391–5

35. Harris R (1967) Iontophoresis. In: Licht S (ed) Therapeutic electricity and ultraviolet radiation. New Haven, Conn

36. Hostyn P, Villain F, Kühne F, Malek N, Parrish RK, Parel J-M (1996) Controlled drug release implant for 5-FU adjuvant therapy in glaucoma. J Fr Ophtalmol 19(2):133–9

37. Hughes L, Maurice DM (1984) A fresh look at ophthalmology. Arch Ophthalmol 102:1825–9

38. Keeley FW, Morin JD, Vesely S (1984) Characterization of collagen from normal human sclera. Exp Eye Res 39:533–42

39. Kimura H, Ogura Y, Hashizoe M, Hishiwaki H, Honda Y, Ikada Y (1994) A new vitreal drug delivery system using implantable biodegradable polymeric device. Invest Ophthalmol Vis Sci 35:2815–19

40. Kimura S, Kobayashi M, Nakamura M, Hirano K, Awaya S, Hoshino T (1995) Immunoelectron microscopic localization of decorin in aged human corneal and scleral stroma. J Electron Microsc (Tokyo) 44:445–9

41. Komai Y, Ushiki, T (1991) The three dimensional organization of collagen fibrils in the human cornea and sclera. Invest Ophthalmol Vis Sci 32:2244–58

42. Kralinger MT, Voigt M, Kieselbach GF, Hamasaki D, Parel J-M (2003) In vivo safety of repetitive Coulomb Controlled Iontophoresis administered Acetylsalicylic acid. Ophthalmic Research 35:102–10

43. Kralinger MT, Hamasaki D, Kieselbach GF, Voigt M, Parel J-M (2001) Intravitreale Applikation von Azetylsalizylsäure mittels Silikonöltamponade. Spektrum Augenheilkd 15(5):194–201

44. Kralinger MT, Kieselbach GF, Voigt M, Parel J-M (2001) Slow release of Acetylsalicylic acid by intravitreal silicone oil. Retina 21:513–20

45. Kralinger MT, Hamasaki D, Kieselbach GF, Voigt MV, Parel J-M (2001) Intravitreal Acetylsalicylic acid in Silicone oil: Pharmacokinetics and evaluation of its safety by ERG and histology. Graefe's Arch Clin Exp Ophthalmol 239:806–16

46. Lam TT, Edward DP, Zhu X, Tso M (1989) Transscleral iontophoresis of dexamethasone. Arch Ophthalmol 107:1368–74

47. Lam TT, Fu J, Chu R, Stojack K, Siew E, Tso MO (1994) Intravitreal delivery of ganciclovir in rabbits by transscleral iontophoresis. J Ocular Pharmacol 10:571–5

48. Lang JC (1995) Ocular drug delivery: conventional ocular formulations. Adv Drug Delivery Rev 16:39–43

49. Larrosa JM, Veloso AAS, Leong FL, Refojo MF (1997) Antiproliferative effect of intravitreal alpha-tocopherol and alpha-tocopheryl acid succinate in a rabbit model of PVR. Curr Eye Res 16:1030–5

50. Lee TW, Robinson JR (2001) Drug delivery to the posterior segment of the eye: some insights on the penetration pathways after subconjunctival injection. J Ocul Pharmacol Ther 17:565–72

51. Lesar TS, Fiscella RG (1985) Antimicrobial drug delivery to the eye. Drug Intell Clin Pharm 19:642–54

52. Lewis H, Kamei M, Skaguchi H, Kaiser P, Zhou T, Schwendeman S (2002) XXIII Club Jules Gonin meeting, Montreux Switzerland 8/31–9/4. Program p 49

53. Lu SX, Anseth KS (1999) Photopolymerization of multilaminated poly (HEMA) hydrogels for controlled release. J Controlled Release 57:291–300

53a. Maurice DM (1986) Iontophoresis of fluorescein into the posterior segment of the rabbit eye. Ophthalmology 93:128–32

54. Maurice DM, Ota Y (1978) The kinetics of subconjunctival injections. Jpn J Ophthalmol 22:95–100

55. Maurice DM, Polgar J (1977) Diffusion across the sclera. Exp Eye Res 25:577–82

56. Meseguer G, Gurny R, Buri P (1994) In vivo evaluation of dosage forms: application of gamma scintigraphy to non-enteral routes of administration. J Drug Targeting 2:269–88

57. Mietz H, Diestelhorst M, Rumpf Af, Theisohn M, Klaus W, Kreigelstein GK (1998) Ocular concentrations of mitomycin C using different delivery devices. Ophthalmologica 212:37–42

58. Miller SC, Donovan MD (1982) Effect of poloxamer 407 gel on the miotic activity of pilocarpine nitrate in rabbits. Int J Pharm 12:147–52

59. Miyamoto H, Ogura Y, Hashizoe M, Kunou N, Honda Y, Ikada Y (1997) Biodegradable scleral implant for intravitreal controlled release of fluconazole. Curr Eye Res 16:930–5

60. Moses R, Hart W (1987) Adler's physiology of the eye: clinical applications, 8th edn. St. Louis: Mosby

61. Nose I, Parel J-M, Lee W, Cohen F, De Kozak Y, Rowaan C, Paldano A, Jallet V, Söderberg PG, Davis J (1996) Ocular Coulomb Controlled Iontophoresis (OCCI). ARVO Invest Ophthalmol Vis Sci 37(3):S41

62. Oakley DE, Weeks RD, Ellis PP (1976) Corneal distribution of subconjunctival antibiotics. Am J Ophthalmol 81:307–12

63. Olsen K, Parel J-M, Lee W, Hernandez E (1989) Biodegradable mechanical retinal fixation: a pilot study. Arch Ophthalmol 107:735–41

64. Parel J-M, Gautier S, Jallet V, Franck Villain (2000) Silicone oils: physico-chemical properties. In: SJ Ryan (ed) Surgical retina, 3nd edn, ch 131. St Louis: CV Mosby Co, pp 2173–94

65. Parel J-M, Behar-Cohen F, Davis J, Murray T, Yoo S (2002) Non-invasive topical drug delivery to retina–choroid via Coulomb Controlled Iontophoresis. XXIII meeting of the Club Jules Gonin, Montreux Switzerland, 8/31–9/4, Program p 24

66. Park K (ed) (1997) Controlled drug delivery challenges and strategies. Washington DC: ACS

67. Perkins SL, Yang CH, Ashton PA, Jaffe GJ (2001) Pharmacokinetics of the silicone filled eye. Retina 21:10–14
68. Robinson JR (1989) Ocular drug delivery mechanisms of corneal drug transport and mucoadhesive delivery systems. S.T.P. Pharm Sci 5:839–46
69. Rootman J, Ostry A, Gudauskas G (1984) Phramacokinetics and metabolism of 5-fluoruracil following subconjuntival versus intravenous administration. Can J Ophthalmol 19:187–91
70. Rozier A, Mauzel C, Grove J, Plazzonnet B (1989) Gelrite: a novel ion activated, in situ gelling polymer for ophthalmic vehicles. Effect of bioavailability of timolol. Int J Pharm 57:163–8
71. Rubsamen PE, Davis PA, Hernandez, et al (1994) Prevention of experimental proliferative vitreoretinopathy with a biodegradable intravitreal implant for the sustained release of fluorouracil. Arch Ophthalmol 112:407–13
72. Rudnick, DE, Noonan JS, Geroski DH, Prausnitz MR, Edelhauser HF (1999) The effect of intraocular pressure on human and rabbit scleral permeability. Invest Ophthalmol Vis Sci 40:3054–8
73. Saettone MF, Chetoni P, Torracca MT, Burgalassi S, Giannaccini B (1989) Evaluation of mucoadhesive properties and in vivo activity of ophthalmic vehicles based on hyaluronic acid. Int J Pharm 72:131–9
74. Sarraf D, Equi RA, Holland GN, Yoshizumi MO, Lee DA (1995) Transscleral iontophoresis of foscarnet. Am J Ophthalmol 115:748–9
75. Sasaki H, Yamamura K, Tei C, Nishida K, Nakamura J (1995) Ocular permeability of FITC-dextran with absorption promoter for ocular delivery of peptide drug. J Drug Target 3:129–35
76. Savic R, Luo L, Eisenberg A, Maysinger D (2003) Micellar nanocontainers distribute to defined cytoplasmic organelles. Science Apr 25:615–18
77. Spector R, Forster R, Rodrigues M, Friedland B, Parel J-M (1984) Improved ocular Natamycin penetration by Iontophoresis. ARVO Invest Ophthalmol Vis Sci 25(3):187
78. Souied EH, Reid S, Nusinowitz S, Kunimura A, Piriev N, Lerner L, Farber DB (2002) Gene transfer into the mouse retina using iontophoresis. ARVO. Invest Ophthalmol Vis Sci, Program summary book. Abstract #2891
79. Souli M, Kopsinis G, Kavouklis E, Gabriel L, Giamarellou H (2001) Vancomycin levels in human aqueous humor after intravenous and subconjunctival administration. Int J Antimicrob Agents 18:239–43
80. Thale A, Tillmann B, Roche R (1996) Scanning electron microscopic studies of the collagen architecture of human sclera – normal and pathological findings. Ophthalmologica 210:137–41
81. Tornquist P, Alm A (1986) Carrier-mediated transport of amino-acids through the blood-retinal and the blood-brain barriers. Graefes Arch Clin Exp Ophthalmol 224:21–5
82. Trier K, Olsen EB, Kobayashi T, Ribel-Madsen SM (1999) Biochemical and ultrastructural changes in rabbit sclera after treatment with 7-methylxanthine, theobromine, acetazolamide or L-ornithine. Br J Ophthalmol 83:1370–5
83. Uhrich K, Cannizzaro SM, Langer RS, Shakesheff KM (1999) Polymeric systems for controlled drug release. Chem Rev 99:3181–98
84. Unlu N, Robinson JR (1998) Scleral permeability to hydrocortisone and mannitol in the albino rabbit eye. J Ocul Pharmacol Ther (1998) 14:273–81
85. Vandamme ThF (2002) Microemulsions as ocular drug delivery systems: recent developments and future challenges. Prog Retinal Eye Res 21:15–34
86. Van Ooteghem (1993) Formulation of ophthalmic solutions and suspensions. Problems and advantages. In: Edman P (ed) Biopharmaceutics of ocular drug delivery. pp 27–42
87. Veloso AMS, Kadrmas EF, Larrosa JM, Sandberg MA, Tolentino FL, Refojo MF (1997) 13-cis-Retinoic acid in silicone-fluorosilicone copolymer oil in a rabbit model of proliferative vitreoretinopathy. Exp Eye Res 65:425–34
88. Vert M, Mauduit J, Li SM (1994) Biodegradation of PLA/GA polymers – increasing complexity. Biomaterials 15:1209–13
89. Voigt M, Kralinger M, Kieselbach G, Chapon P, Hayden B, Anagoste S, Parel J-M (2002) Ocular Aspirin distribution: a comparison of intravenous, topical and Coulomb controlled iontophoresis administration. Invest Ophthalmol Vis Sci 43:3299–306
90. von Sallmann L (1942) Sulfadiazene iontophporesis in pyrocyaneus infection of rabbit cornea. Am J Ophthalmol 25:1292–300
91. Weijtens O, Ferron El, Schoemaker RC, Cohen AF, Lentjes EG, Romijn FP, van Meurs JC (1999) High concentration of dexamethasone in aqueous and vitreous after subconjunctival injection. Am J Ophthalmol 128:192–7

92. Yoo SH, Dursun D, Dubovy S, Miller D, Alfonso EC, Forster RK, Behar-Cohen F, Parel J-M (2002) Iontophoresis for the treatment of Paecilomyces keratitis. Cornea 21:131–2
93. Yoshizumi MO, Dessouki A, Lee DA, Lee G (1997) Determination of ocular toxicity in multiple applications of foscarnet. J Ocular Pharmacol Ther 13:526–36
94. Yang CS, Khawly JA, Hainsworth DP, Chen SN, Ashton P, Guo H, Jaffe GJ (1998) An intravitreal sustained-release triamcinolone and 5-fluoruracil codrug in the treatment of experimental proliferative vitreoretinopathy. Arch Ophthalmol 116:69–77
95. Yasukawa T, Kimura H, Tabata Y, Miyamoto H, Honda Y, Ogura Y (2002) Sustained release of cis-hydroxyproline in the treatment of proliferative vitreoretinopathy in rabbits. Graefes Arch Clin Exp Ophthalmol 240:672–8
96. Zivojnovic R, Mertens DAE, Peperkamp E (1982) Das flüssige Silikon in der Amotiochirurgie II. Berichte über 280 Fälle weitere Entwicklung der Technik. Klin Monatsbl Augenheilkd 181:444–52
97. Zhou T, Lewis H, Foster RE, Schwendeman SP (1998) Development of a multiple-drug delivery implant for proliferative vitreoretinopathy. J Control Release 55:281–95

Correspondence: J.-M. Parel, OBC/BPEI, 1638 NW 10 Avenue, Miami, FL 33136, USA, E-mail: jmparel@med.miami.edu

Minimally invasive vitreoretinal surgery (25-gauge)

E. de Juan Jr., R.R. Lakhanpal, A. Barnes, M.S. Humayun, and G.Y. Fujii

The Retina Institute, Doheny Eye Institute, University of Southern California,
Los Angeles, CA, USA

The 25-gauge Transconjunctival Standard Vitrectomy (25-G TSV) system furthers the trend in ophthalmology towards minimally invasive surgical intervention. Such was the case for phacoemulsification [1–5] as compared to extracapsular cataract extraction in which smaller incision size resulted in faster recovery. The same can be said for 25-G TSV in which smaller self-sealing incisions result in faster patient recovery due to minimal astigmatic effect on the cornea, less ocular discomfort, minimization of the opening and closing portions of the surgery, and less postoperative inflammation due to less ocular trauma.

Previous authors have described methods of creating self-sealing incisions for vitreoretinal surgery [6–11]. Chen [12] described tunnel-based sclerotomies, but the procedure still required performing a conjunctival peritomy and suturing. Numerous complications were also reported using the tunnel-based sclerotomies. Milibák and Süvegas [6] placed sutures in ten of the seventeen cases (59%) performed, and six eyes (35%) exhibited wound leakage after surgery. Jackson and coworkers [9] revealed that ten of their thirty eyes (33%) exhibited wound leakage, two eyes (7%) exhibited vitreous incarceration, and one eye each (3%) exhibited retinal incarceration, wound extension, wound dehiscence, and wound hemorrhage.

Our previous reports from the Doheny Retina Institute (DRI) have outlined the instrumentation and surgical technique associated with the Bausch & Lomb Millennium™ 25-G TSV system [13, 14]. A variety of 25-gauge instruments have been developed over the past few years. One such development is the Entry-Site Alignment System, an integrated cannula system that provides a transconjunctival entry, eliminates the need for conjunctival dissection, and provides a sutureless exit. This allows the non-critical portions of the surgery, the opening and closing, to be minimized. Next, the high-speed vitreous cutter tip mounts to a standard high-speed cutter hand piece with no additional attachments necessary. Experimental studies have shown that the 25-gauge high-speed cutter is capable of removing vitreous at a higher rate than a 20-gauge pneumatic cutter at its standard settings.

Other instruments that have been recently introduced are the following: Endo-Illuminator, Micro Pic Forceps, Vertical Scissors, Extendable Pick, Aspirator, Aspirating Pick, Diathermy Probe, Flexible-Extendable pick, and EndoLaser Probe. The aspirating pick is able to engage membranes and aspirate them into the tip. The vertical acting scissors may be manual actuated or mounted on an automated hand piece. Another new instrument, the flexible-extendable pick, may be used to perform an arteriovenous adventitial sheathotomy without vitrectomy in the case of a branch retinal vein occlusion. The extendable pick allows the curvature to be adjusted and may be fully retracted to facilitate insertion and removal through the Entry-Site Alignment System cannulas. One of the early drawbacks to the system had been that certain procedures required sclerotomy enlargement and introduction of larger instrumentation, such as a Michels' pick for ERM removal or 20-gauge endolaser probe for PDR cases. With the advent of these new instruments, we have the capability of minimal invasive surgery without compromising surgical technique.

We developed the system in such a way that the sclerotomy incisions were small (0.5 mm diameter) as compared to conventional 20-gauge incisions (1.0 mm diameter). Smaller port size with smaller instrumentation results in less ocular trauma and resultant less postoperative inflammation. We found that due to the smaller port size, both the infusion and aspiration rates were less than corresponding 20-gauge systems. On the other hand, the 25-gauge high speed cutter is faster than corresponding 20-gauge systems. The result is a well-balanced infusion/aspiration system that does not prolong vitrectomy time as compared to 20-gauge systems. Complementary vitrectomy time combined with less time for opening and closing steps results in less overall intraoperative surgical time. Also, due to the relative small incision size, most often the sclerotomy sites can be left sutureless [13, 14].

We feel that the 25-G TSV system allows the surgeon to minimize invasiveness while maximizing efficiency in the setting of a large subset of vitreoretinal procedures encountered in everyday practice setting. Such diagnoses include epiretinal membranes (ERM), non-clearing vitreous hemorrhage (NCVH), branch retinal vein occlusion (BRVO), mild tractional retinal detachments (TRD) from proliferative diabetic retinopathy (PDR), macular hole (MH), rhegmatogenous retinal detachment (RRD) in the absence of proliferative vitreoretinopathy (PVR), subretinal neovascular membrane (SRNVM) and pediatric retinopathy surgery such as early retinopathy of prematurity (ROP). These diagnoses are optimal because they do not usually involve aggressive fibrovascular proliferation which may occlude the smaller ports of the 25-Gauge TSV system. Of course, each case should be evaluated carefully because any of these above diagnoses can progress to stages in which dense fibrous tissue may be encountered.

We have recently examined the safety and efficacy of the 25-G TSV system for over one-hundred consecutive primary vitrectomy surgeries at the Doheny Retina Institute (DRI) (*unpublished data*); we found that patients recovered faster due to negligible astigmatic change and minimal inflammation by one week postoperatively. This compared favorably to previous postoperative astigmatic 20-gauge data [15, 16]. Wirbelauer and coworkers [15] found a significant degree of postoperative astigmatism (>1–2 D in many cases) post 20-gauge vitrectomy even after one month. Jampel and coworkers [16] determined that postoperative astigmatism normalized by approximately six to eight weeks post 20-gauge vitrectomy.

Another retrospective study concluded that we have been able to maintain postoperative intraocular pressure in sutureless vitrectomy cases with successively fewer complications, such as blebs and choroidal detachments (*unpublished data*). Furthermore, we are examining comparative data between outcomes of 25-gauge TSV versus standard 20-gauge vitrectomy (*unpublished data*). We intend to examine patient outcomes in these various studies in order to better understand and perfect the system. Further study will continue.

Our ultimate goal is to introduce a system that will allow the surgeon to perform office-based surgery for common vitreoretinal procedures. All surgeries would be under local anesthesia. We are currently examining the feasibility of such an endeavor by providing patients with a detailed questionnaire asking about preferences for sedation during a surgical procedure (*unpublished data*). In this way, we will be able to determine patient preferences for office-based vitreoretinal surgery. Our opinion is that advanced minimally invasive surgical systems utilizing local anesthesia combined with efficient office-based surgical suites may be the next step in vitreoretinal surgery. Further study regarding patient preferences and safety of such an endeavor will be reported upon shortly.

References

1. Cleasby GW (1979) The advantages and disadvantages of Kelman phacoemulsification (KPE). Ophthalmology 86:1973–9
2. Kraff MC, Sanders DR (1982) Planned extracapsular extraction versus phacoemulsification with IOL implantation: a comparison of concurrent series. J Am Intraocul Implant Soc 8:38–41
3. Sanders DR, Spigelman A, Kraff C, et al (1983) Quantitative assessment of postsurgical breakdown of the blood-aqueous barrier. Arch Ophthalmol 101:131–3
4. Kaiya T (1992) Observation of blood-aqueous barrier function after posterior chamber intraocular lens implantation. J Cataract Refract Surg 18:356–61
5. Oshika T, Yoshimura K, Miyata N (1992) Postsurgical inflammation after phacoemulsification and extracapsular extraction with soft or conventional intraocular lens implantation. J Cataract Refract Surg 18:356–61
6. Milibak T, Suveges I (1998) Complications of sutureless pars plana vitrectomy through self-sealing sclerotomies [letter]. Arch Ophthalmol 116:119
7. Kwok AK, Tham CC, Lam DS, et al (1999) Modified sutureless sclerotomies in pars plana vitrectomy. Am J Ophthalmol 127:731–3
8. Schmidt J, Nietgen GW, Brieden S (1999) Self-sealing, Sutureless sclerotomy in pars plana vitrectomy. Klin Monatsbl Augenheilkd 215:247–51
9. Jackson T (2000) Modified sutureless sclerotomies in pars plana vitrectomy [letter]. Am J Ophthalmol 129:116–7
10. Lam DS, Chua JK, Leung AT, et al (2000) Sutureless pars plana anterior vitrectomy through self-sealing sclerotomies in children. Arch Ophthalmol 118:850–1
11. Rahman R, Rosen PH, Riddell C, Towler H (2000) Self-sealing sclerotomies for sutureless pars plana vitrectomy. Ophthalmic Surg Lasers 31:462–6
12. Chen JC (1996) Sutureless pars plana vitrectomy through self-sealing sclerotomies. Arch Ophthalmol 114:1273–5
13. Fujii GY, de Juan, Jr E, Humayun MS, et al (2002) A new 25-gauge instrument system for transconjunctival sutureless vitrectomy surgery. Ophthalmology 109:1807–13
14. Fujii GY, de Juan, Jr E, Humayun MS, et al (2002) Initial experience using the transconjunctival sutureless vitrectomy system for vitreoretinal surgery. Ophthalmology 109:1814–20
15. Wirbelauer C, Hoerauf H, Roider J, Laqua H (1998) Corneal shape changes after pars plana vitrectomy. Graefe's Arch Clin Exp Ophthalmol 236:822–8
16. Jampel HD, Thompson JT, Nunez M, Michels RG (1987) Corneal astigmatic changes after pars plana vitrectomy. Retina 7:223–6

Correspondence: Eugene de Juan, jr, MD, Retina Institute, Doheny Eye Institute, University of Southern California, 1450 San Pablo St, DEI-3600, Los Angeles, CA 90033, USA, E-mail: dejuan@usc.edu

Indocyanine-green enhanced vitreous surgery

A. Abri, S. Binder, A. Assadoullina, and S. Brunner

Department of Ophthalmology, Rudolf Foundation Hospital, Vienna, Austria

Introduction

Direct treatment of macular diseases became possible as vitreous surgery technique improved [1–4]. Thereafter, reports showed that the internal limiting membrane (ILM) could play a major role in the relaxation of macular hole borders [5–7].

Indocyanine green (ICG) is a tricarboncyanin $C_{43}H_{47}N_2NaO_6S_2$ – molecule with a molecular weight of 775 and an absorption maximum of 800 nm. The intra-operative application of ICG may improve visualization and preparation of the ILM and other fine epiretinal membranes.

Purpose

To describe the dosage and technique of the intravitreal use of ICG in a consecutive series of eyes with macular diseases and compare it with a control group in a retrospective study.

Material and methods

A total of 115 eyes underwent vitreoretinal surgery for macular diseases. ICG was used in 42 eyes of 40 patients from March 2001 to March 2002. Indications for surgery were a macular hole (MH) (22 eyes) and macular pucker (MP) (20 eyes) for either direct staining of the ILM or staining of the edges of a vitreoretinal membrane. Patients had complete clinical examinations before and after surgery. In addition, fluorescence angiography, multifocal electroretinography and optical coherence tomography (Fig. 2) were performed in 3 months intervals thereafter. In this study, visual acuity outcome and intra- and postoperative complications were compared with a control group (n = 75) operated in the year before (Tables 1 and 2).

Technique: The filtered and diluted (1.5 mg/ml) ICG is gently injected in the fluid filled vitreous cavity over the retinal surface. Not more than 0.2–0.4 ml of the solution are generally used. After a contact time of 1 minute the ICG is rinsed from the vitreous cavity completely. An endgripping forceps is used to grasp and peel the dyed ILM or edges of the epiretinal membrane as complete as possible (Fig. 1).

Results

Macular pucker
Visual acuity improved in 90% of patients of the ICG group, but only in 73% of non-ICG controls (Table 3). It deteriorated in only 5% of patients treated with ICG and in 20% of controls, which seems to be a substantial difference.

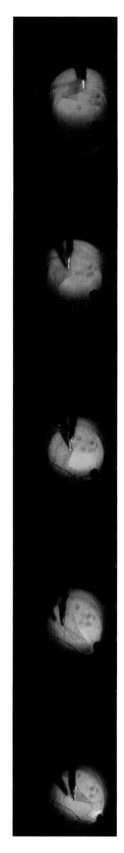

Fig. 1. Intra-operative peeling of ICG stained membrane

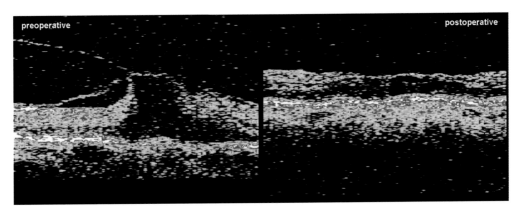

Fig. 2. OCT imaging (patient 5) in case of stage II macular hole with vitreous traction

Table 1. Macular pucker

	with ICG	without ICG
Patients	20 (8 f, 12 m)	57 (32 f, 25 m)
Eyes	20	57
Age (mean)	69,9	69,3
Anamnesis:		
idiopathic	13 (65%)	43 (74%)
St. p. detachment	1 (5%)	4 (7%)
St. p. laser	3 (15%)	5 (8,5%)
Myopia alta	–	2 (3,5%)
Synchisis. sc.	–	2 (3,5%)
Retinoschisis	–	1 (1,8%)
St. p. uveitis	1 (5%)	–
St. p. ppV	1 (5%)	–
St. p. CVT	1 (5%)	–

Table 2. Macular hole

	with ICG	without ICG
Patients	22 (15 f, 7 m)	16 (12 f, 4 m)
Eyes	22	18
Age (mean)	71	69
Anamnesis		
idiopathic	18 (81,8%)	16 (89%)
St. p. laser	2 (9,1%)	–
Synchisis. sc.	–	1 (5,5%)
St. p. ppV	2 (9,1%)	1 (5,5%)
Stages of macular hole:		
I	–	–
II	1 (4,55%)	1 (5,5%)
III	10 (45,5%)	10 (55%)
IV	11 (50%)	7 (39,5%)

Macular hole

Visual acuity improved in 63.6% of the ICG group compared to 55.5% of non-ICG controls (Table 4). It deteriorated in 9% of the ICG group, but in 22.5% of controls.

It was interesting to observe that the predominant macular hole stage (staging after Gass [11]) was stage IV in the ICG group and stage III in the non-ICG group (Table 2).

Table 3. Outcome of patients with macular nuclear

	VA ↑	VA →	VA ↓
ppV + ICG	18 (90%)	1 (5%)	1 (5%)
ppV	43 (73%)	4 (7%)	11 (20%)

VA visual acuity

Table 4. Outcome of patients with macular hole

	VA ↑	VA ↔	VA ↓
ppV + ICG	14 (63,6%)	6 (27,3%)	2 (9,1%)
ppV	10 (55,5%)	4 (22,5%)	4 (22,5%)

VA visual acuity

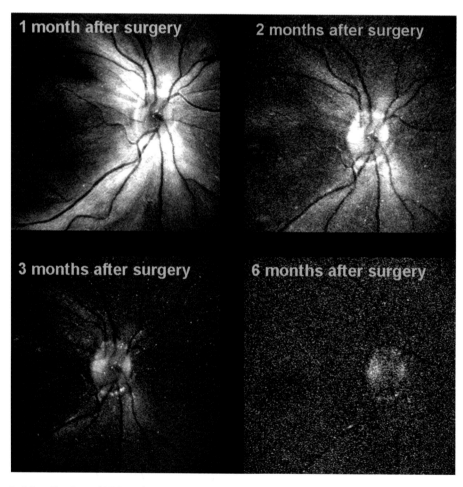

Fig. 3. Visualization of ICG in the neuroretina of an operated eye (for up to 6 months after surgery)

Conclusion

Peeling of the internal limiting membrane (ILM) is a highly sophisticated surgical skill. The visualization of the ILM or overlying structures (e.g. epiretinal membranes or parts of the posterior vitreous body) can be improved by intra-operative staining with Indocyanine green (ICG) [8–10]. This procedure may help surgeons to shorten peeling time for a fine removal of the ILM and other epiretinal membranes, thereby also reducing light toxicity.

Based on our first results we believe that the current procedure with the dosage described is safe. Dying of transparent membranes is clearly helpful in the understanding of the pathomechanism of the vitreoretinal interface and leads to lesser surgical trauma with more complete removal of the tissue. Better functional outcomes were found in our series, when compared with a control group. However, only long-term observation and controlled randomized studies will give us the final information.

In our patients, we have observed that ICG may be visualized in the neuroretina of operated eyes for up to 6 months after surgery (Fig. 3). Therefore, many questions remain unanswered for the moment, concerning toxicity, type of application, or concentration and osmolarity of ICG.

References

1. Michels RG (1984) Vitrectomy for macular pucker. Ophthalmology 91:1384–1388
2. Kelly NE, Wendel RT (1991) Vitreous surgery for macular holes. Results of a pilot study. Arch Ophthalmol 109:654–9
3. Smiddy WE, Michels RG, Glaser BM, de Bustros S (1988) Vitrectomy for macular traction caused by incomplete vitreous separation. Arch Ophthalmol 106:624–8
4. Kampik A, Green WR, Michels RG, Nase PK (1980) Ultrastructural features of progressive idiopatic epiretinal membrane removed by vitreous surgery. Am J Ophthalmol 90:797–809 t
5. Eckhardt C, Eckhardt U, Groos S, et al (1997) Entfernung der Membrana limitans interna bei Maculalöchern. Klinische und morphologische Befunde. Ophthalmologe 94:545–51
6. Park DW, Sipperley JO, Sneed SR, et al (1999) Macular hole surgery with internal-limiting membrane peeling and intravitreous air. Ophthalmology 110:610–8
7. Brooks HL Jr (2000) Macular hole surgery with and without internal limiting membrane peeling. Ophthalmology 107:1939–48
8. Kim U, Clark J (1999) ICG as an aid to membrane peeling in macular hole surgery (scientific poster 349, AAO 1999, Orlando)
9. Kadonosono K, Itoh N, Uchio E, Nakamura S, Ohno S (2000) Staining of internal limiting membrane in macular hole surgery. Arch Ophthalmol 118:1116–8
10. Gandorfer A, Messmer EM, Ulbig MW, Kampik A (2001) Indocyanin green selectively stains the internal limiting membrane. Am J Ophthalmol 131:387–8
11. Gass JD (1995) Reappraisal of biomicroscopic classification of stages of development of macular hole. Am J Ophthalmol 119:752–9

Correspondence: Dr. Ali Abri, Department of Ophthalmology, Rudolf Foundation Hospital, Juchgasse 25, A-1030 Vienna, Austria, E-mail: ali.abri@kar.magwien.gv.at

Epi-retinal prosthesis

E. de Juan Jr, J. D. Weiland, M. S. Humayun, and G. Y. Fujii

The Retina Institute, Doheny Eye Institute, University of Southern
California, Los Angeles, CA, USA

Introduction

Retinitis pigmentosa (RP) and age-related macula degeneration (AMD) lead to the degeneration of photoreceptors, resulting in a significant visual deficit for the afflicted individual [1]. Research is proceeding to investigate the feasibility of replacing the function of the photoreceptors with an electronic device [2, 3]. The photoreceptors initiate a neural signal in response to light. The experiments to be discussed investigate the possibility of using electrical signals (generated by a retinal prosthesis) to initiate a neural response in the remaining cells of the retina. Results from both animal and human research conducted over the past decade have established the following: Intraocular stimulating electrodes can evoke focal responses that correlate with the stimulus position and timing [4–6], the inner retina in RP and AMD is relatively unharmed even when the outer retina is severely degenerated [7–9], and a device can be implanted on the surface of the retina without causing significant damage to the retina [10, 11]. Based on these preliminary trials, an FDA approved clinical trial was intiated to assess safety of implantation of an epiretinal device in humans blind from retinitis pigmentosa. 2 human volunteers have used permanently implanted devices to detect ambient light and sense motion. Based on these encouraging results, the current focus is being shifted from feasibility studies to the development of an implantable, electronic device, which will be capable of stimulating the retina at hundreds of individual points.

Background

A retinal prosthesis system consists of several elements (Fig. 1). A video camera will capture an image and convert it to an electric signal. The electric signal will be appropriately coded and then sent via telemetry to an implanted receiver. The receiver will decode the signal and generate the desired current pulse pattern for the stimulating array. The engineering of the system, while seemingly daunting, is considered feasible.

Our approach is analogous to that of the cochlear implant. The cochlear implant electrically stimulates the auditory nerve, bypassing damaged cochlear hair cells, to produce the sensation of sound. Using only six electrical inputs to the auditory nerve, which contains approximately 30,000 fibers, the cochlear implant can produce sound perception with sufficient fidelity to enable a deaf individual to speak on an ordinary telephone [12]. Additionally, cochlear implant patients improve their ability to hear with practice. This suggests that the brain can adapt to the reduced input and, with training, restore significant sensory function. Research in the visual system has shown that reducing visual input to a 25×25 array of pixels still allows a good degree of mobility [13]. These are encouraging examples when one considers that a retinal implant will provide input to a system designed to process information from 1 million ganglion cells.

Previous experiments show that electrical stimulation of the visual system produces the perception of vision (as opposed to tactile or pain sensation). Stimulation of the visual

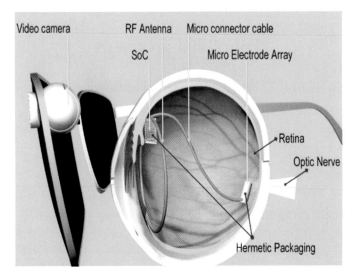

Fig. 1. Retinal prosthesis concept. A video camera mounted in glasses will capture an image. Video processing electronics will convert the image into a radio frequency signal which is transmitted to an implanted device. The conceptual drawing shown here places the entire device inside the eye. The prototype device currently under test has part of the implanted device extraocular due to the size of the device

cortex has been shown to produce phosphenes [14, 15]. In our lab, human volunteers are evaluated prior to surgery with electrical stimulation of the globe with a contact lens electrode. The subjects have been able to "see flashes" when the electrical current is applied.

The feasibility of a retinal prosthesis is supported by several studies. Morphometric analyses in post-mortem eyes with almost complete photoreceptor loss either due to RP or AMD have shown as many as 90% of the inner retinal neurons remain histologically intact [7, 8, 9, 16, 17]. In tests where electrical stimulating devices were temporarily positioned on the retina, blind subjects reported seeing percepts that corresponded in time and location to the electrical stimulus [4–6]. Several research groups have investigated various aspects of retinal prosthesis, ranging from electrical stimulation of retinal neurons to surgical implantation methods [18–20]. Two distinct retinal prosthesis efforts have materialized depending on the position of the stimulating electrode array. In the first, the electrodes are positioned on the ganglion cell side of the retina (epiretinal approach), [19, 21] whereas, in the second the electrodes and most of the electronics are placed between the retina and the retinal pigment epithelium (subretinal approach) [22]. Both approaches have advantages and disadvantages. The device developed for this study has a 16 electrode stimulating array positioned on the epiretinal surface, an electronic implant positioned outside the eye to generate stimulation pulses, and an external system for image acquisition, processing, and wireless communication (to the implanted unit).

Material and methods

Subject selection

The study was approved by the United States Food and Drug Administration and the University of Southern California Institutional Review Board. Two subjects with bare or no light perception secondary to photoreceptor loss were enrolled in the study. Subjects with

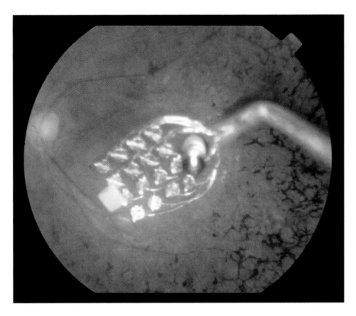

Fig. 2. Fundus photo is subject 2, 2 months post operative. Retinal blood vessels are noted under the array and no gross damage to the retina is evident

visual loss due to all other causes were excluded. The electronic device implanted was developed by our group in conjunction with Second Sight, LLC™ (Valencia, CA). It consists of an implanted and an external unit. The external unit consists of a small camera worn in the glasses that connects to a belt-worn visual processing unit. The electronic implant was secured to the skull in similar fashion to cochlear implants. The cable was routed to the orbit and then into the eye through a 5 mm circumferential scleral incision placed 3 mm posterior to the limbus. Prior to introduction of the implant, the majority of the vitreous gel was removed. The electrode array was then positioned just temporal to the fovea and a single retinal tack (Second Sight Retinal Tack) was inserted through the electrode array and into the sclera. At the end of the implant procedure, the device was tested electrically to assure that all wires were intact.

Results

Two subjects with bare or no-light perception were implanted with the Model 1 Retinal Stimulator subjects had bare light perception or no-light perception in the implanted eye. The surgical implantation was without any complications (Fig. 2). Electrical stimulation testing focused on two main areas: percepts from single electrode activity (stimulus pattern controlled by computer) and percepts from multiple electrode activity (stimulus pattern controlled by the camera).

Single electrode studies focused on determining the amount of electrical energy required to reliably produce a percept reported by the subject. This level of electrical stimulus is called the stimulus threshold. The timing of the pulse was typically a biphasic current pulse, 1 ms/phase with a 1 ms intraphase delay. These numbers were chosen based on prior studies that suggest a stimulus impulse longer than 0.5 ms can target bipolar cells. The stimulus threshold for subject 1(S1) ranged from 28–1.3 mA and for subject 2(S2) ranged from 43–679 µA. Subjects reported false positive less than 5% of the time. The test subjects reported seeing small spots or half circles that were typically white or yellow. In

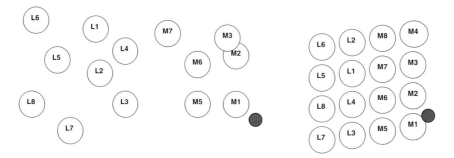

Patient Reported Locations

Expected Results based on Retinal Location of Electrode

Fig. 3. Spatial map reported by Subject 1. Red dot indicates the estimated center of vision based on the location of fovea. The array was positioned temporal to the fovea in the right eye, so most of the subject percepts were to the left

both subjects, the reported spatial location of the percept in general corresponded to the retinal location of the stimulating electrode. The implant in S1 was temporal to the fovea in the right and thus all percepts appeared to the left (Fig. 3). In S2, the electrodes were on either side of the fovea and percepts were reported on both the left and right.

Both subjects demonstrated the ability to use a head-mounted video camera to detect ambient light, to locate and count objects, and to distinguish the direction of motion of objects. Testing was done in a double masked fashion after training the subject. The tests were forced choice tests. For example, in an pattern recognition task, the subject was asked to describe the orientation of a tumbling L, which was presented in 1 of 4 orientations (Fig. 4). The results are presented as a percentage or fraction based on thee number of correct response and the total number of tests. Both subjects demonstrated the ability to detect room lights on or off with 100% accuracy (10/10 and 10/10). The subjects are able to count and localize up to two objects: 60% (12 in 20 for S1) and 90% (9 in 10 for S2). Using the camera, S1 could correctly identify the orientation of a tumbling L (four alternative, forced choice) in 15 of 20 attempts (75%) (Fig. 4). Both subjects could identify object movement directions (S1: 4/5 correct, S2 7/10 correct).

Summary

Retinitis pigmentosa afflicts 1/4000 and a large number of these patients become legally blind in their 5th decade. An even greater number of people lose vision due to photoreceptor loss in age related macular degeneration (AMD). Although some treatments to slow the progression of AMD are available, no treatment exists that can replace the function of lost photoreceptors. We have summarized our results from 2 test subjects implanted with an electronic retinal prosthesis Electrical stimulation results in the subjects seeing spots of light (phosphenes) that are both reliable and reproducible with respect to the spatial location of the stimulating electrodes on the retina and the stimulating electrical current. Currently, the subjects can determine some directional movement and perform object recognition tasks. Further training and testing will be necessary to determine the maximum effectiveness of this type of treatment for restoring vision that would allow

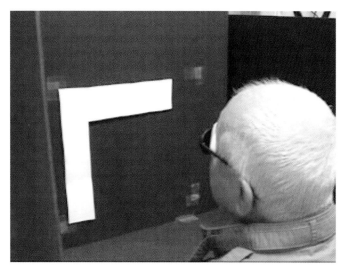

Fig. 4. Pattern recognition task. Subject used a head mounted video camera to determine the orientation of the tumbling L. Responses were limited to 4 choices. Subject could successfully identify the orientation of the L 75% of the time

mobility and recognition of more complex objects. The next generation electronic retinal prosthesis is expected to provide higher number of electrodes and more complex stimulation control capability.

References

1. Heckenlively JR, Boughman J, Friedman L (1988) Diagnosis and classification of retinitis pigmentosa. In: Heckenlively JR (ed) Retinitis pigmentosa. Philadelphia, PA: JB Lippincott, 21
2. Zrenner E (2002) Will retinal implants restore vision? Science 295(5557):1022–5
3. Margalit E, Maia M, Weiland JD, Greenberg RJ, Fujii GY, Torres G, et al (2002) Retinal prosthesis for the blind. Surv Ophthalmol 47(4):335–56
4. Humayun MS, de Juan EJ, Weiland JD, Dagnelie G, Katona S, Greenberg RJ, et al (1999) Pattern electrical stimulation of the human retina. Vision Research 39:2569–76
5. Weiland JD, Humayun MS, Dagnelie G, de Juan JE, Jr., Greenberg RJ, Iliff NT (1999) Understanding the origin of visual percepts elicited by electrical stimulation of the human retina. Graefes Arch Clin Exp Ophthalmol 237(12):1007–13
6. Rizzo J, Wyatt J, Loewenstein J, Kelly S (2000) Acute intraocular retinal stimulation in normal and blind humans. ARVO abstracts [532]
7. Stone JL, Barlow WE, Humayun MS, de Juan EJ, Milam AH (1992) Morphometric analysis of macular photoreceptors and ganglion cells in retinas with retinitis pigmentosa. Arch Ophthalmol 110(11):1634–9
8. Santos A, Humayun MS, de Juan EJ, Greenburg RJ, Marsh MJ, Klock IB, et al (1997) Preservation of the inner retina in retinitis pigmentosa. A morphometric analysis. Arch Ophthalmol 115(4):511–15
9. Kim S, Sadda S, Pearlman J, Humayun M, de Juan EJ, Melia M, et al (2001) Morphometric analysis of the macula in eyes with disciform age-related macular degeneration. Arch Ophthalmol (Submitted)
10. Majji AB, Humayun MS, Weiland JD, Suzuki S, D'Anna SA, de Juan JE Jr (1999) Long-term histological and electrophysiological results of an inactive epiretinal electrode array implantation in dogs. Invest Ophthalmol Vis Sci 40(9):2073–81
11. Margalit E, Fujii G, Lai J, Gupta P, Chen S, Shyu J, et al (2000) Bioadhesives for intraocular use. Retina 20:469–77

12. House WF (1976) Cochlear implants. Ann Otol Rhinol Laryngol 85 [Suppl 27](3Pt2):1–93
13. Cha K, Horch K, Normann RA (1992) Simulation of a phosphene-based visual field: visual acuity in a pixelized vision system. Ann Biomed Eng 20(4):439–49
14. Veraart C, Raftopoulos C, Mortimer JT, Delbeke J, Pins D, Michaux G, et al (1998) Visual sensations produced by optic nerve stimulation using an implanted self-sizing spiral cuff electrode. Brain Res 813(1):181–6
15. Schmidt EM, Bak MJ, Hambrecht FT, Kufta CV, O'Rourke DK, Vallabhanath P (1996) Feasibility of a visual prosthesis for the blind based on intracortical microstimulation of the visual cortex. Brain 119(Pt 2):507–22
16. Butler LD, Stieglitz TL (1993) Contagion in schizophrenia: a critique of Crow and Done (1986). Schizophr Bull 19(3):449–54
17. Blau A, Ziegler C, Heyer M, Endres F, Schwitzgebel G, Matthies T, et al (1997) Characterization and optimization of microelectrode arrays for in vivo nerve signal recording and stimulation. Biosens Bioelectron 12(9–10):883–92
18. Thielecke H, Stieglitz T, Beutel H, Matthies T, Ruf HH, Meyer JU (1999) Fast and precise positioning of single cells on planar electrode substrates. IEEE Eng Med Biol Mag 18(6):48–52
19. Rizzo J, Wyatt J (1997) Prospects for a visual prosthesis. Neuroscientist 3:251–62
20. Zrenner E, Miliczek KD, Gabel VP, Graf HG, Guenther E, Haemmerle H, et al (1997) The development of subretinal microphotodiodes for replacement of degenerated photoreceptors [see comments]. Ophthalmic Res 29(5):269–80
21. Eckmiller R (1997) Learning retina implants with epiretinal contacts. Ophthalmic Res 29(5):281–9
22. Chow AY, Chow VY (1997) Subretinal electrical stimulation of the rabbit retina. Neurosci Lett 225(1):13–16

Correspondence: Eugene de Juan, Jr, MD, The Retina Institute, Doheny Eye Institute, University of Southern California, 1450 San Pablo St, DEI-3600, Los Angeles, CA 90033, USA, E-mail: dejuan@usc.edu

The subretinal implant – present status of the German Research Group

H. G. Sachs and V.-P. Gabel

University Eye Clinic, Regensburg, Germany

The presentation summarizes the experience of the German Subretinal Implant Research Group and gives an overview of the present status.

The key questions in the subretinal implant project is how to replace degenerated photoreceptors by a safe subretinal Micro-Photodiode Array that provides sufficient spatial resolution and contrast vision in natural ambient light levels.

The subretinal concept

- the function of the degenerated photoreceptors is substituted in their physiologic original position by an electronic implant
- the remaining neuronal structure is used for signal transduction
- a fixation of the prosthesis in the subretinal space does not result in difficulties
- PVR risk seems minimal for the subretinal attempt
- there is no need for an external camera like in the epiretinal concept
- the built-in circuits allow a stimulation over a wide range of luminance
- the eye movements can be used to follow objects

The consortium first started to develop a passive Micro-Photodiode-Array (MPDA) (see Fig. 1)

- this MPDA uses the available light to stimulate the retina
- there are good manageable modified surgical standard procedures (e.g. modified standard 3 port vitrectomy)
- there are no fixation problems
- stable retinal conditions are established by long term follow up (up to 3 years) in the minipig model.

The prototype of this implant consisted of 7000 pixels (micro photo diodes)

What could be learned from this passive implants (MPDA's) in in vivo animal experiments (cat and minipig)?

- that the proof of cortical activation (optical imaging) is only possible with this type of implant when using unphysiologically bright light levels (that means we had to expose the subretinal implant to a laser light to demonstrate a cortical activation; with ambient light levels no cortical response was detectable)
- there is obviously and requirement of an additional energy supply of an subretinal implant:
  - the passive MPDA (alone) did not evoke cortical responses in the cat and minipig in ambient light conditions
  - there is a necessity for additional energy supply for subretinal stimulation

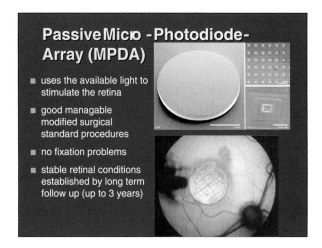

Fig. 1

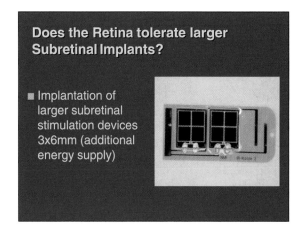

Fig. 2

The question which was to answer was: Does the retina tolerate larger subretinal implants which allow an additional energy supply in form of infrared energy in long term follow up? (see Fig. 2)

– implantation of larger subretinal stimulation devices (3 × 6 mm) which aloud an additional energy supply were carried out with prototypes.

Results of the implantation of complex stimulation structures

• good toleration of the complex implants in the follow up period of up to 1 year in the minipig model (see Fig. 3)
• no adverse events especially no retinal detachment in the follow up period
• no dislocation and encouraging histological findings in the minipig model

Design of the current prototype

– active implant with the stimulation chip and the subretinal localized IR-receiver and an additional extraocular part of electronic components. (see Fig. 4)

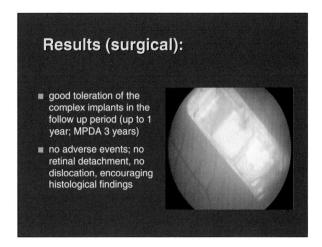

Fig. 3

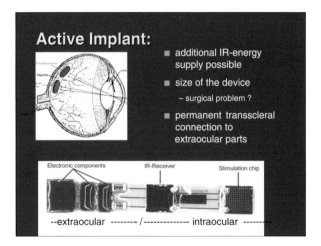

Fig. 4

Surgical aspects

– this complex structures could be handled with our modified implantation procedure
– feasibility of permanent transscleral connection to extraocular parts

The different implantation strategies

– three different way's to implant subretinal structures (see Fig. 5)
– ab interno procedure were the implant is inserted during a modified standard 3-port vitrectomy
– ab externo version were an transscleral access is used to place the subretinal device (was successfully demonstrated in rabbits)
– combined ab interno and transsclerel access (in this procedure the retina is detached during a pars plana vitrectomy like in macular translocation surgery and an additional safe transscleral access is used for the implantation of the foil bound active devices under the detached retina)

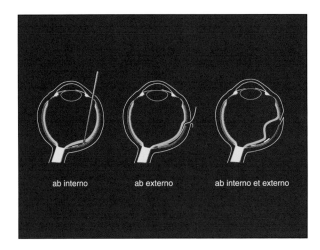

Fig. 5

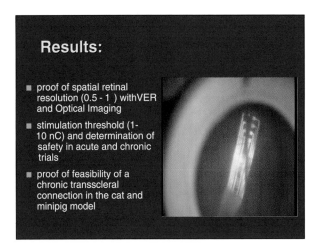

Fig. 6

Steps in the development of the subretinal prosthesis

- determination of stimulation parameters with stimulation foils
- determination of thresholds and spatial resolution with foil-stimulators (the foil-stimulators had a contact plate outside of the eye, which was connected during the trials)
- function testing with multi-electrode matrices from the cat brain in the Department of Physics at the University of Marburg
- proof of a spatial resolution of about one degree visual angle for the cat eye
- optical imaging as alternate procedure to demonstrate the topographical specifity (applied at the University of Bochum

Results of the stimulation experiments (see Fig. 6)

- proof of spatial resolution of the retina of about 0.5–1° with VEP and Optical Imaging.
- the stimulation threshold was determined with 1–10 nC

– determination of safety thresholds in acute and chronic trails
– proof the feasibility of a chronic transscleral connection in the cat and minipig model.

Conclusion

The principle feasibility of the subretinal approach has been shown in electrophysiological experiments. The chronic tolerance of larger subretinal implants was shown. The concept of an additional energy supply for a subretinal implant was evaluated making this type of active prosthesis applicable for ambient light conditions.

Acknowledgements

Professor Zrenner from the University Eye Hospital in Tuebingen coordinates the German Subretinal Implant Research Group. In this cooperation the University Eye Clinic in Regensburg is developing the surgical access for the subretinal implants. The implant is developed by the Natural Science Institute (NMI) of the University of Tuebingen, in Reutlingen, the Institute of Physics and Electronics (IPE) of the University of Stuttgart and the Institute of Microelectronics (IMS) in Stuttgart. Other project partners are the Institute of Neurophysiology at the University Bochum and the Institute of Neurophysics at the University of Marburg were the electrophysiological examinations are done.
Grant: German Ministry of Research (BMBF)

Correspondence: Dr. Helmut G. Sachs, University Eye Clinic, Franz Josef Strauss Allee 11, D-93042 Regensburg, Germany, E-mail: sachs@eye-regensburg.de

Index

SpringerOphthalmologie

Spektrum
der Augenheilkunde

Zeitschrift der Österreichischen
Ophthalmologischen Gesellschaft – ÖOG

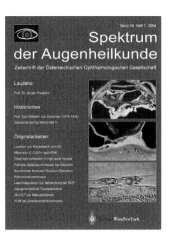

Bezugsbedingungen
2004. Bd. 18 (6 Hefte)
ISSN 0930-4282, Titel–Nr. 717
EUR 179,– plus Versandkosten

Herausgegeben von:
S. Binder, Wien (verantwortlich)
J. Faulborn, Graz
W. Göttinger, Innsbruck

Schriftleitung:
P. Drobec, Wien

Fachbeirat:

H. Busse, Münster
J. Draeger, Hamburg
V. P. Gabel, Regensburg
H. D. Gnad, Wien
G. Grabner, Salzburg
A. Huber, Zürich
V. Huber-Spitzy, Wien
P. Kroll, Marburg
O. E. Lund, München
M. Mertz, München
K. Ossoinig, Iowa City

H. Remky, München
G. Richard, Hamburg
R. Rochels, Kiel
K. W. Ruprecht, Homburg
K. Schirmer, Montreal
H. Slezak, Wien
P. Speiser, St. Gallen
W. Stark, Baltimore
J. Stepanik, Wien
F. Todter, St. Pölten
R. Winter, Hannover

Spektrum der Augenheilkunde ist eine Fortbildungszeitschrift für Ophthalmologen in Klinik und Praxis. Sie erscheint sechsmal jährlich und publiziert Übersichten (Reviews), Originalarbeiten, Editorials, Kasuistiken und Analysen über Innovationen auf dem Geräte- und Instrumentensektor. Leserbrief, Gastkommentare, Buchbesprechungen, Literaturübersichten, Produktinformationen und ein Kongresskalender ergänzen das Informationsspektrum.

Spektrum der Augenheilkunde informiert somit den Augenarzt aktuell über neue Entwicklungen in Klinik und Forschung, die für seine Praxis Relevanz besitzen. Die fachliche Kompetenz der Herausgeber und des Fachbeirates garantieren eine ausgewogene inhaltliche Gestaltung.

SpringerWienNewYork

P.O. Box 89, Sachsenplatz 4–6, 1201 Wien, Österreich, Fax +43.1.330 24 26, e-mail: books@springer.at, **springer.at**
Haberstraße 7, 69126 Heidelberg, Deutschland, Fax +49.6221.345-4229, e-mail: orders@springer.de, springer.de
P.O. Box 2485, Secaucus, NJ 07096-2485, USA, Fax +1.201.348-4505, e-mail: orders@springer-ny.com
Eastern Book Service, 3–13, Hongo 3-chome, Bunkyo-ku, Japan, Tokyo 113, Fax +81.3.38 18 08 64, e-mail: orders@svt-ebs.co.jp
Preisänderungen und Irrtümer vorbehalten.

SpringerPsychologie

Josef Grünberger

Pupillometrie in der klinisch-psychophysiologischen Diagnostik

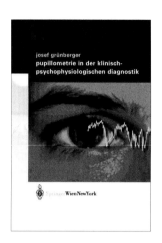

2003. XVI, 249 Seiten. 72 Abbildungen.
Text: deutsch/englisch
Broschiert **EUR 44,95**, sFr 68,–
ISBN 3-211-83854-6

Die Pupille gilt als das Fenster zur Seele. Starke Gefühle, Erregungen oder Gefühlsregungen führen zu einer Erweiterung der Pupille. Die objektive und ökonomische Messung der Pupillenreaktion als Parameter der vegetativen Erregung hat in den letzten Jahren zunehmend an Bedeutung gewonnen, da sowohl die Aufnahme- als auch die Auswertungstechniken wesentlich verbessert werden konnten.

Der Autor gibt einen Überblick über die computergesteuerte statische und dynamische Pupillenmessung an Patienten mit verschiedenen psychosomatischen Krankheitsbildern, wie beispielsweise Ulcus, Colitis, Herzneurose, Anorexie und Asthma.

Der Einsatz und die Bedeutung der statischen Messung bei gesunden jungen und älteren Menschen in der Psychopharmakologie und bei psychischen Störungen wird erläutert. Weiters werden die dynamischen Pupillenreaktionen auf verschiedene sensorische Stimuli (optische und akustische) verglichen.

„... bietet einen ineressanten Einblick in ein neues Feld der medizinischen Diagnostik."

Hausarzt

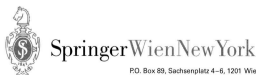

SpringerWienNewYork

P.O. Box 89, Sachsenplatz 4–6, 1201 Wien, Österreich, Fax +43.1.330 24 26, e-mail: books@springer.at, **springer.at**
Haberstraße 7, 69126 Heidelberg, Deutschland, Fax +49.6221.345-4229, e-mail: orders@springer.de, springer.de
P.O. Box 2485, Secaucus, NJ 07096-2485, USA, Fax +1.201.348-4505, e-mail: orders@springer-ny.com
Eastern Book Service, 3–13, Hongo 3-chome, Bunkyo-ku, Japan, Tokyo 113, Fax +81.3.38 18 08 64, e-mail: orders@svt-ebs.co.jp
Preisänderungen und Irrtümer vorbehalten.

SpringerOpthalmologie

Josef Zihl,
Siegfried Priglinger

Sehstörungen bei Kindern

Diagnostik und Frühförderung

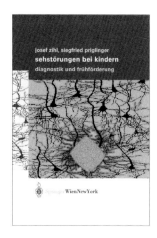

2002. XI, 183 Seiten. 21 Abbildungen.
Broschiert **EUR 29,–**, sFr 49,50
ISBN 3-211-83608-X

Dieses Buch beschäftigt sich mit der Entwicklung und den Störungen der visuellen Wahrnehmung bei Kindern. Die einzelnen Kapitel befassen sich mit der Organisation und Funktionsweise des Zentralnervensystems, insbesondere des visuellen Systems und der Okulomotorik, der Entwicklung der verschiedenen Teilleistungen, ihren Störungen, Aspekten der Sehbehinderung sowie der Diagnostik und Dokumentation von Funktionsstörungen. Im lezten Kapitel werden die diagnostischen und therapeutischen Vorgehensweisen beispielhaft an vier Einzelfällen dargestellt.

Ein umfangreiches Literaturverzeichnis sowie zahlreiche Abbildungen und Tabellen vervollständigen das Buch. Die Besonderheiten dieses Buches liegen in der empirisch fundierten Darstellung der visuellen Teilleistungen und ihrer Störungen auf dem Hintergrund der zentralnervösen Organisation von Kognition, Erleben und Handeln sowie in der Anwendung neuer wissenschaftlicher Erkenntnisse in Diagnostik und Behandlung bzw. Frühförderung von Kindern mit Sehstörungen.

„... Den Autoren ist eine Überblicksdarstellung visueller Teilleistungen, ihrer Störungen[,] sowie deren Diagnostik und Therapie unter Einbeziehung neuester wissenschaftlicher Erkenntnisse als auch praktischer Gesichtspunkte gelungen ... für alle mit kindlichen Sehstörungen beschäftigten Berufsgruppen ein lohnendes Buch zum Einstieg in die Problematik."

Klinische Monatsblätter für Augenheilkunde

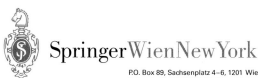

Springer Wien New York

P.O. Box 89, Sachsenplatz 4–6, 1201 Wien, Österreich, Fax +43.1.330 24 26, e-mail: books@springer.at, **springer.at**
Haberstraße 7, 69126 Heidelberg, Deutschland, Fax +49.6221.345-4229, e-mail: orders@springer.de, springer.de
P.O. Box 2485, Secaucus, NJ 07096-2485, USA, Fax +1.201.348-4505, e-mail: orders@springer-ny.com
Eastern Book Service, 3–13, Hongo 3-chome, Bunkyo-ku, Japan, Tokyo 113, Fax +81.3.38 18 08 64, e-mail: orders@svt-ebs.co.jp
Preisänderungen und Irrtümer vorbehalten.

Springer-Verlag
und Umwelt

ALS INTERNATIONALER WISSENSCHAFTLICHER VERLAG sind wir uns unserer besonderen Verpflichtung der Umwelt gegenüber bewusst und beziehen umwelt-orientierte Grundsätze in Unternehmensentscheidungen mit ein.

VON UNSEREN GESCHÄFTSPARTNERN (DRUCKEREIEN, Papierfabriken, Verpackungsherstellern usw.) verlangen wir, dass sie sowohl beim Herstellungsprozess selbst als auch beim Einsatz der zur Verwendung kommenden Materialien ökologische Gesichtspunkte berücksichtigen.

DAS FÜR DIESES BUCH VERWENDETE PAPIER IST AUS chlorfrei hergestelltem Zellstoff gefertigt und im pH-Wert neutral.